MOTOR BEHAVIOR:
From Learning to Performance

Darlene A. Kluka, Ph. D.
Associate Professor
Grambling State University, Grambling, Louisiana

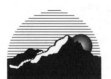

Morton Publishing Company
925 W. Kenyon Ave., Unit 12
Englewood, Colorado 80110
http://www.morton-pub.com

Book Team

Publisher	Doug Morton
Managing Editor	Ruth Horton
Copy Editor	Keith Campbell
Editorial Assistant	Dona Mendoza
Production Manager	Joanne Saliger, Ash Street Typecrafters, Inc.
Cover Design	Bob Schram, Bookends
Design & Typography	Ash Street Typecrafters, Inc.
Photo Models	Mohammed Ali, Jody Conradt, Jackie Joyner-Kersee, Marc Maurer, Michelle Smith, Bill Pink, Theresa Weatherspoon, Angela Lawson, Heather Sipe, Shawn Peterson

Special Photo Credits:

	Pages
Photo courtesy of AP/Wide World Photos, used with permission	61
Photos courtesy of Bill Scherer	51, 161
Photo courtesy of Clint Carlton	14
Photos courtesy of Darlene A. Kluka, Ph.D.	6, 19, 22, 23, 45, 113, 127, 128, 129, 148, 175, 213, 222, 230, 251, 253, 265, 275
Photos courtesy of Fitness & Wellness, Inc., Boise, ID © 1998	13, 27, 94, 107, 173, 231, 261, 277
Photo courtesy of Grambling State University	217
Photo courtesy of Lafayette Instrument Company. Used with permission.	139
Photo courtesy of Mike Powell/Allsport USA. Used with permission.	87
Photo courtesy of Mike Strawn, UAB Photography	287
Photo courtesy of National Federation of the Blind. Used with permission.	99
Photo courtesy of Rafael "Boy" Inocentes, Philippine Sports Commission	287
Photo courtesy of University of Texas Sports Photography Department. Used with permission.	211

Printed in the United States of America

By Morton Publishing Company, 925 W. Kenyon Ave., Unit 12, Englewood, CO 80110

10 9 8 7 6 5 4 3 2 1

ISBN: 0-89582-386-1

About The Author

Darlene A. Kluka earned her Ph.D. in physical education, with a major emphasis in motor learning and a minor emphasis in biomechanics, from Texas Woman's University. She has taught undergraduate and graduate courses in motor learning for the past twelve years at The University of Alabama at Birmingham, the University of Central Oklahoma, and Grambling State University. During her university-level career, she has been director of the Human Performance Center at Grambling State University, founding director of a Motor Behavior/Sports Vision Laboratory at The University of Alabama at Birmingham, and departmental graduate studies coordinator at the University of Central Oklahoma. She is currently associate professor of physical education and coordinator of health and physical education in the Department of HPER at Grambling State University.

Additionally, she now serves as a charter member of the USA Volleyball Sports Medicine and Performance Commission; vice president of Member Relations and Human Resources for USA Volleyball; vice president for research on the International Academy of Sports Vision's Executive Committee; as the Founding Editor of the *International Journal of Volleyball Research*; on the editorial board of the International Council for Sports Science and Physical Education ICSSPE); as the general review editor for the internationally refereed journal, *Women in Sport and Physical Activity;* and as a reviewer for *JOPERD Coaching Volleyball Journal, The Physical Educator,* and *Strategies.* She recently completed a seven-year tenure as founding co-editor of the *International Journal of Sports Vision.*

She is an AAHPERD Research Consortium fellow in the area of motor behavior. In 1995, she was honored with the ICHPERSD Distinguished Scholar in Sport Science and the Olympic Movement Award for her work in the areas of sports vision and women in sport; she was also the recipient of the University of Central Oklahoma's Distinguished Scholar Award in 1997 and most recently was honored with USA Volleyball's Leader in Volleyball Award for her contributions over the past twenty-five years (1998).

The author has been published in the *Journal of the American Optometric Association, Journal of Vision Development, Medicine and Science in Sports and Exercise, Pediatric Exercise Science Journal, International Journal of Sports Vision, Perceptual and Motor Skills, International Journal of Volleyball Research, ICHPERSD Journal, JOPERD, Strategies, Coaching Volleyball Journal, Coaching Women's Basketball Journal, LAHPERD, OAHPERD,* and *SCAHPERD Journals.* She has presented at international conferences on topics relating to the text in the Czech Republic, Germany, Philippines, Australia, Finland, Switzerland, and the United States. She has presented nationally at over 25 AAHPERD, AOA - SVS, CLAO, COVD, NASPSPA, AVCA, WBCA, and NSCA conventions on topics related to the content of the text.

ICHPERSD (International Council for Health, Physical Education, Recreation, Sport and Dance)

JOPERD (Journal of Physical Education, Recreation and Dance)

LAHPERD (Louisiana Association for Health, Physical Education, Recreation and Dance)

OAHPERD (Oklahoma Association for Health, Physical Education, Recreation and Dance)

SCAHPERD (South Carolina Association for Health, Physical Education, Recreation and Dance)

AAHPERD (American Alliance for Health, Physical Education, Recreation and Dance)

AOA - SVS (American Optometric Association - Sports Vision Section)

AVCA (American Volleyball Coaches Association)

CLAO (Contact Lens Association of Optometry)

COVD (College of Optometrists in Vision Development)

NSCA (National Softball Coaches Association)

WBCA (Women's Basketball Coaches Association)

To those who have always believed in my worth:

Annie and Alois Petrasek; Bernice, John, Ray and Dave Kluka; Emily Liphardt; Marie Knez; Phyllis Love, Kay Covington, Coni Staff, Gerry Staab, Ginny Crafts, Phebe Scott; Sue Schafer, Carolyn Mitchell, Sylvia Stroops, Dong Ja Yang, Willie Daniel, Doris Corbett, Gudrun Doll-Tepper, Dick Jones, Peter Dunn; Jean Pyfer, Bettye Myers, Aileene Lockhart, Jane Mott, Claudine Sherrill; Linda Bunker, Peggy Kellers; Carole Tabor, Joe Andera, Sandy Vivas, Debbie Hunter and Gerry Denk.

— D. A. K.

Acknowledgments

As with any project of this magnitude, much is owed to many. My parents, Aloysius and Lillian Kluka, provided me with an environment that was constantly dynamic and challenging; Dr. Aileene Lockhart provided me with opportunities to grow and believe in my ability to communicate through print; Dr. Bettye Myers provided experiences for me to continue to develop communication skills via thoughts and words; Dr. Joan Vickers, Dr. Linda Bunker, Dr. Peggy Kellers, and Dr. Gib Darden provided professional insight and perspective on a variety of topics throughout recent years included in this text; Dr. Paul Salitsky and Dr. Geraldine Van Gyn provided informative and helpful suggestions as reviewers of this text; and Dr. Phyllis Love, Ruth Horton, Dona Mendoza, and Joanne Saliger provided conceptual and technical expertise as well as unconditional support that was deeply appreciated, particularly when the creative candle flickered and nearly extinguished.

Additionally, thousands of high school (Fenton High School, Bensenville, IL; New Trier East High School, Winnetka, IL; Illinois Valley Central High School, Chillicothe, IL), undergraduate (Newberry College, South Carolina; The University of Alabama at Birmingham, University of Central Oklahoma, Edmond, OK; and Grambling State University, LA) and graduate students (The University of Alabama at Birmingham, University of Central Oklahoma, and Grambling State University) have helped me to realize that strong educational foundations based upon the quest for and acquisition of conceptual understanding and application are the roots from which we grow. Their enthusiasm to learn, their eagerness to find solutions to challenges, and their sparks of excitement to ask questions, search for answers, and formulate new questions to increase the body of knowledge known as motor behavior represent the hope of the profession.

Finally, those who capture the essence of motor behavior through photographs have provided texture for the pages of this textbook. Their contributions are acknowledged within this text, and they have graciously allowed their perceptual expertise to be included. I have also, throughout the last two decades, thoroughly enjoyed capturing moments of human movement through the lens and hope the reader will glean additional understanding and insight into motor behavior from a photographic perspective.

Contents

Section I   Motor Behavior Perspectives   1

Section III   Learning Perspectives   87

Preface

This textbook was conceived for upper-division undergraduate students whose interest in human motor behavior was initiated by their own involvement in sport and physical activity. This is their first opportunity to be introduced to the body of knowledge known as motor behavior. The basic constructs of motor behavior and their relationship to human movement are presented in an easy-to-understand format so that more in-depth pursuit of the discipline can subsequently be undertaken. The undergraduate students may ultimately choose professions as physical educators, sport-specific coaches, strength coaches, athletic directors, sport or exercise psychologists, athletic and personal trainers, physical and dance therapists, biomechanists, exercise physiologists, exercise scientists, corporate fitness managers, recreation specialists, or human factors engineers.

The learning and performance of motor skills become the cornerstones from which concepts, processes, and strategies are built. This textbook seeks to provide students with a basic understanding of the discipline and to provide experiences that will enhance their understanding and application of motor behavior perspectives in a variety of environments.

The text is divided into five sections: Motor Behavior Perspectives, Biological Perspectives, Learning Perspectives, Social Perspectives and Performance Perspectives. Embedded in selected chapters are activities that enable students to better understand concepts and perspectives. Some experiences require specific answers, while others involve several possibilities. Professors may use the learning experiences to generate discussions during class or students may use them as examples. Discussion questions and additional reading suggestions at the end of each chapter are presented along with a glossary, textbook references, author index, and subject index to complete the text.

One of the important components of an introductory undergraduate course in motor behavior involves experiences that underscore basic concepts and principles. When there are no sophisticated motor behavior laboratory facilities available, the field-based laboratory experiences in this text can be used to provide a better understanding of motor behavior. Each of the experiences selected for inclusion in this text is intended to serve as a means for understanding specific perspectives in motor behavior. The equipment required to conduct each experience, where appropriate, is inexpensive and easy to construct. It should also be noted that because each experience uses small samples, the results may not be similar to those of controlled research investigations.

Because this is an introductory text in motor behavior, from learning to performance, students are encouraged to read, think, ask questions, learn, apply, and integrate motor behavior into their own lifestyles and into the lifestyles of those whose lives they touch. They are also asked to continue to be life-long learners through sport science to more completely understand, appreciate, and integrate the vitally important role motor behavior has in the total perspective of human movement.

Finally, the professor is provided with a PowerPoint computer diskette and test bank that can be used to enhance learning from the text. The colorful PowerPoint display and creatively designed format should prove to be a useful tool in communicating motor behavior perspectives during class presentations. The professor can easily make additions to the PowerPoint presentation with comments, overhead transparencies, or slides. The test bank should provide the professor with choices for the assessment of students in motor behavior classes.

The area of motor behavior continues to be a dynamic interrelationship of disciplines and topics focusing on the learning and performance of human movement in varying environmental conditions. I hope that the material selected for inclusion in this introductory text is interesting and enriching to those who read it.

—D. A. K.

Motor Behavior Perspectives

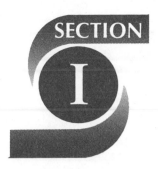

Marie, now a freshman middle hitter on the university's volleyball team, enmeshed herself in a hitting/blocking drill during an early August practice. As a junior and senior in high school, she had made first team all-state. She was one of the tallest young women in the state (six feet, 5 inches) and had a vertical jump of twenty-five inches. She was confident . . . until now. She suddenly found that she was being stuff-blocked by every junior and senior on the team. It seemed that each of them knew where she would be coming from, where she was hitting to, and when she would be arriving. The approach, jump, and arm swing she used automatically no longer seemed effective. What has happened to Marie? What are some of the variables that have affected her hitting?

Motor Behavior and Its Meaning

*W*hat does the term Motor Behavior mean? **Motor behavior** can be considered the study of executed human performances and postures that are the result of integrated internal processes that lead to a relatively permanent change in performance (an act at a moment in time). Motor behavior, then, includes all human movements and postures that are performed; it also includes the processes that lead to relatively permanent changes in performance.

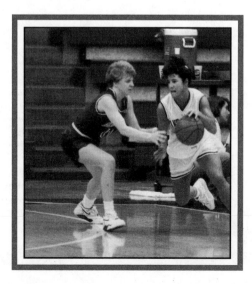

Motor behavior
all human movements and postures; also, the processes that lead to relatively permanent changes in performance

Motor control
human performance and postures and the internal processes that command them

Motor learning
a multifaceted set of internal processes that effect relatively permanent change in human performance through practice, provided the change cannot be attributed to a human's maturation, temporary state, or instinct

The study of motor behavior can be divided into two subfields: *motor control* and *motor learning*. **Motor control** refers to the study of human performances and postures and the internal processes that command them. This implies that there are mechanisms that guide muscles and joints. **Motor learning** can be defined as a multifaceted set of internal processes whereby relatively permanent changes occur in human performance through practice, provided the change cannot be attributed to a human's maturation (i.e., the growth of the body from ages two to twelve), temporary state (i.e., use of performance-enhancing drugs; motivation; excitation; arousal), or instinct. Learning implies that there is a change in behavior that is more or less permanent. Figure 1.1 displays motor behavior and its subfields of study. Learning continues over time and may be slow. Learning is a direct result of practice.

Figure 1.2 indicates that motor behavior is the observable outcome of motor control and motor learning. It also displays the relationships of other disciplines with motor behavior and human movement.

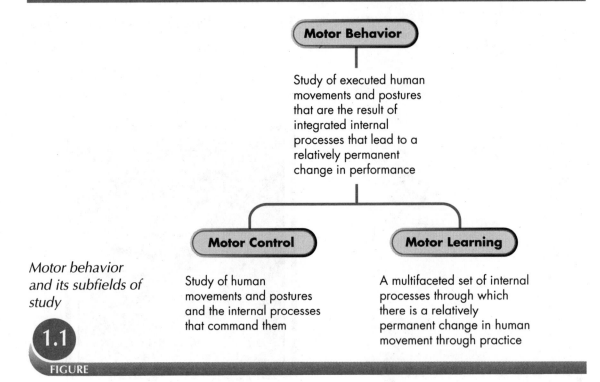

Motor Behavior

Study of executed human movements and postures that are the result of integrated internal processes that lead to a relatively permanent change in performance

Motor Control

Study of human movements and postures and the internal processes that command them

Motor Learning

A multifaceted set of internal processes through which there is a relatively permanent change in human movement through practice

Motor behavior and its subfields of study

1.1

FIGURE

MOTOR SKILLS

Motor skills are a vital part of the discussion involving motor control and motor learning through motor behavior. The definition of *skill* depends upon the context in which it is used. It has a different meaning when used as an adjective (e.g., a *skilled performer* in golf) than when used as a noun (e.g., the *skill* of putting, chipping, or swinging that contributes to the skilled performance in golf).

A motor **skill**, then, may be defined as a voluntarily controlled body/limb action or task that is goal-directed. Whatever the skill, there is an implication that the motor skill must be learned in order to be performed. The skill of bull riding has as its goal to successfully remain on the back of an untamed bull for a specific number of seconds. This requires finger, palm, hand, arm, torso, leg, foot, and toe movement to accomplish the goal of the skill. Bull riding has a goal, requires body/limb movement, and is voluntarily controlled.

Skill
a goal-oriented action; a qualitatively assessed performance

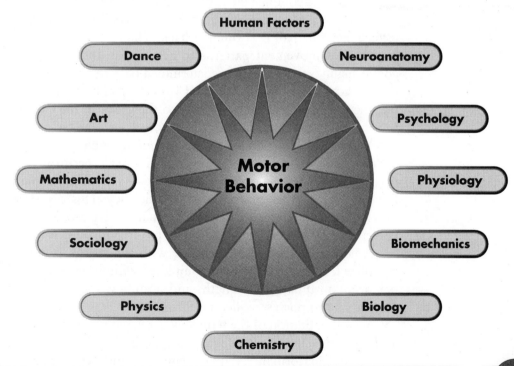

Relationships of other disciplines with motor behavior on human movement

1.2
FIGURE

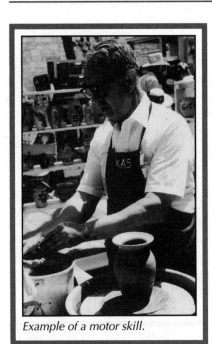

Example of a motor skill.

On the other hand, reading, math calculation, and foreign language comprehension are also skills. They are not motor skills, because they do not require body and/or limb movement. They are, however, goal-directed. These types of skills are referred to as cognitive skills.

Because motor control and motor learning processes are dynamic, it is sometimes difficult to understand when motor behavior can be considered motor learning and when it can be considered motor control. One of the central characteristics of skill from motor learning and motor control perspectives involves action. Skill and action can be used interchangeably. What is important is that a variety of skills or movement patterns contribute to particular actions. Specifically, if the goal is to score a touchdown in American football, the quarterback has a variety of choices in the accomplishment of the goal; if the decision is to complete a running play over the goal line, then the quarterback gets the ball to a running back. The running back combines a variety of movement patterns to accomplish the task. When the goal is highly specific, with predetermined patterns of movement, the skill or action may contain limited variety of movement. For example, the golf shot from the rough onto the green to the cup requires specific limited movement patterns to accomplish the task.

A second definition of the term *skill* involves a quantitative and/or qualitative assessment of an individual's performance skill. An individual who is a skilled performer has reached a particular level of performance that indicates proficiency. This determination may be quantitative or qualitative. A quantitative assessment might be determined by making eight out of ten free throws. A qualitative assessment relates to the technique with which the free throw is completed. If the free throw is completed with appropriate rhythm, balance, coordination, strength, and accuracy, then the individual may be said to possess skilled performance.

A third definition of the term *skill* is related to performance characteristics. The use of meaningful cues, the ability to determine in advance what performance requirements are, and actual performance consistency comprise this third definition of skilled performance. When waiting to receive a volleyball serve, a skilled individual gains meaningful cues from the server's stance, the ball's toss, the position of the hand upon contact, and the first one-third of the ball's trajectory. The unskilled receiver will be unable to discern similar meaningful cues. In ice hockey, the skilled goalie can successfully anticipate the trajectory of an oncoming puck prior to the shot, while the unskilled goalie must wait until the puck is hit. Finally, a batter is said to be skilled when his or her batting average is over .300. The batting average is determined by repeated trials over an extended period of time. The batting average represents a profile of responses to a variety of conditions, including various pitchers, pitches, and game situations.

Another meaningful term in the discussion of motor skills and motor behavior is *motor ability*. This refers to an individual's general capacity in the performance of motor skills (Fleishman, 1978; Magill, 1993). A person who possesses high motor ability in a wide variety of motor skills that are required in an activity or sport has a greater potential for success. For example, the person who possesses agility, coordina-

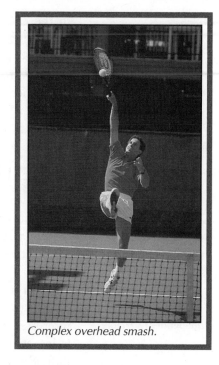

Complex overhead smash.

tion, and quickness has the potential of being successful in tennis, soccer, badminton, and fencing. Agility, coordination, and quickness are important for success in these sports.

To help us to understand motor control and motor learning, researchers have developed theories and models systematically that provide direction for the field of interest. Motor control theories have permeated the last century of scientific thinking, while motor learning theories and models have been devised over the past half century. The concepts of theories, models, and research designs will be discussed first, followed by theories of motor control and motor learning. The section will close with a discussion of scientific measurement and motor behavior.

THE THEORY

Through observation that is scientifically based, statements can be made about the behavior that has occurred. Motor behavior can also be explained and predicted. One of the first questions asked when discussing theories of motor behavior is: "What is a theory?"

Theory
a succinct way of explaining a concept

Hypothesis
an "educated guess" designed to be logically developed to predict the change in outcome

Variable
that portion in an experimental investigation which needs to be controlled to determine the effect of the experiment

Independent variable
the variable in a research design that is manipulated or changed (in contrast to the dependent variable)

Dependent variable
the variable that is measured in an experimental investigation (in contrast to the independent variable, which is not)

Basic research
an experiment to determine additional information to contribute to a theory

Applied research
an experiment to determine an answer to a specific question for the field-based professional

Theoretical model
a succinct way of explaining a concept

In the case of motor behavior, a **theory** can be a succinct way of explaining why behavior happens.

Theories present opportunities for an "educated guess," or **hypothesis,** to be logically developed and tested. The hypothesis seeks to predict the change in outcome as a result of the theoretical perspective. To test a hypothesis, one designs an experiment. An experiment can take many forms.

THE EXPERIMENT

One of the most important constructs used to determine scientific observation is the experiment. The experiment's goal is to control as many variables as possible so that those variables being investigated are relatively pure. A **variable** is that portion which needs to be controlled. Typically, the investigator measures the effect of one variable on another one by manipulating or providing some type of change to the original variable. The variable that the investigator is interested in is referred to as the **independent variable.** This variable is intentionally changed for different groups of individuals. If some individuals receive a reward for running a figure eight pattern and others do not, the presence of a reward becomes the independent variable. The variable that is measured is known as the **dependent variable.** An example of a dependent variable could be performance measurements used in the experiment, such as the number of minutes it takes for an individual to learn to run a figure eight pattern in the experiment, regardless of conditions. If there is a change in the outcome of the dependent variable, it is understood to be the result of what was done to the independent variable.

If the purpose of the experiment is to determine additional information to contribute to theory, the research is considered **basic research.** If the purpose of the experiment is to answer a specific question for the field-based professional, the research is considered **applied research.**

THE THEORETICAL MODEL

Those who are interested in studying motor behavior have also developed **theoretical models.** A model is a pictorial or schematic representation of a process or a theory. Figure 1.3 is an example of a theoretical taxonomy model in motor behavior. Theoretical models are generally developed through basic research experiments.

Example of a theoretical model (Internal feedback provided by the individual learner's sensory receptors)

1.3

FIGURE

THE RESEARCH DESIGN

A research design that is often used in motor behavior research involves two groups: an **experimental group** and a **control group**. Individuals are placed in one or the other group randomly, so that each person has an equal chance of being put into either group. Both groups are then tested to achieve a baseline measurement. The control group is also used as the "measuring stick" for both groups, because only the experimental group will have a variable changed during the experiment. Other than the one variable being manipulated, all conditions for both groups during the experiment must remain constant in order to determine the effect of manipulating the variable. For example, sixty college-aged students in a novice tennis class are randomly assigned to two groups, a control and an experimental (Figure 1.4). What effect does the additional racket weight have on forehand stroke efficiency. After an initial skill test for both groups with standardized rackets, those in the control group continue to use standardized rackets, while those in the experimental group use weighted rackets. Skill/drill presentations and practice remain the same for both groups throughout the semester. Both groups are then skill tested at the end, using standardized rackets.

When experiments are concerned with the relationship of independent and dependent variables, the relationship is referred to as a causal relationship. In the previous example, the goal is to determine cause and effect. In other words, the goal was to determine the

Experimental group
the component of a research design that is given a treatment to determine the effects of that treatment

Control group
a group designated in a research design that is given no treatment

effect of additional racket weight on forehand stroke efficiency. If differences occur between the standardized racket and the weighted racket groups, the performance difference is a result of the difference in racket weights. This determination is referred to as the conclusion of the investigation.

This and other types of research designs provide interesting data that present a generalization about each group, made from each group's average score. What happens when one person's results are compared with the hypothesis? It could be that the person's scores are higher or lower than the group's average. In other words, on

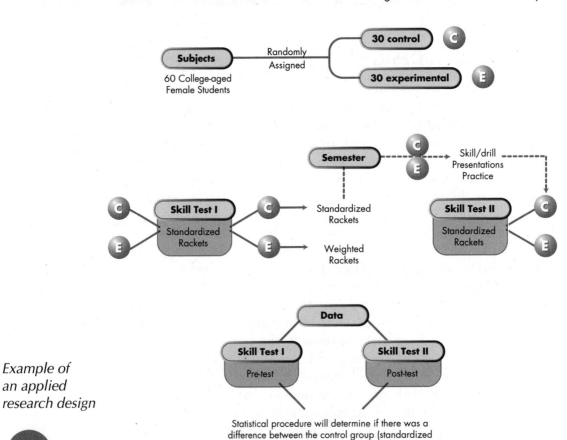

Novice Tennis Class – Effect of additional racket weight on forehand stroke efficiency

*Example of
an applied
research design*

Statistical procedure will determine if there was a difference between the control group (standardized racket) and the experimental group (weighted racket)

1.4

FIGURE

average, the group performed in a particular way, and individuals in the group may have scored higher or lower than the average.

We must generalize the information so that we can apply it. Generalizations can be made from multiple experiments, based upon similarities between findings. Without similar research-based findings, generalizations could not be made; without generalizations, predictions would be difficult to make. Please note that human motor behavior is dynamic. Predictions cannot be made with absolute certainty. With reasonably controlled experiments, motor behavior research can be used to answer real-world questions as well as contribute to its theoretical base.

KEY POINTS

- Motor behavior is considered the study of executed human movements and postures that result from integrated internal processes that lead to a relatively permanent change in performance.

- Motor behavior can be divided into two subfields: motor control (study of human movements and postures and the internal processes that command them) and motor learning (a multifaceted set of internal processes through which there is a relatively permanent change in human action through practice, provided the change cannot be attributed to human maturation, temporary states, or instinct.

- Processes are dynamic; therefore, it is sometimes difficult to understand when motor behavior can be considered motor learning and when it can be considered motor control.

- Theories and models are developed to explain phenomenon and to provide direction for thought and research.

- A theory can be a succinct way of explaining why and how behavior happens.

- A hypothesis ("educated guess") seeks to predict changes in performance outcomes.

- Basic research determines additional information to contribute to theory.

- Applied research helps to answer a specific question for the field-based professional.

- A model is a pictorial or schematic representation of a process or a theory.
- A control group is used as the "measuring stick" for these groups in an experiment, because only the experimental group will have a variable changed during the experiment.

DISCUSSION QUESTIONS

1. Determine the definitions of skill and ability. Provide three examples of each in motor behavior.

2. Compare and contrast the concepts of motor control and motor learning.

3. Describe how motor behavior is interconnected with other sport science disciplines.

4. Cite two examples of theories and explain why they qualify as theories.

5. Describe two examples of basic research as defined in the text; describe two examples of applied research as defined in the text.

6. What is one example of a typical applied research design, using experimental and control groups?

ADDITIONAL READINGS

Abernethy, B., & Sparrow, W. A. (1992). The rise and fall of dominant paradigms in motor behaviour research. In *Approaches to the study of motor control and learning*, Ed. J. J. Summers, pp. 3–45. North-Holland: Elsevier Science Publishers B. V.

Adams, J. A. (1987). Historical review and appraisal of research on the learning, retention, and transfer of human motor skills. *Psychological Bulletin, 101,* 41–74.

Pew, R. W. (1972). Levels of analysis in motor control. *Brain Research, 71,* 393–400.

REFERENCES

Fleishman, E. A. (1978). Systems for describing human tasks. *Ergonomics, 21,* 1007–1019.

Magill, R. (1993). *Motor learning: Concepts and applications.* (4th ed.). Madison, WI: Brown & Benchmark.

Theories of Motor Control

CHAPTER FOCUS

- Contributions by motor behavior professionals throughout history
- Motor control theories as they relate to motor behavior
- Motor control theories, their commonalities, and their uniquenesses
- Motor control theories and how they have shaped motor behavior research

*B*efore we discuss motor behavior theories, it will be helpful to think about what a motor control theory is. What are the characteristics of motor control theories? To provide some perspective, Sheridan (1984) has suggested that four characteristics of skilled movement in any theory of motor control must account for: (1) the flexibility of movement skill; (2) the uniqueness of movement skill; (3) consistency of movement skill; and (4) modifiability of movement skill (Figure 2.1).

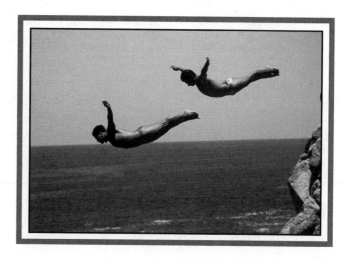

13

Flexibility of movement
the ability to accomplish a task using a variety of musculoskeletal resources

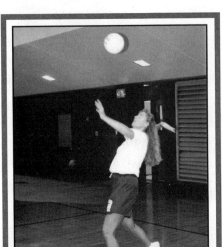
Volleyball serve.

Flexibility of movement, in Sheridan's explanation, is not concerned with the range of motion within joints, but rather with a person's ability to accomplish a task using a variety of musculoskeletal resources. For example, if the goal is to get a volleyball across the net legally, the player may use the head, shoulder, elbow, or knee to hit the ball over, or the hands or forearms in a pass. The idea of flexibility of movement, then, is to be able to move in a limited variety of ways to accomplish the same goal. Each movement skill incorporates a number of degrees of freedom of movement. *Degrees of freedom* refers to the limited number of possibilities available within the system to perform a movement. In essence, by restricting available possibilities, the system can be channeled to produce goal-directed behavior appropriate to environmental demands. In the volleyball example, there are six ways to accomplish the goal, all with different degrees of freedom.

Even if several slow-motion video recordings are taken of the javelin throw for distance, no two throws will be exactly alike when the tapes are

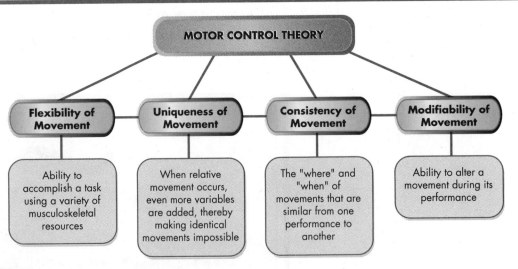

MOTOR CONTROL THEORY

Flexibility of Movement	**Uniqueness of Movement**	**Consistency of Movement**	**Modifiability of Movement**
Ability to accomplish a task using a variety of musculoskeletal resources	When relative movement occurs, even more variables are added, thereby making identical movements impossible	The "where" and "when" of movements that are similar from one performance to another	Ability to alter a movement during its performance

2.1 *Four characteristics of movement which must be accounted for in any theory of motor control*
FIGURE

analyzed. **Uniqueness of movement** must also be addressed in any theory of motor control. When the individual is moving and the object is stationary; when the object is moving and the individual is stationary; or when both the individual and the object are moving (referred to as *relative movement*), even more variables are added, thereby making identical movements impossible.

Consistency of movement refers to the *where* (spatial characteristics) and the *when* (temporal characteristics) of movements that are similar from one performance to another. For example, an experienced softball batter can "groove the swing" by displaying the temporal characteristics of when to swing the bat, with spatial characteristics of where to swing the bat repeatedly.

Finally, the explanation for a person's ability to modify a movement during its performance is the final characteristic of a motor control theory offered by Sheridan (**modifiability of movement**). A gymnast performing a back walkover, back handspring, back handspring tumbling pass on the balance beam can literally alter the direction of the second back handspring by adjusting hand placement. The ability to make such adjustments at high speed is particularly valuable for performers and motor behavior professionals.

In the motor behavior theory literature, several paradigms have influenced the study of motor control. They have emerged in three basic categories: theories involving reflexes (involuntary rapid responses to stimuli), theories based on the hierarchy of the central nervous system, and, the most recent, dynamic systems theory.

Generally, early theories of motor control are worth reexamining. These early theories provide for experiments that, at first glance, seem rather simplistic by present-day research standards. This is the case with those who developed **reflex theories** of motor control, as will be seen after reading the next section.

REFLEX THEORIES

Sherrington, specializing in neurophysiology (1906), Thorndike, specializing in behavioral psychology (1927), and Skinner, specializing in behavioral psychology (1938) hypothesized that movement was controlled by reflexes. Ultimately, an action was the culmination of a series of reflexes that were linked together to produce a reaction. Basically, it was suggested that reflexes at the spinal cord level were stimulated by sensory receptors; they gleaned information from the environment, so that muscles were stimulated to respond.

Uniqueness of movement
the relative movement occurs, even more variables are added, thereby making movements identical impossible

Consistency of movement
close similarity over a series of performances

Modifiability of movement
the explanation for a person's ability to alter a movement during its performance

Reflex theories
paradigms that explain behavior as the use of stereotyped, involuntary, and rapid responses to stimuli

Early researchers, using a procedure known as deafferentation, performed many of their experiments on rats, mice, and cats by severing their spinal cords just under the brain. For two decades (1920s and 1930s), behaviorists like Thorndike and Skinner, who focused on studying observable behavior, hypothesized that reflexes, linked together, produced observable performance. They also believed that habits, through conditioning, were the key to motor control. The general idea was that a response that occurred naturally at the reflex level could be related to a stimulus that would eventually get the response as a result of practice. One of the most famous experiments was conducted in the late 1800s by Pavlov, who successfully paired the stimulus of a bell ringing to a dog's salivation.

Reflex theories were designed to explain motor behavior that was observable. Unfortunately, the depth of the explanation was limited to stimulus-response and did not account for goal-directed performance. For example, the theory did not explain movements that occurred when the individual made choices in behaviors to be performed. Nowadays, reflex theories, although instrumental to the thinking of early motor control theorists, no longer seem relevant to explain voluntary movement control. As knowledge of the nervous system has increased, more sophisticated theories have been required to explain the area of motor control.

HIERARCHICAL THEORIES

The evolution in theories of motor control next manifested itself through the idea of a hierarchy of central nervous system functioning. According to this view, all component portions of movement planning and execution are designated in one or more centers of the cortex within a hierarchy of the central nervous system. Based on a hierarchical or top-down approach to command, which began with the brain and its neocortex, theorists believed that the brain commanded all parts of decision making and performance. This theory was referred to as the **hierarchy theory** of motor control. The brain was the "supreme commander," having all of the necessary information for all motor behavior; it operated in a hierarchical fashion to orchestrate lower areas of the central nervous system in the performance.

It was originally hypothesized (Woodworth, 1899) that information was sent in only one direction. This model, with input originating from the top (the brain) and descending to the bottom (the

Hierarchy theory
a concept of motor control based on a hierarchy that begins with the brain and its neocortex and operates in a hierarchical fashion to orchestrate lower areas of the central nervous system in performance

muscles), resembled business models in the 1950s through the 1980s. The commander (president/brain) made the decisions and charted the course for movement (company/body), allowing no communication back to the commander (president/brain) from the musculature (company/body). By the 1970s (Greene, 1972; Thach, 1978), initial hierarchical theory was modified to include the idea that the brain communicates with lower levels of the central nervous system during motor performance through various forms of feedback. In either case, investigators espousing hierarchical theory associated the brain and descending nervous system with the initiation and regulation of motor control.

A conceptual model of human performance, known as the **motor program**, was initially devised in the 1960s (Keele, 1968; Henry & Rogers, 1960). It provided a means for understanding how movements could be planned in advance. The model is based on the premise that plans (programs) are created in advance, stored in the brain, and processed through the rest of the system, uninterrupted. This is performed through an open-loop system, involving two levels: an **executive level** and an **effector level**. Figure 2.2 indicates diagrammatically the open-loop system. Open loop refers to the generation of action plans by a central executive in the cerebral cortex. The action is completed without additional sensory feedback.

The executive level of the open-loop system determines which movement to make, which muscles contract, when they contract, and in what order they contract. Theoretically, it contains all of the necessary information for the effector level to perform the movement to completion. The effector level organizes the muscles and joints to produce the preplanned movement. For example, a gymnast performing a tumbling pass (roundoff, back handspring, whip back, back handspring, full twisting back somersault) uses the executive level (decision-making stage) to determine what pass sequence to perform and when to begin it. As the pass begins, the effector level controls the movement.

To help establish the viability of this line of thought, researchers during the late 1960s and 1970s conducted deafferentation investigations on animals (Taub & Berman, 1968; Grillner, 1975). The surgical procedure of deafferentation involves cutting nerves that enter the spinal cord so that information from the periphery cannot be received. Interestingly, animals, after the procedure, were still able to use gross motor movements to play, climb, and feed

Motor program
a plan or program determined in advance, stored in the brain, and run through the rest of the body system

Executive level
one of two levels in an open-loop system, which determines the movement to make, which muscles to contract, when they contract, and in what order they contract

Effector level
one of two levels in an open-loop system that organizes the muscles and joints to produce the preplanned movement

The Open-Loop System

2.2 FIGURE

themselves, but they lacked precision accuracy. This line of investigation provided proof that sensory information is not necessary for all motor movements to occur.

The generalized motor program paradigm developed by Schmidt and associates (Schmidt, 1975; Schmidt, 1976; Schmidt, 1978; Shapiro, 1978; Schmidt & Young, 1987) sought to group motor programs into larger generalized parts, as it did not seem plausible to store literally thousands of individual motor programs in memory for each specific motor behavior. The generalized motor program paradigm is rather abstract. There is, according to Schmidt (1991), a general movement representation stored in memory to be controlled. The program controls groups of movements. In this way, movements can be easily modified or changed to meet environmental demands. These environmental demands might include the timing necessary for the movement to occur, the space needed to perform it, the overall force needed to execute it, and the flow of the movement as it relates to spatial and temporal demands. This generalized representation of movement stored in memory helps to explain the idea of making similar general movement patterns using different musculature to accomplish the movements. In an aerobics class, for instance, a person performs the general movement sequence of stepping in place, from barely getting the heels off the floor to marching in place with knees high, all performed to the same musical beat.

Hierarchical theories of motor control continued to evolve through the 1970s and early 1980s to account for the generation of the concept of *novel* motor behaviors. Attempting to juggle three tennis balls simultaneously for the first time can be considered a *novel* task.

In general, positions taken in hierarchical theories of motor control have also been questioned by other researchers (Bernstein, 1967; Gibson, 1966; Kelso 1982; Kelso & Kay, 1987; Kugler & Turvey, 1986) representing the fields of psychology, neuroscience, physics, and physical education. This has led to another possible explanation of motor behavior through motor control.

Dynamic systems theory a paradigm that describes the control of coordinated movement and its dynamic relationship between the environment and the individual

DYNAMIC SYSTEMS THEORY

Leading theorists using this approach to explain motor behavior would deny the existence of a "supreme commander" to describe control. A more representative explanation, they contend, is the **dynamic systems theory** (also known as the ecological theory or action systems theory). Placed at its core is the dynamic relationship between the individual and the environment. The theory establishes the environment as the source from which to glean information that is needed to perform a movement. All information for movement is found in the environment and can be directly perceived by the individual. Theorists (Bernstein, 1967; Gibson, 1966; Kelso & Tuller, 1984; Kugler & Turvey, 1987; Reed, 1982) advocate that there is an integrated interaction of smaller systems (e.g., biological, muscular, skeletal, neurological, cardiorespiratory) cooperatively functioning to meet the environmental demands. This cooperation of smaller systems has no "supreme commander"; rather, it derives its prioritization from the characteristics of the information gleaned from the environment. The interaction (or

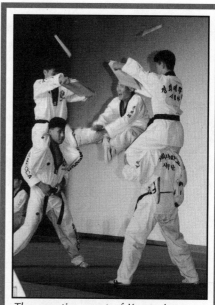

The coactive sport of Karate is an example of Dynamic Systems Theory.

Self-organization
the interaction or coordination of smaller systems within dynamic systems theory

coordination) of smaller systems can be referred to as **self-organization.** For example, if an individual plans to throw a ball to a target five meters away, the muscles and joints of the body act together (even though muscles function as pairs in opposition) to meet the goal, throwing the ball to a target five meters away. Specific body parts will begin and end their movements based upon the dynamics (degrees of freedom) of range of motion, tension, gravity, equilibrium, and so on as they relate to the goal and the environment. Put another way, the performance is affected by what the individual intends to do as well as by what is environmentally controlled. Additionally, as the smaller systems coordinate throughout the body, minor adaptations in movement can be easily and quickly made. These are based on sensory feedback or short feedback loops to adjust for unique situations.

A typical mechanical representation of this theory is found in a neighborhood grocery store. When one goes to the store to buy fruit, often the store has a scale in the form of a basket suspended from a spring weight. Once the fruit is weighed, the basket returns to its normal balancing point because of its original mechanical properties involving the spring's flexibility and tensile strength. The mass-spring model (Figure 2.3) illustrates this theory. When one performs a leg extension, the weight is against the ankle/foot. The knee is extended, making the quadricep muscles one set of springs and the hamstring group another set in opposition. The lower leg/foot comes to extension at the knee (the desired position), no matter what position the ankle/foot started from. The quadricep

LAB EXERCISE

THEORIES OF MOTOR BEHAVIOR

Objective: To determine the model used to explain the movement.

Equipment and Preparation: Partner; school desk; blindfold; chalkboard eraser.

Experience: With a partner who is blindfolded and seated in the desk, place the eraser on the desk in front of the partner. Ask the partner to pick up the eraser. As the individual picks up the eraser, remove the blindfold. Observe the action.

Assignment: Describe the movement that occurred as the blindfold was being removed. Determine what part of the movement was voluntarily controlled. Explain, based upon theories of motor behavior, what occurred. Develop a model to represent that which occurred.

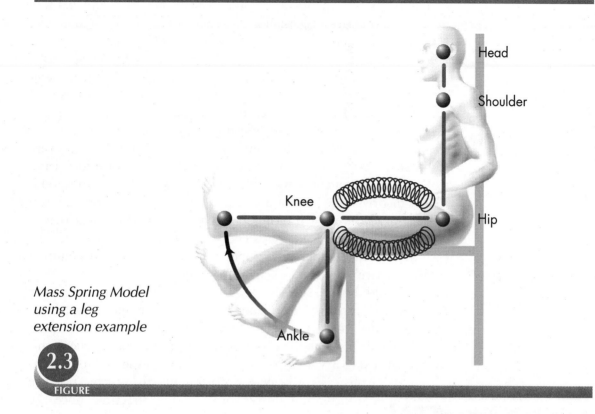

Mass Spring Model using a leg extension example

2.3
FIGURE

group becomes the prime mover and the hamstring group becomes the antagonist. The theory infers that the lower leg/foot will move to the specific desired point because of the flexibility and tension of the springs (muscles) involved in the movement.

Additional paradigms continue to be explored to explain motor behavior and its bases for motor control. Recent attempts have come from neuroscience, psychology, vision science, and the sport sciences. Included in these attempts are those involving neural network theory (Gowitzke & Milner, 1988; Horridge, 1987) and parallel processing theory (Trachtman & Kluka, 1993; Mather & Fisk, 1985). Both of these categories of theories seek to provide additional insight into the nervous system's connection with psychological parameters that organize human motor behavior. The notion that movements either descend from the central nervous system (as in hierarchical theories) or are reflexive in nature (as in reflex theories) or are dynamically interactive between the individual and environmental demands (as in dynamic systems theory) is most similar to a dynamic systems theory approach. Neural network and parallel processing theories suggest that a variety of areas throughout the central nervous and musculoskeletal systems choreograph movements.

To conclude this chapter of the Motor Behavior Perspectives section, we consider how reflex theories, hierarchical theories, and dynamic systems theories compare to the four characteristics suggested by Sheridan (1984). Clearly absent from reflex theories is the explanation of uniqueness of movement and repetition of performances. It was suggested that reflexes at the spinal cord level were stimulated by sensory receptors and that they gleaned information from the environment so that muscles were stimulated to respond. Reflex theorists also cannot account for adjustments (modifiability) in the execution of each motor performance. Finally, reflex theory could be used to explain consistency of performance as it related to each movement's spatial and temporal characteristics by accounting for the "where" and the "when" of movement.

It should be no surprise that as researchers explored other theories and provided different perspectives on motor behavior through motor control, theories became better at meeting the four characteristics that Sheridan has suggested. In the original hierarchical model, using a variety of musculoskeletal resources to accomplish a task was not difficult to justify; because information flowed only in one direction, once the choice was made about the movement, the execution of the movement began uninterrupted. Hierarchical theorists, through the concept of generalized motor programs, easily addressed the notion of flexibility of movement by adding different goals to the task. For example, although an individual may never have played Takarow, its juggling footwork is similar to the juggling footwork in soccer, so therefore, the motor program that was developed for soccer juggling is adjusted for initial success in Takarow. Continuing this line of thought, when the timing of sensory feedback is possible, movements can be adjusted during their execution, as in the case of a gymnast on rings who adjusts his grip while he approaches the bottom of a giant swing. Also, the uniqueness and consistency of motor behavior can also be accounted for by the motor program paradigm. Although no two movements may be identical, the time, space, force, and flow

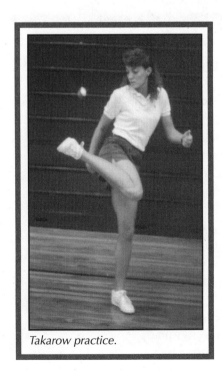

Takarow practice.

of the movements closely resemble one another. This, then, combines the uniqueness of the movement with the individual's ability to execute similar movements at a particular level of expertise.

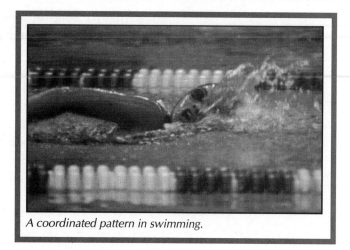

A coordinated pattern in swimming.

The dynamic systems theory approach also includes the four characteristics determined by Sheridan. Because the dynamic interaction between the individual and the environment is placed at the theory's core, flexibility of movement and the altering of movement are inherent in the approach. The prioritization of the information obtained from the environment by the individual (self-organization) is key. Uniqueness of performance and consistency of movement can also be explained through dynamic systems thought: Because muscles of the body function together to meet the goals of the movement, yet work in opposition, they help to provide the individuality of each movement while also providing overall similarity of movement patterns in differing environmental situations. When swimming the crawl two lengths of the pool recreationally, the arms, legs, torso, and head move in a coordinated pattern; when swimming the crawl two lengths of the pool in a timed event, the arms, legs, torso, and head move in a similar coordinated pattern, while altering the time between strokes and the force applied in the stroke. In other words, even after changing the goal of the task from leisurely swimming two lengths of the pool to competitively swimming two lengths of the pool, the synchronization of the patterns is similar.

It seems that both the dynamic systems theory and the hierarchical theories of motor behavior through motor control satisfy some of the characteristics of motor control offered by Sheridan: flexibility of movement, uniqueness of movement, consistency of movement, and modifiability of movement. The hierarchical theories more adequately account for the characteristics: flexibility of movement occurs by increasing movement parameters to a generalized motor program; uniqueness of movement can also be accounted for by a generalized motor program. Although both of these paradigms, inherently different from one another, attempt to explain human movement, nothing to date can account for all human movements.

These two paradigms, along with those offered by theorists advocating neural network and parallel processing theories, may increase our understanding of the nervous system's connection with the psychological parameters that organize human motor behavior. With increasingly advanced technology to investigate both the nervous system and the psychological parameters, theorists with an interest in motor control are destined to find even more satisfying explanations of motor behavior. Magnetic resonance imaging (MRI), for example, will provide interesting insight into the brain and real-time assessment of the brain's activity involvement in motor control.

KEY POINTS

- Sheridan (1984) suggested that four characteristics should be included in any theory of motor control: flexibility of movement, uniqueness of movement, consistency of movement, and modifiability of movement.

- Reflex theories were designed to explain motor behavior that was observable.

- Hierarchical theory of motor control was based on the notion that the brain controlled all parts of decision-making and performance.

- The motor program provided a means for understanding how movements could be planned in advance.

- Hierarchical theories of motor control continued to evolve through the 1970s and early 1980s to account for the concept of new, different, or novel motor behaviors.

- The dynamic systems theory is also known as the ecological theory or action systems theory.

DISCUSSION QUESTIONS

1. Compare and contrast theories of motor control according to the characteristics of motor control devised by Sheridan (1984).

2. Compare/contrast hierarchical theory with dynamics systems theory.

3. Why has hierarchical theory been questioned by researchers?

4. Compare/contrast the notion that movement either descends from the central nervous system or is dynamically interactive between the individual and environmental demands.

ADDITIONAL READINGS

Kugler, P. N., & Turvey, M. T. (1987). *Information, natural law and the self-assembly of rhythmic movement.* Hillsdale, NJ: Erlbaum.

Schmidt, R. A. (1985). A schema theory of discrete motor skill learning. *Psychological Review, 82,* 225–60.

Sherrington, C. S. (1906). *The integrative action of the nervous system.* New Haven, CT: Yale University Press.

Taub, E., & Berman, A. J. (1968). Movement and learning in the absence of sensory feedback. In S. J. Freedman (Ed.), *The neuropsychology of spatially oriented behavior* (pp. 173–192). Homewood, IL: Dorsey Press.

REFERENCES

Bernstein, N. (1967). *The coordination and regulation of movements.* Oxford, England: Pergamon Press.

Gibson, J. J. (1966). *The senses considered as perceptual systems.* Boston: Houghton Mifflin.

Gowitzke, B. A., & Milner, M. (1988). *Scientific bases of human movement.* (3rd ed.). Baltimore: Williams & Wilkins.

Greene, P. H. (1972). Problems of organization of motor systems. In R. Rosen & F. M. Snell (Eds.), *Progress in theoretical biology* (vol. 2). New York: Academic Press.

Grillner, S. (1975). The role of muscle stiffness in meeting the postural and locomotor requirements for force development by the ankle extensors. *Acta Physiologica Scandinavia 86,* 92–108.

Henry, F. M., & Rogers, D. E. (1960). Increased response latency for complicated movements and a memory drum theory of neuromotor reaction. *Research Quarterly, 31,* 448–458.

Horridge, G. A. (1987). The evolution of visual processing and the construction of seeing systems. London: *Proceedings of the Royal Society, 230,* 279–292.

Keele, S. W. (1968). Movement control in skilled motor performance. *Psychological Bulletin, 70,* 387–403.

Kelso, J. A. S. (Ed.) (1982). *Human motor behavior: An introduction.* Hillsdale, NJ: Erlbaum.

Kelso, J. A. S., & Kay, B. A. (1987). Information and control: A macroscopic analysis of perception-action coupling. In H. Heuer & A. F. Sanders (Eds.), *Perspectives on perception and action* (pp. 3–32). Hilldale, NJ: Erlbaum.

Kelso, J. A., & Tuller, B. (1984). A dynamical basis for action systems. In M. S. Gazzaniga (Ed.), *Handbook of cognitive neuroscience* (pp. 321–356). New York: Plenum Press.

Kugler, P. N., & Turvey, M. T. (1986). *Information, natural law, and the self-assembly of rhythmic movement.* Hillsdale, NJ: Erlbaum.

Mather, J. A., & Fisk, J. D. (1985). Orienting to targets by looking and pointing: Parallels and interactions in ocular and manual performance. *Quarterly Journal of Experimental Psychology, 37A,* 315–338.

Reed, E. S. (1982). An outline of a theory of action systems. *Journal of Motor Behavior, 14,* 98–134.

Schmidt, R. (1991). *Motor learning and performance: From principles to practice.* Champaign, IL: Human Kinetics Books.

Schmidt, R. (1978). *Motor control and learning: A behavioral emphasis.* (2nd ed.). Champaign, IL: Human Kinetics.

Schmidt, R. (1976). Control processes in motor skills. *Exercise and Sport Sciences Reviews, 4,* 229–261.

Schmidt, R. (1975). A schema theory of discrete motor skill learning theory. *Psychological Review, 82,* 225–260.

Schmidt, R. A., & Young, D. E. (1987). Transfer of motor control in motor skills learning. In S. M. Cormier & J. D. Hagman (Eds.), *Transfer of learning* (pp. 47–79). Orlando, FL: Academic Press.

Shapiro, D. C. (1978). *The learning of generalized motor programs.* Unpublished doctoral dissertation, University of Southern California, Los Angeles.

Sheridan, M. G. (1984). Planning and controlling simple movements. In M. M. Smyth and A. L. Wing (eds.), *The psychology of movement* (pp. 47–82). London: Academic Press.

Sherrington, C. S. (1906). *The integrative action of the nervous system.* New Haven: Yale University Press.

Skinner, B. F. (1938). *The behavior of organisms: An experimental analysis.* New York: Appleton.

Taub, W. T., & Berman, A. J. (1968). Movement and learning in the absence of sensory feedback. In S. J. Freedman (Ed.), *The neuropsychology of spatially oriented behavior* (pp. 173–192). Homewood, IL: Dorsey Press.

Thach, W. T. (1978). Correlation of neural discharge with pattern and force of muscular activity, joint position, and direction of the intended movement in motor cortex and cerebellum. *Journal of Neurophysiology, 41,* 654–676.

Thorndike, E. L. (1927). The law of effect. *American Journal of Psychology, 39,* 212–222.

Trachtman, J. N., & Kluka, D. A. (1993). Future trends in vision and peak sport performance. *International Journal of Sports Vision, 1*(1), 1–6).

Turvey, M. T. (1990). Coordination. *American Psychologist, 45,* 938–953.

Woodworth, R. S. (1899). The accuracy of voluntary movement. *Psychological Review, 3*(Suppl. 2), 1–114.

Theories of Motor Learning

- Degrees of freedom as they relate to motor behavior

- Coordination in skilled motor behavior

- Practice and experience in motor skill acquisition

- Motor learning theories as they relate to motor behavior

- Motor learning theories, their commonalities and their uniquenesses

- Motor learning theories and how they have shaped motor behavior

A *brief discussion of the concepts of skill development, coordination and movement control as they relate to motor behavior provides an entree to theories of motor learning. The issue of skilled motor behavior and its development will be discussed in detail later in this part of the textbook. Inherent in that discussion is the notion of **degrees of freedom**, derived from dynamic systems theorists. This relates to the limited number of independent parts of the human body that can be used within the environment to produce*

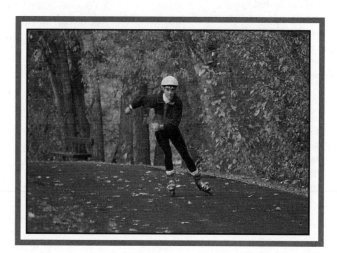

Degrees of freedom (of movement)
the options or possibilities available within the human body to perform a movement

the movement. A specific performance, narrowed from a range of possibilities, becomes skilled performance when the body is directed into appropriate performance. The pushoff in rollerblading, for instance, contains degrees of freedom. The joints of the foot, lower and upper leg, hip, spine, hands, lower and upper arms, and skull, as well as the muscles involved, comprise segments. They provide many degrees of freedom that must be constrained to produce the most effective and efficient movement.

Each of the joints and muscles involved produces an overall effect for human movement. Borrowing from Gestalt psychology, "the whole is greater than the sum of its parts," and applying this to motor control, total movement is more than the summation of those parts called into play to comprise a single performance. Movement is influenced by mechanical properties manifested throughout the musculoskeletal system. As an illustration of this, consider the children's game "crack the whip." The goal is to get the last person in the line to move as fast as possible without breaking the connection created by holding hands. The linkage produces more force than that which could be created by each person individually.

The development of skilled performance, then, contains the elements of coordination and control as well as sensory mechanisms (discussed in Section III). Skilled motor performance implies that the individual effectively and efficiently organizes body segments to accomplish a specific goal. **Coordination** has been defined succinctly by Turvey (1990) as a patterning of body movements that effectively and efficiently interacts with the patterning of environmental objects and events. Sparrow (1992) has also defined coordination as the process used to condense the available degrees of freedom into the smallest necessary to achieve the goal of the skill. Perhaps a combination of the two definitions is best: Coordination is the process of effectively and efficiently patterning body movements by constraining the available degrees of freedom to achieve the goal of the skill.

Coordination
effectively and efficiently patterning body movements by constraining the available degrees of freedom to achieve the goal of the skill

Control
arriving at total body movement based upon the degrees of freedom for each segment

Control, for several theorists (Kugler, Kelso, & Turvey, 1990; Newell, 1985; Turvey, 1990), provides a somewhat different perspective than that of coordination. **Control** involves the way in which total body movement is arrived at based upon the degrees of freedom for each segment. Control is based on movement parameters describing the body's total action: How much force was generated? What was the linear displacement of the movement? What was the angular displacement? What was the distance traveled?

Skilled motor behavior, then, is a performance in which environmental parameters have been selected and degrees of freedom have been condensed to produce an appropriate performance. A **motor skill** is a performance with a goal that is accomplished by voluntary body movement. Magill (1993) suggests that there are three characteristics of a motor skill: (1) there must be an achievable goal; (2) it must be voluntarily performed; and (3) body movement is required to achieve the goal. These three characteristics, when combined, imply that motor skills have purpose, they involve the interaction of nervous and musculoskeletal systems, and they are learned. Figure 3.1 represents these characteristics diagrammatically.

Skilled motor behavior
a performance wherein environmental parameters have been selected and degrees of freedom condensed to produce an appropriate action

Motor skill
a performance with a goal accomplished by voluntary body movement

THEORIES OF MOTOR LEARNING

Motor learning theories offer a clearer understanding of the processes involved in learning motorically. These theories also support the idea of creating optimal learning environments to enhance effectiveness and efficiency in performance. As we saw earlier, *motor learning* is a multifaceted set of internal processes that result in relatively permanent change in human movement through practice, provided the change cannot be attributed to maturation, temporary states, or instinct. Schmidt (1991), Magill (1993), Rose (1997), and Hilgard and Bower (1975) suggest three assumptions that characterize motor learning theories: (1) motor learning is a process within the individual that results in a relatively permanent change to en-

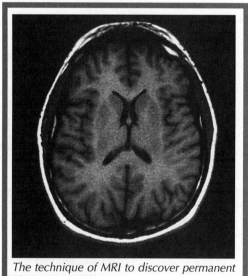

The technique of MRI to discover permanent change in the brain.

hance motor performance; (2) the process is not directly observable; and (3) the enhanced motor performance is a result of practice and

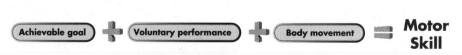

Three characteristics of a motor skill

3.1
FIGURE

experience rather than maturation, temporary states, or instinct. Figure 3.2 brings these components together.

Researchers have uncovered permanent changes in the neurological structures of the brain. Through the technique of MRI (magnetic resonance imaging), researchers were able to capture the brain activity of children raised in Eastern European orphanages (Jarvis, Smith, & Kozelsky, 1996). These youngsters were limited in motor, social, and emotional experiences from birth to three years of age. They were compared to youngsters raised with families in the United States. Those who were raised with families displayed increased cortical activity, particularly in the motor cortex area. As a result, it appeared that neural connections made early in the life cycle are critical to the development of the nervous system and its interaction with movement, so that the necessary structures are created to build subsystem connections for future learning.

No technology now exists to enable us to directly observe motor learning. As a result, motor learning can only be observed through repeated performances. Over time, the acquisition of skilled performance can be assessed and learning implied.

Practice and experience play key roles in motor skill acquisition. Maturation, temporary states (alteration of motivation or use of hypnosis; use of performance-enhancing drugs; physical training

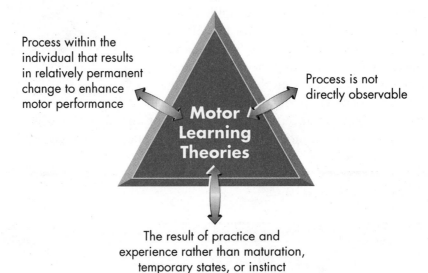

Assumptions underlying motor learning theories

FIGURE

LAB EXERCISE

THEORIES OF MOTOR BEHAVIOR

Objective: To determine theories used to explain the movement.

Equipment and Preparation: Partner. Stand upright, with arms hanging by the side of the body, straight elbows.

Experience: Eyes open, standing and facing a partner, from the position described above, flex the elbow of the preferred arm 30 degrees. Then, with eyes closed, simulate the movement again.

Assignment: Determine a plausible explanation using motor behavior theories about the results when sighted and the results when unsighted.

effects), and instinct (an infant suckling) cannot be considered learning. When an offensive lineman in American football is in the locker room during halftime, the coach may use a mythical motivational technique of "rattling the lockers," in which the lineman literally rattles the lockers by banging them with both fists, kicking and bumping against the lockers while yelling. The effectiveness of this technique remains undocumented. The use of anabolic steroids to enhance motor learning also remains undocumented. Although steroid use can produce short-term enhanced performance, it also has serious side effects. When an individual improves cardiovascular strength and endurance, muscular strength and endurance, flexibility, agility, and/or power, performance can temporarily be enhanced. If there is a loss in any of these training effects, performance can diminish.

Sheffield (1961) was one of the first to investigate how motor skills were learned. His perspective was through observational learning. Using the latest technology available in the early 1960s, he devised a theory (contiguity-mediational) to explain how filmed demonstrations and learning serial motor skills were related. An individual, by observing someone else performing a skill, formed a "blueprint" that served as a perceptually coded guide for the individual to follow in order to reproduce the skill. Sheffield's work formed the basis of others' works in the 1970s. The two most prominent theories were proposed by Adams (1971) and Schmidt (1975).

In chapter 2 we discussed an open-loop system of motor control. The open-loop system features a control center, referred to as the executive level, which initiates movement commands to the effector level. Muscles and joints are controlled by the effector level, which is responsible for carrying out the movement. In this model, feedback is not needed to produce motor behavior. The exclusion of feedback from motor skill learning however, was unsatisfactory to theorists.

Adams wondered what was being used in the detection and correction of performance errors. By basing a model on simple movements that were self-paced and on previously conducted research using arm and leg positioning, he devised a model that included feedback and could be generalized to all types of movements. It was labeled **closed-loop theory.** Figure 3.3 serves as a model for the theory. He provided a unique perspective that included the presence of two memory mechanisms: **memory trace** and **perceptual trace.** The memory mechanism used to select and initiate a movement was referred to as *memory trace.* The *perceptual trace,* developed from practice and sensory feedback, was the mechanism used to compare the movement being performed with its internal memory reference. He reasoned that if either of the memory mechanisms was diminished, learning was less than optimal.

As one of the contemporary pioneers in motor learning theory, Adams's perspectives gave impetus to others to conduct research using the paradigm (Adams & Goetz, 1973; Newell, 1976). Among those who became troubled by the closed-loop theory of motor behavior was Schmidt.

After having published work related to Adams's theory (Schmidt & White, 1972), Schmidt encountered difficulty explaining how every symbolic representation of movement in every situation was

Closed loop theory
a paradigm that compares feedback against a reference to explain human movement

Memory trace
the memory mechanism that selects and initiates movements

Perceptual trace
the mechanism used to compare the movement being performed with its internal memory reference

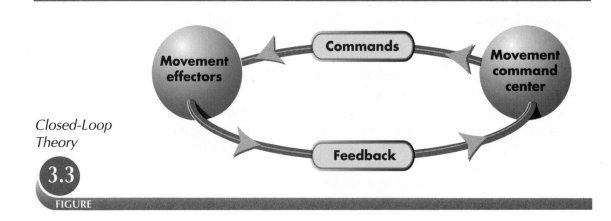

Closed-Loop Theory

3.3

FIGURE

stored in memory. It seemed that matching memory trace to every movement ever made would be an insurmountable (and time-consuming) task. He also wondered how memory trace could account for movements never made or seen before.

By 1975, Schmidt published his perspective on motor skill acquisition. He called it **schema theory**. A *schema* is a set of rules that guide decision-making about the goal of the skill. Schmidt suggested that once a performance is made, information is grouped and stored in memory in four general areas: (1) the environmental conditions as movement begins (e.g., body position, temperature); (2) the specific requirements of the movement (e.g., speed, time, space, force); (3) the outcome of the movement and its knowledge of results (e.g., comparing the actual outcome with the intended outcome); and (4) sensory information relating to the movement (e.g., how the movement felt, appeared, sounded). Learning is optimized if the grouped information is stored. Building upon Adams's ideas of the two memory mechanisms, he devised *recall* and *response recognition schemas* to facilitate information storage. A **recall schema** provides parameters for specific movement and initiates the goal-directed performance. For example, for a shortstop in baseball or softball, environmental conditions are such as to get the ball to the player covering second in order to turn the double play. For a play in which the distance from the shortstop to second base is only six feet, the shortstop chooses to scoop and backhand flick the ball. Once the generalized motor program has been selected and the movement has been performed, A **response recognition schema** is used to assess and compare the outcome with the parameters selected, using sensory information to store future corrections. Through additional practice and sensory feedback, the player can refine performances in a variety of environmental conditions using grouped information, whether the information received is appropriate or inappropriate. Figure 3.4 provides graphic insight into the theory.

In our discussion of the hierarchical theory of motor control in chapter 2, Schmidt's notion of a generalized motor program was discussed. It is central to his perspective on how individuals learn motorically. Succinctly, the **generalized motor program** is symbolically

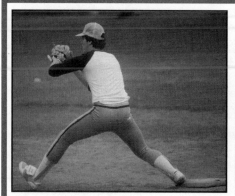

Shortstop in baseball uses a schema to guide performance.

Schema theory
a paradigm that explains the rules governing movement

Recall schema
a set of rules that selects parameter values for specific movement and initiates the goal-directed performance

Response recognition schema
a set of rules used to assess and compare the outcome with parameters selected, using sensory information to store future corrections

Generalized motor program
program that produces novel and flexible movement in various dimensions

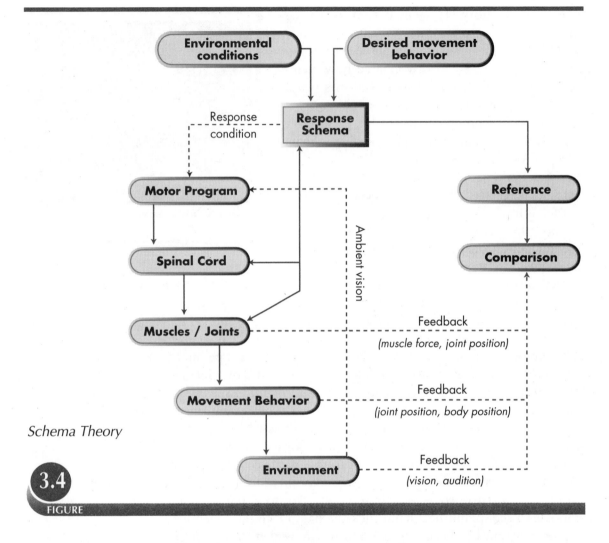

Schema Theory

3.4

FIGURE

stored in memory and controls groups of movements. The motor program is developed from every experience the individual has that is similar. Kicking experiences are grouped to form a general motor program for kicking which, when selected to be used to meet the goal of the skill, can be quickly and easily modified to meet environmental conditions. Once the relationships of responses are put together, the schema is devised.

Despite Schmidt's meticulous attempt to explain how motor skills are learned, it has not provided a complete understanding. It has, however, provided insight into learning through both appropriate and inappropriate performances — that learning can occur from both. It also provided questions for 1980s researchers (Goode, 1986; Goode & Magill, 1986; Goode & Wei, 1988) to investigate: Assuming that a generalized motor program exists, can practice conditions be varied to enhance learning? If so, to what extent can they be varied to enhance learning? If not, why not?

ECOLOGICAL THEORY: PERCEPTION AND MOVEMENT

By the 1970s, theorists began to wonder what the relationships between human groups and their physical and social environments were. This type of thought has been referred to as *human ecological theory*. Those who were instrumental in the application of human ecological theory to human perception and movement were Turvey and Carello, (Turvey, 1974; Turvey & Carello, 1988). They formulated an **ecological theory** of motor learning as it related to the learning of motor skills through coordination. They incorporated the work of Gibson (Gibson, 1979) and Bernstein (1967) to include a dynamic systems approach, whereby the individual, through movement, interacts with the environment, and the interaction of the individual with the environment is based upon the individual's perception. Their theory embodied both a dynamic systems approach and the perception of the individual, making it learner-centered. The person searches the environment proactively, establishing concepts that enhance the learning of motor skills and assist in the identification of information that inhibits the learning of motor skills.

Newell (1991) and Schmidt (1991) discussed several difficulties with traditional motor learning theories and the ecological theory:

1. Traditional theorists have been unable to justify the way in which new coordinated behaviors are acquired.
2. Traditional theorists have not elaborated on how individuals make small adjustments in a dynamic environment. Perception and movement-based ecological theory seems to provide a more plausible understanding of why movements can be changed once movement has begun, as in a well-executed overhead drop shot in badminton that can be held until the last moment and appropriately placed on the court.

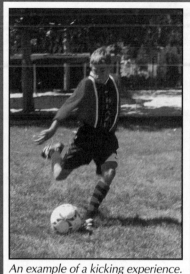

An example of a kicking experience.

Ecological theory
a paradigm explaining human movement in which the individual interacts with the environment and that interaction is based upon the individual's perception

THEORIES OF MOTOR BEHAVIOR

Objective: To determine theories used to explain the movement.

Equipment and Preparation: Partner; golf ball. Stand upright, with one arm by the side of the body, the other flexed at 90 degrees at the elbow, palm up; eyes closed. Upon the command, "now," the individual opens the eyes and attempts to catch the ball that is dropped a distance of two feet.

Experience: With the eyes closed, standing and facing a partner, the other partner says "now." The partner immediately drops the golf ball into the other's hand.

Assignment: Determine explanations for what was observed.

3. Ecological theorists diminish the role of memory (or memory trace) in motoric learning. Traditional theorists argue that without knowledge, reasoning, and judgment about rules or about the goal of skills used in specific games, the individual would be hard-pressed to select the appropriate motor behavior.

4. Ecological theorists continue to provide limited explanations for the notion of a generalized motor program (advocated by Schmidt, 1975). They contend that the generalized motor program lacks flexibility for a variety of environments, such as jai alai, where ball speeds have been recorded in excess of 120 mph, or slow-moving Nintendo computer games that require interception skills at speeds of less than 1 mph.

It remains to be seen whether or not ecological theory will continue to provide meaningful information to the theories of motor behavior. Further investigations are necessary to help us more fully understand the complexity of the theory's meaning and its contribution to the understanding of motor behavior through motor learning.

KEY POINTS

- Degrees of freedom relates to the number of independent components of the human body that are available to be used within the environment to produce the movement.

- Coordination and control as well as sensory mechanisms are involved in the development of skilled performance.

- Coordination is the process of effectively and efficiently patterning body movements by constraining the available degrees of freedom to achieve the goal of the skill.

- Control is based on movement parameters describing the body's total action.

- Magill (1993) suggests three characteristics of a motor skill: (1) must be an achievable goal; (2) must be voluntarily performed; and (3) body movement is required to achieve the goal.

- Learning is not directly observable.

- The open-loop system features a control center that initiates movement commands to the effector level.

- If either the memory trace or the perceptual trace is diminished, learning is less than optimal.

- A schema is a set of rules that guide decision-making about the goal of the skill.

- A recall schema selects parameter values for specific movement and initiates the goal-directed performance.

- A response recognition schema is used to assess and compare the outcome with parameters selected, using sensory information to store future collections.

- The generalized motor program is symbolically stored in memory and controls groups of movements.

DISCUSSION QUESTIONS

1. Describe the notion of degrees of freedom and its relationship to motor behavior.

2. Describe the fundamental tenets of schema theory. What unique qualities does this theory provide to understanding motor learning?

3. Identify the components of the closed-loop theory. How does this theory compare with the open-loop theory?

4. Define ecological theory. How does it relate to the learning of motor skills through coordination?

5. Compare/contrast ecological theory with schema theory and closed-loop theory.

ADDITIONAL READINGS

Gentile, A. M. (1987). Skill acquisition: Action, movement, and neuromotor processes. In *Movement science foundations for physical therapy*, eds. J. Carr, R. Shephard, J. Gordon, A. M. Gentile, & J. Held, pp. 93–130. Rockville, MD: Aspen.

Newell, K. M. (1985). Coordination, control and skill. In D. Goodman, R. B. Wilberg, and I. M. Franks (eds.), *Differing perspectives in motor learning, memory, and control* (pp. 295–317). Amsterdam: North-Holland.

Schmidt, R. A. (1988). Motor and action perspective on motor behavior. In O. G. Meijer and K. Roth (eds.), *Complex movement behaviour: "The" motor-action controversy* (pp. 3–44). Amsterdam: North-Holland.

REFERENCES

Adams, J. A. (1971). A closed-loop theory of motor learning. *Journal of Motor Behavior, 3*, 111–150.

Adams, J. A. & Goetz, E. T. (1973). Feedback and practice as variables in error detection and correction. *Journal of Motor Behavior, 5*, 217–224.

Bernstein, N. (1967). *The coordination and regulation of movements*. Oxford, England: Pergamon Press.

Gibson, J. J. (1979). *The ecological approach to visual perception*. Boston: Houghton Mifflin.

Goode, S. L. (1986). *The contextual interference effect in learning an open motor skill*. Unpublished doctoral dissertation, Louisiana State University, Baton Rouge, LA.

Goode, S. L., & Magill, R. A.(1986). The contextual interference effect in learning three badminton serves. *Research Quarterly for Exercise and Sport, 57*, 308–314.

Goode, S.L. & Wei, P. (1988). Differential effects of variations of random and blocked practice on novice learning an open motor skill. In D.L. Gill and J.E. Clarke (Eds.), *Abstracts of research papers, 1988* (p. 80). American Alliance for Health, Physical Education, Recreation and Dance Annual Convention, Kansas City, MO Reston, VA: AAHPERD.

Hilgard, E & Bower, G. (1975). *Theories of learning.* Englewood Cliffs, NJ: Prentice Hall.

Jarvis, P. T., Smith, A. S., and Kozelsky, J. S. (1996). The effects of isolation on occipital development in children. *Vision Science, 65,* 234–239.

Kugler, P. N., Kelso, J. A. S. & Turvey, M. T. (1982). On the control and coordination in naturally developing systems. In J. A. S. Kelso and J. E. Clark (Eds.), *The development of movement control and coordination.* (pp.5–78). New York: Wiley.

Magill, R. (1993). *Motor learning: Concepts and applications.* (4th ed.) Madison, WI: Brown & Benchmark Publishers.

Newell, K.M. (1991). Motor skill acquisition. *Annual Review of Psychology, 42,* 213–237.

Newell, K. M. (1985). Coordination, control and skill. In D. Goodman, R. B. Wilberg, and I. M. Franks (Eds.), *Differing perspectives in motor learning, memory, and control* (pp. 295–317). Amsterdam: North-Holland.

Newell, K. M. (1976). Motor learning without knowledge of results through the development of a response recognition mechanism. *Journal of Motor Behavior, 8,* 209–217.

Rose, D. (1997). *A multilevel approach to the study of motor control and learning.* Boston, MA: Allyn and Bacon.

Schmidt, R. (1991). Motor learning and performance: From principles to practice. Champaign, IL: Human Kinetics Books.

Schmidt, R. (1975). A schema theory of discrete motor skill learning theory. *Psychological Review, 82,* 225–260.

Schmidt, R. A. & White, J. L. (1972). Evidence for an error-detection mechanism in motor skills: A test of Adams' closed-loop theory. *Journal of Motor Behavior, 4,* 143–153.

Sheffield, F. N. (1961). Theoretical considerations in the learning of complex sequential tasks from demonstrations and practice. In A.A. Lumsdaine (Ed.), *Student response in programmed instruction* (pp. 13–32). Washington, DC: National Academy of Sciences, National Research Council.

Sparrow, W. A. (1992). Measuring changes in coordination and control. In J. J. Summers (Ed.), *Approaches to the study of motor control and learning,* pp. 147–162. North Holland: Elsevier Science Publishers.

Turvey, M.T. (1990). Coordination. *American Psychologist, 45,* 938–953.

Turvey, M. T. (1974). Preliminaries to a theory of action with reference to vision. In R. Shaw. & J. Bransford (Eds.), *Perceiving, acting and knowing* (pp. 211–265). Hillsdale, NJ: Erlbaum.

Turvey, M.T., & Varello, C. (1988). Exploring a law-based ecological approach to skilled action. In A.M. Coley and J.R. Beech (Eds.), *Cognition and action in skilled behavior* (pp. 247–253). Amsterdam: North-Holland.

Basic Tenets of Motor Learning

CHAPTER FOCUS

- Theoretical models that provide the architecture for stages in motor learning

- Evolution of motor learning theories as it relates to the progress of logical thought on questions of interest

- Classifications of motor behavior and their relationship to one another

- Influence of transfer on the learning of motor skills

Theoretical models serve as basic tenets upon which we can build motor skill acquisition descriptions. They provide a "road map" where certain markers or behaviors can be used to chart progress in the learning of motor skills. These markers or behaviors can be considered stages in the motor learning process. Several stage models have been developed (Vereijken, 1991; Gentile, 1972; Adams, 1971; Fitts & Posner, 1967).

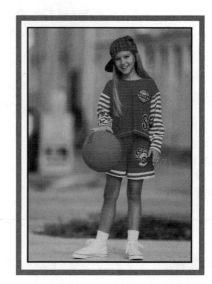

Cognitive stage of learning
level at which learners initially attempt to form the overall concept of a specific motor skill by gaining information through the senses in the form of sensory feedback by observing, getting verbal feedback from others, or through muscle spindles that detail each movement internally

The first theoretical model developed and published by any researcher generally becomes the classic. Fitts and Posner (1967) devised the classic three-stage model for the learning of a motor skill (Figure 4.1). In the first stage, referred to as the **cognitive stage**, learners initially try to form the overall concept of a motor skill by gaining information through the senses (vision, audition, kinesthesis) by observation, verbal feedback from others, or through muscle spindles that detail each movement internally. The learner is trying to define the goal and the general methods for achievement. Enormous amounts of information are gleaned from the environment, modified and/or discarded. Frequent errors make performances quite variable. The learner senses that the behavior does not produce the desired outcome but does not know what to do or how to do it differently to enhance the quality of each performance.

Three-stage model for the learning of a motor skill

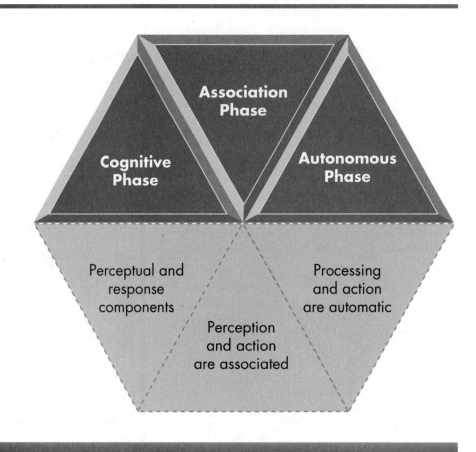

FIGURE

Because of limited performance success and high variability rates, the learner discovers many dimensions of time, space, force, and flow relative to the movement.

The second stage, the **associative stage**, is characterized by consistency of performance as one of the markers of skill development. The learner seemingly comprehends how parts of the movement relate to one another; movements begin to appear biomechanically efficient to the motor behavior professional; errors are fewer; and quality practice produces refinement of skill. The learner also develops the ability to identify inappropriate performances and to attempt solutions in subsequent trials of the skill in dynamic environments.

Associative stage of learning
the level at which performance becomes consistent

In the final stage, known as the **autonomous stage**, changes in performance over time become less noticeable. The learner's movements appear automatic, stable, and somewhat effortless. Automaticity of performance in a variety of settings becomes the marker of this stage. This automaticity provides the learner with the ability to focus attention on other details of the environment (e.g., the velocity and trajectory of the ball; the defensive alignment; the placement of the shot). The ability to self-correct and make minute adjustments are also inherent in this stage, particularly by those who are elite athletes.

Autonomous stage of learning
the level at which a learner's movements appear automatic, stable, and somewhat effortless

This classic model of how motor skills are acquired provides a basis for those in field-based motor behavior professions (e.g., physical educators, coaches, therapeutic recreation specialists, occupational, rehabilitative, and physical therapists) to aid them in the development of instructional strategies that are appropriate for effective and efficient learning.

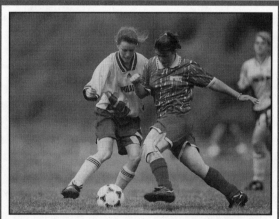

Playing the game of soccer requires stages of learning.

Once the Fitts and Posner model was published in 1967, subsequent models rapidly followed. In 1971 Adams proposed a two-stage model. In this model, the first stage was referred to as the **verbal/motor stage**. Essentially, this stage combined the cognitive and associative stages from the Fitts and Posner model, while acknowledging an association between the cognitive and motor aspects in the initial stage of learning. The second and final stage, the

Verbal/motor stage of learning
the cognitive and associative stages were combined from the Fitts and Posner model, while divulging an association between the cognitive and motor aspects in the initial stage of learning

Motor stage of learning
autonomous stage in the Fitts and Posner model of 1967

"Getting the idea" stage of learning
the phase at which the learner understands how the movement must be organized to accomplish the goal of the skill

motor stage, rather simplistically included all that was included in the 1967 model's autonomous stage.

Gentile's (1972) two-stage model of learning (Figure 4.2) was meaningful to two groups: those who were learning *and* field-based motor behavior professionals. The first stage, identified as the **"getting the idea of the movement"** stage, encompassed the general concept of organizing movement to accomplish the goal of the skill. The learner must determine the relevance of information that will regulate (or influence) the movement during performance. For example, if the goal of the movement is to score a goal by kicking the soccer ball from within the circle, regulatory conditions might include the speed of the ball, its trajectory, the direction from which it approaches, and its spin. Irrelevant information might include the goalie's initial posture prior to the kick, the placement of the defending team's offense, and such other distractions as a spectator

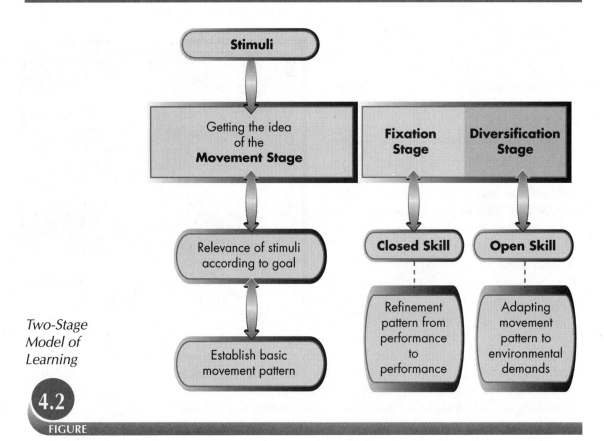

Two-Stage Model of Learning

4.2

FIGURE

standing behind the goal cage and waving a brightly colored towel. When practice is introduced in this stage, its goal is to develop the overall movement pattern sufficiently to achieve the goal of the skill in response to the regulatory information.

The second stage proposed by Gentile, the **fixation/diversification stage**, suggests two ways in which skill learning may proceed based on the demands of the task. If it is a closed skill that requires consistent repetition of the same action, then it is considered *fixation*. If it is an open skill that requires variability of action, then it is considered *diversification*. If the individual is performing the first half of a parallel bar routine, the movement pattern must have increasingly less variability through numerous attempts, which requires consistent repetitions of the same action (fixation). Practice conditions must be structured to model consistency of variables. For example, parts of a luge run must be repeatedly simulated in order to eliminate variability in performance effectiveness and efficiency. If, however, a tennis player is trying to learn to hit a forehand drive out of reach of an opponent's backhand, diversification of the movement occurs by varying the angles at which the ball is contacted relative to the placement of both players, the net, and the ball. By varying the practice conditions, the movement pattern becomes more varied, and the player will ultimately perform more flexibly to meet dynamic environmental demands. Yet another approach, however, has more recently been offered from an ecological viewpoint that focuses on the containment of variables in behavior.

In 1991, Vereijken developed a three-stage model based on Bernstein's (1967) work. Bernstein conceived the notion of degrees of freedom, which refers to the amount of flexibility within the human movement system. Essentially, the more degrees of freedom available within the system, the greater the opportunity for ineffective and inefficient movement. Bernstein believed that the ultimate challenge was the containment of as many degrees of freedom as possible in motor skill performance. Based on this notion, Vereijken's model (Figure 4.3) included a **novice stage,** in which the person tries to reduce the degrees of freedom issue and simplify the

Fixation/diversification stage of learning the level at which the movement is consistent within the presented environments (fixation) and adapting (diversification) the movement enough to perform successfully in the environment

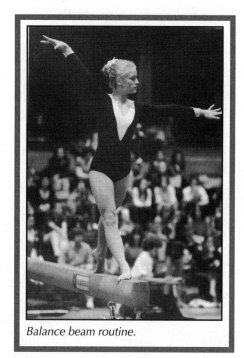

Balance beam routine.

Novice stage of learning the phase at which individuals try to simplify the degrees-of-freedom issue by increasingly reducing them

*Ecological
Three-Stage
Model of
Learning*

Novice Stage	**Advanced Stage**	**Expert Stage**
GOAL OF EACH STAGE:		
Reduce degrees of freedom of joint movement	Release/reinstate degrees of freedom of joint movement	Release/reorganize degrees of freedom of joint movement

4.3
FIGURE

Advanced stage of learning
the level of freedom at which joints and body segments are most coordinated

action. Vereijken uses the term *freezing out* to refer to joints and body segments that appear stiff, rigid, forced, and mechanical when in action. For example, when riding a horse at a trot for the first time, a person literally stiffens the hips, torso, shoulders, and arms, thereby creating dysfunctioning segments that contribute to a dysfunctioning unit. What is needed is to reintroduce more degrees of freedom so that the rider's body synchronizes with the horse's rhythm, and horse and rider appear as one. In the second stage, the **advanced stage**, additional degrees of freedom are added so that joints and body segments become more coordinated. Through increased coordination, the movement becomes more synchronized and effective. A simple equation can be used to remember these stages:

NOVICE STAGE OF MOVEMENT = FREEZING OUT − DEGREES OF FREEDOM

ADVANCED STAGE OF MOVEMENT = FREEZING OUT + DEGREES OF FREEDOM

Expert stage of learning
the level at which the movement produces efficiency as well as effectiveness through reorganization and addition of degrees of freedom

The final stage is the **expert stage**. Efficiency as well as effectiveness are attained by the reorganization and addition of degrees of freedom until efficiency is produced in the movement. Additionally, the individual can consider and adjust to external forces exerted on the body during the performance of the movement based upon a perception of what is necessary to accomplish the goal of the skill. A simple equation can be devised to remember this stage:

EXPERT STAGE = INDIVIDUAL PERCEPTION + WHAT IS NEEDED TO ACCOMPLISH GOAL + REORGANIZATION OF DEGREES OF FREEDOM

The models presented by Fitts and Posner, Gentile, and Vereijken represent stages of motor learning that have direct practical implications. They each contribute to an understanding of the learning process that characterizes motor learning. Each presents a different perspective: Both the Fitts and Posner model and the Gentile model helped field-based motor behavior professionals to structure practice for success in motor skill acquisition. Fitts and Posner emphasized cognitive and performance perspectives to understand learning progression, while Gentile offered strategies for the organization of practice to enhance the learning process. Both Gentile and Vereijken emphasize the role of the environment in the learning of motor skill acquisition. Implicit in all three of the models is the uniqueness of the individual, which must be considered in creating instructional strategies for motor behavior success.

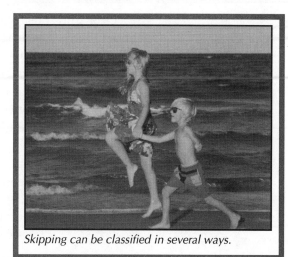

Skipping can be classified in several ways.

CLASSIFICATION OF MOTOR BEHAVIOR

It is important in the discussion of basic tenets of motor behavior to include ways in which motor skills are classified. Taxonomies (classifications) have been developed for a number of areas: Bloom's taxonomy classifies thought processes in a hierarchical fashion; muscle fiber types have been classified into slow- and fast-twitch fibers; visual skills for sport have been classified into focal/ambient and magno/parvo. In motor behavior, classification in terms of movement characteristics, goal of the skill, use of the body as a projectile, or shape and effort promotes a better understanding about commonalities, differences, and uniqueness.

Fitts (1964) was one of the first to classify motor skills. A **discrete skill** is one in which the movement has both a specific beginning and an ending (e.g., baseball pitch; ring toss; basketball free throw). A **continuous skill** involves a series of movements that are repeated or linked together with other parts of skills to achieve a goal. Continuous skills can include running a 50-meter sprint, swimming a 100-meter freestyle, rowing in a sprint event, and cross-country skiing.

Discrete skill
a skill in which the movement has a specific beginning and a specific ending

Continuous skill
a series of movements that are repetitive or linked with other parts of skills to achieve a goal

Fitts and Posner (1967) also developed a two-dimensional model that focused on two performance factors, (1) the individual and (2) the environment. Figure 4.4 organizes the environment from *stable* to *in motion* and the individual from *at rest* to *in motion.* When the individual is at rest, the environment is stable; when the individual is in motion, the environment can be either stable or in motion; when the environment is moving, the individual is also in motion.

In 1963, Knapp devised a classification of motor skills based upon the environmental demands in sport. He classified motor skills along a continuum. At one end, habit and stable or closed environments played a substantial role in performance success. At the other,

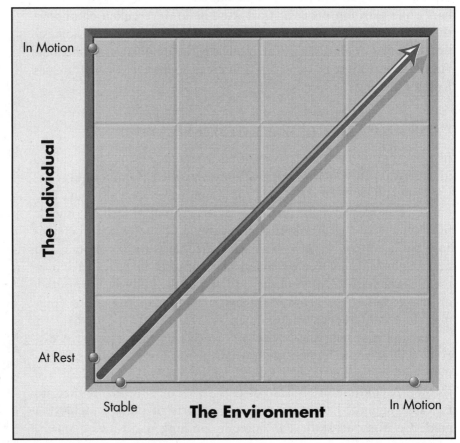

Two-dimensional model of learning (Relationship of individual to the environment)

4.4

FIGURE

the perceptual adaptability of the performer and the flexibility of dynamic or open environments played a substantial role. A closed environment meant that a number of variables were controlled or stabilized for performance consistency. An open environment meant that many variables were present that produced variability of performance. Figure 4.5 illustrates Knapp's classification.

Broer (1966) classified motor skills by purpose. Skills either provided support (sitting, standing, balancing), suspension (hanging, dangling), motion (running, skipping, hopping), moving external objects (throwing, hitting, pushing, pulling), or force reception (catching) (Figure 4.6). Each category contained many solutions for accomplishing the purpose of the skill. For example, moving a ball could be accomplished by throwing overarm, sidearm, underarm, or flicking it laterally. This classification could be used by field-based professionals in motor behavior to develop movement exploration challenges or basic motor skills competency checklists.

A proponent of motor control, Konorski (1969) devised a classification that also specified purpose. Classification focused upon locomotor behavior (jumping, running, sliding), isolated limb movement (throwing, kicking, dribbling), and postural movement (standing). Included in the classification was the designation of neurological control centers for each category; postural movement is controlled by "older" neurological structures of the brain, whereas isolated limb movement and the interaction of object and limb require "newer" neurological control mechanisms of the brain. Konorski suggested

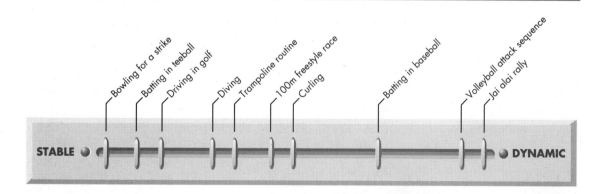

STABLE ●————————————————————————————————————● DYNAMIC

Bowling for a strike
Batting in teeball
Driving in golf
Diving
Trampoline routine
100m freestyle race
Curling
Batting in baseball
Volleyball attack sequence
Jai alai rally

Knapp's (1963) classification of motor skills based upon sporting environmental demands

4.5
FIGURE

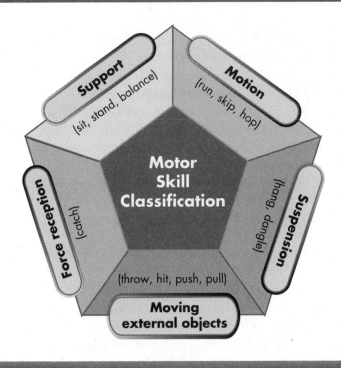

Classification of motor skills by purpose

4.6

FIGURE

that postural and locomotor classifications preempt those of isolated limb movement and object/limb interaction, since it is necessary for the person to become competent in bipedal posture (standing upright) and in basic locomotor movements before isolated limb movement and object/limb interaction can occur successfully. Those field-based motor behavior professionals who devise programs for elementary school–aged children may find this classification system helpful because it places postural and basic locomotor skills activities ahead of limb movement and object/limb interaction tasks in learning sequences.

Whiting (1969) classified the learning of motor skills through the use of an object, specifically a ball: (1) acquiring an object in flight (e.g., in a softball glove; from a pass in basketball with the hands; in lacrosse with the crosse); (2) acquiring an object in flight and redirecting it toward a goal or target (e.g., batting in baseball; fielding in field hockey; passing in volleyball); and (3) directing an already-acquired object toward a goal or target (e.g., golf tee shot; field hockey penalty stroke; faceoff in ice hockey). This type of classification, although meaningful as it relates to objects such as balls, pucks, shuttlecocks, pins, and hoops, is highly specific. Those field-based professionals who deal specifically with object acquisition–type sports should find this helpful for creating conceptual instructional strategies.

In 1970, Logan and McKinney developed a classification of motor skills by the type of joint movement that was used in their performance. Movement terms were used to describe the movement of body segments: flexion/extension, depression/elevation, circumduction, abduction/-adduction, medial/lateral rotation, etc. Professionals in the areas of physical therapy, rehabilitative counseling, therapeutic recreation, and occupational therapy may find this classification helpful.

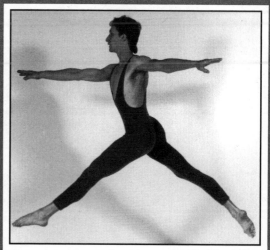

Dance movements have been classified by Laban Notation.

In contrast, Laban (Dell, 1970) developed a unique method of classifying movements specifically used in dance, called **Laban Notation**. Space outside the personal reach of the body was **general space**. Space within personal reach of the body was referred to as the **kinesphere**. The body was considered capable of moving in twenty-six directions from the body's center. The twenty-seventh "direction" was the kinesphere. Movements were classified according to the type of exertion or effort and the type of spatial adaptation or shape used (Figure 4.7). Movement qualities were further classified in "shorthand" to describe movement. For example, sustained/explosive (sudden), light/heavy (strong), free/bound were used as subclassifications. Spatial adaptation (shape) subclassifications included advancing/retreating, growing/shrinking, or rising/sinking. Categories could be used to describe motor skills as well as variations in movement quality, depending on the purpose of the skill. This form of notation might prove helpful for field-based motor behavior specialists who design movement exploration experiences, particularly for people with disabilities, youth, or seniors, because specific movements can be detailed.

An integration of the notions devised by Laban and Broer might provide a new and interesting opportunity for field-based motor behavior professionals to develop creative instructional strategies that

Laban Notation
a classification system of movement according to the type of exertion or effort and the type of spatial adaptation or shape used

General space
in Laban Notation terms, space that is outside the personal reach of the body

Kinesphere
in Laban Notation, space within personal reach of the body

Movement Qualities

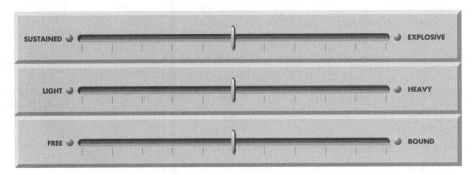

Spatial Adaptations

Laban Notation: A unique method of classifying movements specifically used in dance

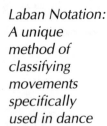

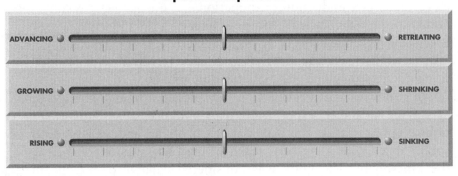

would enable people to experience the joy of movement through time, space, force, and flow components. Broer's classification provides purposes of skills, while Laban's classification provides variations in shape, effort, and movement technique as they relate to experiencing and learning through motor behavior.

One of the most inclusive taxonomies of motor skills was that devised by Gentile (1972), who built upon a classification system initially proposed by Poulton (1957). Gentile developed a two-dimensional model that focused on environmental conditions and relative movement. Figure 4.8 shows the relationship: When there is a stable environment, little change in environmental conditions exists; therefore, the individual is in control of the spatial environment. Beginning and ending movements (which are temporal considerations) are at the discretion of the individual, as is the performance

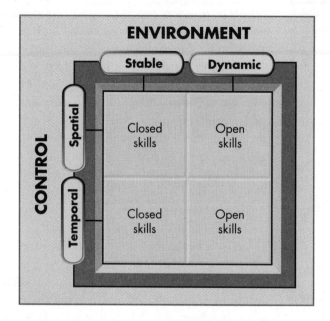

Two-dimensional model focusing on environmental conditions and relative movement

4.8

FIGURE

through direction and position of the movements. These types of movements, which are under spatial control, are considered **closed skills**. Examples of these types of skills include batting from a tee, driving off the tee in golf, bowling for a strike, and performing a tumbling pass in a floor exercise routine. When there is change in the relationship between the environment and the individual or object, both spatial and temporal control are involved. The individual must determine the spatial and temporal demands and match them with the environment. Motor skills such as catching a fish when fly casting, tackling during a field hockey match, calf roping, and performing a backhand drive from a tennis serve can be considered **open skills**.

Gentile (1972) and colleagues (1975) have developed a most comprehensive and inclusive motor skill classification system. This system should provide the field-based professional with a theoretical model whereby methods and skill progressions can be devised to set the stage for optimum learning. Instructional strategies should be in harmony with that which is necessary for movement success. For example, the successful incorporation of a double toe loop in figure skating requires consistent movement within a stable environment

Closed skills
skills characterized by a stable environment, little change in environmental conditions, and the individual's control of the spatial environment

Open skills
skills in which the relationship between the environment and the individual or object changes; the individual must determine the spatial and temporal demands and match them with the environment

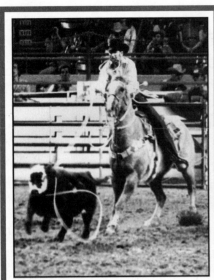

Calf roping utilizes motor skills that are rather unique in purpose.

and the use of kinesthetic feedback to monitor and regulate movement. Success in volleyball, on the other hand, also requires control of temporal dimensions, which include the estimation of time, space, force, and flow as they relate to the speed of the ball, the direction of the attack, the anticipation of ball-to-hand contact in the block, and the appropriate response within the dynamic environment of the rally. By establishing the content, structure, and environmental demands of the game within the practice setting, the field-based professional is best able to create an environment that enables players to learn.

The classifications of motor skills as they relate to motor behavior have provided interesting perspectives on the learning process. The model of Fitts (1954) describes learning progressions with learning stages, based upon cognitive and behavioral mechanisms. Theorists who followed found merit in grouping motor skills by purpose, use of an object, environmental demands, type of joint movement produced, or core body movement as a prerequisite to limb/object interaction. Laban further illuminated the contributions of effort and shape to the classification and description of motor skills. Gentile introduced the aspect of environmental contributions to the learning of motor skills. Each of these classifications provides better insight into how we learn motor skills. The extent to which each one provides value to the field-based professional will depend upon the specific needs, desires, and abilities of learners.

MOTOR BEHAVIOR AND ITS TRANSFER

Based upon motor learning theories, is there any benefit to organizing skills in sequence in order to facilitate learning? If one skill in a classification is learned, what importance does it have on learning another skill?

Transfer
the influence of one skill on the learning of another

This importance or influence is referred to as **transfer,** or the amount of influence the learning of one skill has on the learning of another skill. The transfer can have a positive, negative or neutral influence. Once an overarm throw for distance is learned in baseball, its basic components can be used to throw a softball from deep left field to second base, to throw a twenty-yard pass to a receiver in football, or to shoot for goal over defenders in team handball. These are examples of *positive transfer*, in which the learning of a skill facilitates the learning of another skill.

There may be situations where transfer occurs negatively, producing dissonance between the previously learned skill and the newly learned skill. *Negative transfer* occurs when the learning of one skill interferes with the learning of another. The research indicates very little long-term negative transfer. It may exist initially, but it disappears as skills are made distinct. For example, if a person learns the squash forehand, the learning of the racquetball forehand and the handball forehand may prove to be challenging. Although similar in purpose, the practicing of the squash, racquetball, and handball forehands may provide a temporary period of negative transfer and frustration for the learner. Each of the surfaces to contact the ball is different in shape and size; each requires a different distance from the ball at contact; each requires different angular velocities. Although the environmental demands of each sport differ somewhat, the negative transfer should be temporary and dissipate with practice.

When one learned skill has no influence upon the learning of another skill, it is referred to as *neutral transfer*. There seems to be no transfer of learning between an overarm throwing pattern for distance in baseball and learning to drive a manual transmission car, because completely different parts of the body are used to accomplish the tasks.

THEORIES OF TRANSFER

Theoretical models of transfer were constructed as early as 1901. Thorndike and Woodworth (Thorndike & Woodworth, 1901; Thorndike, 1914) were the first to provide published perspectives on the topic. The major premise of the **identical elements theory** was that learning was quite specific, based upon components of the learning that were exact (elements that were identical). In order for the transfer of motor skill learning to occur, portions of the skill already learned had to be present within the skill being learned. Thorndike believed that actual brain cells, brain activity, and behavior used in one skill were used identically in the other skill.

Several generations later, Osgood (1949) and Holding (1976) provided slightly different perspectives of the identical elements

Identical elements theory
a concept holding that learning is quite specific based upon components of the learning that were exact

theory. Osgood proposed the notion that the direction and amount of positive transfer of verbal skills were similar in the stimulus and response of the two skills. The *size* of the "transfer surface" determined the amount of transfer to be made. Holding furthered Osgood's ideas by linking the physical components of the skills together. The more surface (or exact elements), the more positive transfer would occur; the less surface, the less positive transfer would occur.

Additional perspectives were postulated in the next wave of those interested in transfer. As was the case with Osgood, verbal skills were focused upon by Bransford and others (Morris, Bransford, & Franks, 1977; Bransford, Franks, Morris & Stein, 1979). The basic premise of the *transfer-appropriate processing model,* however, related the *cognitive processing* of characteristic similarities rather than identical physical elements: the more similar the cognitive processing characteristics of the initially learned skill to the one being learned, the more positive the transfer.

A slightly different perspective of the transfer-appropriate processing model, an adaptation to motor skills, was published by Lee in 1988. Focusing upon movement skills, the premise holds that positive transfer should occur by practicing skills that are cognitively similar, even though they are not physically similar. The transfer arises from the cognitive activity and is specific to cognitive processes. For example, the American Red Cross uses land-based swimming and rescue drills. Although these movement skills are not exactly similar to those performed in the water, the cognitive processes used are similar enough for positive transfer of cognitive aspects to occur. Additionally, the diver who practices for a double full-twisting back somersault with the use of a trampoline and twisting harness is practicing similar cognitive processing skills. These skills are not exactly identical to those used on the diving board and in the water; they can, however, provide cognitive processing transfer.

The field-based professional in motor behavior, with an understanding of the theories of transfer, can construct a learning environment conducive to the positive transfer of skills, thereby contributing to learning efficiency. For instance, the construction of sequentially related movement drills would facilitate positive transfer: handstand/forward roll, step out to cartwheel, rather than handstand, then forward roll, then step out, then cartwheel. This can also be done by creating a learning environment that closely simulates the actual performance environment. The use of driving simulators before actually driving a car might prove helpful, or the use of a pitching machine on the field during batting practice rather than only in the batting cage or indoors. The field-based professional must also understand that when a person is faced with learning a new skill, regardless of similarity or uniqueness, there will be some decrease in initial performance. Once an individual has learned to deliver a straight ball in bowling, respectable scores can be achieved. In order for the individual to be able to bowl the "perfect game," however, he or she must learn to deliver a hook ball so that appropriate pin action can be achieved to knock down all of the pins each time. When the individual is required to make a new response (the hook) to an old stimulus (the pin configuration), the previously learned straight ball will derail the individual's score temporarily.

Additionally, dynamic practice settings have been shown to improve opportunities for positive transfer to occur (Christina & Bjork, 1991; Sherwood, 1988). First, the use of contextual interference (Battig, 1972) in an instructional strategy facilitates the learning process. Briefly, using **contextual interference** in an instructional strategy involves devising a practice environment in which several skills are practiced in differing environments. The unpredictability of skill presentation in and out of context provides solid development of realistic cognitive strategies in dynamic environments.

Contextual interference the use of different contexts through practice

Second, variations using the same skill can be provided. Structuring a soccer practice session that includes dribbling around cones, around people who are stationary, around people who are moving, dribbling, then doing a pushup, dribbling again, and dribbling around hoops and flags can create variety and facilitate transfer.

Third, support for the notion of "paralysis by analysis" has been referred to in research. Too much external feedback can lead to the individual relying upon that feedback rather than developing cognitive processing and internal mechanisms for feedback. External feedback is information provided to the individual by someone else that gives meaning to the performance. In the practice environment, it is important to provide enough external feedback to provide goal-direction of motor behavior for the individual, but not so much that the individual relies on the external feedback to the detriment of needing it to perform. By reducing the frequency of feedback, the individual can develop cognitive processing that facilitates transfer.

Finally, the combination of making the practice setting more difficult by using contextual interference, drill variations, and reducing feedback within the same practice setting could be incorporated by the field-based professional. This would produce a collection of instructional strategies that should benefit individuals in the learning process.

KEY POINTS

- Fitts and Posner's classic three-stage model for learning a motor skill includes a cognitive stage, an associative stage, and an autonomous stage.

- The transfer-appropriate processing model is based on similarities between cognitive processing characteristics rather than identical physical elements.

- The transfer-appropriate processing model focuses upon movement skills: the premise holds that positive transfer should occur by practicing skills that are cognitively similar, even though they are not physically similar.

- Contextual interference refers to devising a practice environment whereby several skills are practiced in several different situations or contexts.

DISCUSSION QUESTIONS

1. Describe the three classifications of motor skills.

2. Cite examples of how each classification could be used to learn the concept it represents.

3. Compare the two-stage models of motor learning. Describe their similarities and their differences.

4. Select one of the theories of motor learning described in this chapter. Explain its practical use for learning a specific skill in a specific activity.

5. What are the similarities between theories of transfer? Where do they differ?

6. Select a practice setting in a specific sport. In this practice environment, list two specific drills that can lead to positive transfer. In what types of situations can negative transfer occur?

ADDITIONAL READINGS

Adler, J. (1981). Stages of skill acquisition: A guide for teachers. *Motor Skills: Theory into Practice, 5,* 75–80.

Annett, J., & Sparrow, J. (1985). Transfer of training: A review of research and practical implications. *Programmed Learning and Educational Technology, 22,* 116–24.

Block, B. A. (1998). Keep them in their "place": Applying Laban's Notation of kinesphere and place in teaching scientific concepts. *JOPERD, 69*(3), 43–47.

REFERENCES

Adams, J. A. (1971). A closed-loop theory of motor learning. *Journal of Motor Behavior, 3,* 111–150.

Battig, W. F. (1972). Intertask interference as a source of facilitation in transfer and retention. In R. F. Thompson and J. F. Voss (eds.), *Topics in learning and performance.* (pp.131–159). New York: Academic Press.

Bernstein, N. (1967). *The coordination and regulation of movements.* Oxford: Pergamon Press.

Bransford, J. D. Franks, J. J. Morris, C. D., & Stein, B. S. (1979). Some general constraints on learning and memory research. In L. S. Cermak and F. I. M. Craik (Eds.), *Levels of processing in human memory.* (pp. 331–354). Hillsdale, NJ: Erlbaum.

Broer, M. R. (1966). *Efficiency of human movement.* Philadelphia: W. B. Saunders.

Christina, R. W., & Bjork, R. A. (1991). Optimizing long-term retention and transfer. In D. Druckman and R. A. Bjork (Eds.), *In the mind's eye: enhancing human performance* (pp. 23–56). Washington, DC: National Academy Press.

Dell, C. (1970). *A primer for movement description.* New York: Dance Notation Bureau, Inc.

Fitts, P. M. (1954). The information capacity of the human motor system in controlling the amplitude of movement. *Journal of Experimental Psychology, 47,* 381–391.

Fitts, P. M. (1964). Perceptual-motor skill learning. In W. Melton (Ed.), *Categories of human learning.* New York: Academic Press.

Fitts, P. M., & Posner, M. E. (1967). *Human performance.* Belmont, CA: Brooks/Cole.

Gentile, A. M. (1972). A working model of skill acquisition with application to teaching. *Quest, 17*, 3–23.

Gentile, A. M., Higgins, J. R., Miller, E. A., and Rosen, B. M. (1975). The structure of motor tasks. *Mouvement, 7*, 11–28.

Holding, D. H. (1976). *The principles of training.* Oxford: Pergamon Press.

Knapp, B. (1963). *Skill in sport.* London: Routledge and Kegan Paul.

Konorski, G. (1969). *Integrative activity of the brain.* Chicago: University of Chicago Press.

Logan, G. A., & McKinney, W. C. (1970). *Kinesiology.* St. Louis, MO: W. C. Brown.

Morris, C. D., Bransford, J. D., & Franks, J. J. (1977). Levels of processing versus transfer appropriate processing. *Journal of verbal learning and verbal behavior, 16*, 519–533.

Osgood, C. E. (1949). The similarity paradox in human learning: A resolution. *Psychological Review, 56*, 132–143.

Poulton, E. C. (1957). On prediction in skilled movements. *Psychological Bulletin, 54*, 467–478.

Sherwood, D. E. (1988). Effect of bandwidth knowledge of results on movement consistency. *Perceptual and motor skills, 66*, 535–542.

Thorndike, E. L. (1914). *Educational psychology: Briefer course.* New York: Columbia University Press.

Thorndike, E. L., & Woodworth, R. S. (1901). The influence and improvement in one mental function upon the efficiency of other functions. *Psychological Review, 8*, 247–261.

Vereijken, B. (1991). *The dynamics of skill acquisition.* Unpublished dissertation, Free University, Netherlands.

Whiting, H. T. A. (1969). *Acquiring ball skill.* Philadelphia, PA: Lea & Febiger.

Biological Perspectives

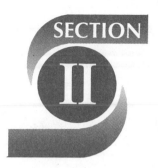

The 1996 Centennial Olympic Games, held in Atlanta, were most impressive. The lighting of the Olympic flame was particularly meaningful at the opening ceremonies of this Olympiad. Muhammad Ali, 1960 Olympic gold medalist in heavyweight boxing, was selected by the Atlanta Organizing Committee to receive the torch to light the huge cauldron that stood in the massive stadium. While more than one billion people watched their televisions throughout the world, they saw, in real time, the historical event. Muhammad Ali, as a charismatic young man, dazzled the world in 1960 with his agile footwork, his lightning fists, and his use of prose. Now thirty-six years older, he held the lighted torch, his hands trembling, his gaze steady. Ever so slowly he struggled to reach forward to ignite the flame. The once lightning-fast Ali, now with Parkinson's disease, experienced yet another proud moment when he successfully passed the fire from the torch to the Olympic flame. What happened to Muhammad Ali's lightning-fast abilities since his diagnosis of Parkinson's disease?

Central Nervous System

CHAPTER FOCUS

- Neural basis of motor behavior
- Basic neuroanatomy and its contributions to motor control and motor learning
- Basic organization of the neuromuscular system and its relationship to motor behavior
- Musculoskeletal system and its contributions to force production

*S*keletal muscles are controlled by the *central nervous system* (CNS), which consists of the brain and spinal cord. This system determines which muscles will contract, when, how fast, to what degree, and what changes in force from moment to moment will occur. Central nervous system function involves the cooperation of the brain and spinal cord to produce coordinated and skilled motor behavior. This cooperation occurs as a

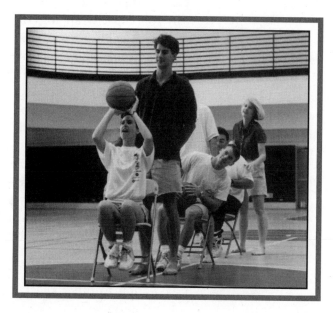

Central nervous system
the brain and spinal cord of the human body, composed of two types of cells: neurons and neuroglia

Neuron
an elongated cell designed to transmit excitation by receiving and conducting impulses

Soma
a cell body of a neuron

Axon
a transmitting pole of a neuron

Dendrite
a receiving pole of a neuron

Myelination
a protective sheath of myelin that insulates each axon from other neural paths

result of feedback loops. Feedback loops connect, consult, compare, adjust, correct, and fine-tune impulses throughout the CNS.

CELL STRUCTURE

Basically, the nervous system is composed of two types of cells: neurons and neuroglia. For purposes of motor behavior/motor control, the **neuron** is the functional unit. Neuroglia are those cells that serve as the "glue" between neural networks and other neurons. A neuron is an elongated cell that is designed to transmit excitation by receiving and conducting impulses. It has a receiving pole (dendrite), a transmitting pole and conducting segment (axon), and a cell body (**soma**). Figure 5.1 shows the composition of a neuron. Axon diameters range from 0.5 microns in unmyelinated fibers — those without a protective sheath of myelin which insulates each axon from other neural parts — to 22 microns in the largest myelinated fibers. Some are over one meter long. Axons are usually single and long. Dendrites are generally multiple, short, and highly branched. The **axon** transmits impulses to other cells. **Dendrites** generally receive impulses from adjacent cells.

NEURAL TRANSMISSION

Each axon is enclosed in a cellular (myelin) sheath of lipid material that insulates the axon from other neural parts. The sheath is formed by concentric wrappings of oligodendrocytes (sheath cells) in the CNS and Schwann cells in the peripheral nervous system (PNS). Those fibers having numerous layers are called **myelinated** fibers. Unmyelinated fibers are those that have only a single layer of sheath cells. The myelin sheath of larger axons (1 to 2 mm) contain segments separated by short unmyelinated gaps called nodes of Ranvier. These myelinated axons can transmit neural messages up to 400 feet per second by jumping from one node to the next; unmyelinated axons transmit messages up to three feet per second (Noback & Demarest, 1972).

It is important to have a basic understanding of the neurophysiology that occurs as messages are sent from the brain and spinal cord to the muscles that control actions. Following is a summary of the process of nerve cell transmission that should serve as a review or as an introduction.

The primary function of a nerve cell is to transmit an impulse or excitation to other cells. It performs this by switching on and off.

The on or off position (or state) is determined by the distribution of charged particles (ions). Ions, having positive and negative charges, surround the inside and outside of each cell. When the charges on one side of the membrane are unbalanced from those on the other side, tension is caused across the cell membrane, creating a membrane potential. The electrical potential difference between the inside and the outside of the membrane of an unexcited cell is called its *resting potential*, and it ranges from 40 to 90 mV. The resting

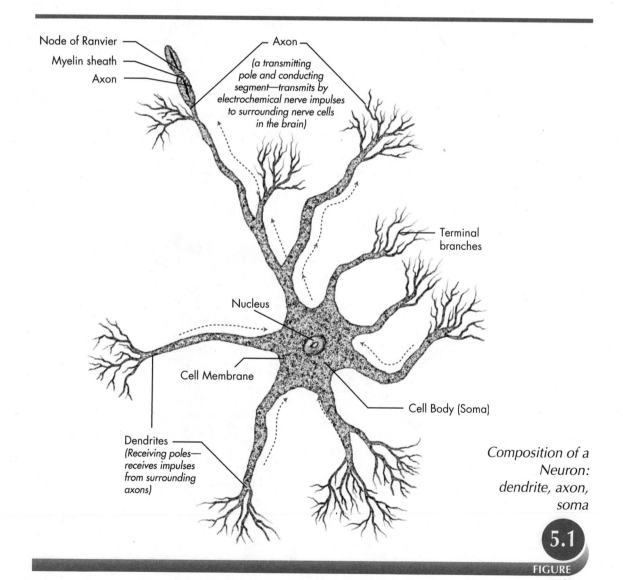

Node of Ranvier
Myelin sheath
Axon

Axon
(a transmitting pole and conducting segment—transmits by electrochemical nerve impulses to surrounding nerve cells in the brain)

Terminal branches

Nucleus

Cell Membrane

Cell Body (Soma)

Dendrites
(Receiving poles—receives impulses from surrounding axons)

Composition of a Neuron: dendrite, axon, soma

5.1
FIGURE

state is also known as a state of *polarization*. An action potential (or depolarization state) is created when sodium (Na⁺) rushes in so that the membrane potential passes beyond zero and the polarization is reversed. The membrane becomes more negative outside and positive inside at the point of excitation. This point of instantaneous firing is known as the **action potential**. Figure 5.2 illustrates this occurrence. The axon membrane, for example, in its resting state, is polarized as a result of the distribution of ions on the two sides of the membrane. Potassium (K^+), sodium (Na^+), and chloride (Cl^-) ions are distributed so that high concentrations of K^+ are on the inside of the cell (cytoplasm), while high concentrations of Na^+ and Cl^- are on the outside of the cell (extracellular fluid). The resting membrane potential is at least ten times more permeable (this refers to how easily a substance can pass through the cell membrane) to K^+ and Cl^- than to Na^+ ions. Na^+, therefore, passes with difficulty. Once the Na^+ leaks into the cell's cytoplasm, it is immediately ejected from the cell by a mechanism known as the sodium pump. At the

Action potential
the point of instantaneous firing of neurons

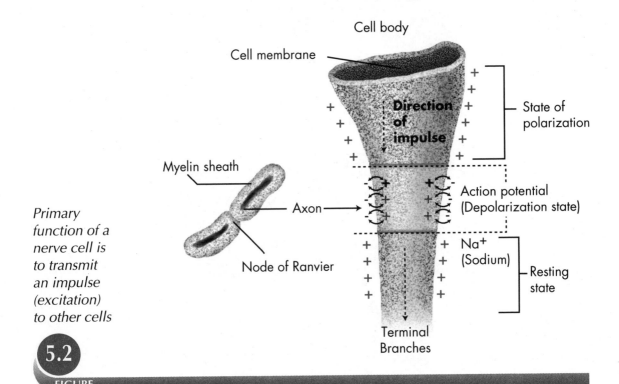

Primary function of a nerve cell is to transmit an impulse (excitation) to other cells

Cell body

Cell membrane

Cell body

Direction of impulse

State of polarization

Myelin sheath

Axon

Action potential (Depolarization state)

Node of Ranvier

Na⁺ (Sodium)

Resting state

Terminal Branches

5.2

FIGURE

same time, it withdraws potassium ions from the extracellular fluid. Before a neuron can fire again, the resting membrane potential must be reestablished. It must be repolarized. The outflow of K^+ ions repolarizes the cell membrane.

No action potential occurs unless it reaches its threshold. A threshold is the size of the smallest stimulus needed to trigger an action potential. Once the threshold is reached, polarization occurs in an all-or-none manner. The message is consistently sent with the same form and amplitude. Once a nerve impulse is initiated in the axon, it is conducted to the end of the axon with the same intensity.

SYNAPTIC TRANSMISSION

To transmit neural impulses from one cell to another to a target site, the action potential reaches a junction, or **synapse**. The journey through a series of these neural chains is referred to as synaptic transmission. The synapse is where the modification of communication occurs; without the synapse, there would be no integrated responses between neurons. At the synapse, there is not an all-or-none transmission. The transmission may be blocked, reduced, amplified, or changed.

Synapse
the junction between two neurons involved in transmitting action potentials

The synapse (Figure 5.3) consists of an axon terminal button of the transmitting neuron (presynaptic neuron), a fluid-filled space (synaptic cleft), and a membrane of the receiving neuron (postsynaptic neuron). Within the presynaptic neuron's terminal button are vesicles that release chemical transmitters as a result of the impulse's arrival. These transmitters influence the communication of the neural impulse. A transmitter is excitatory if it has a depolarizing effect on the postsynaptic membrane. It is inhibitory if it decreases the possibility of firing.

Motor neuron
a type of neuron that carries messages from the brain and spinal cord and innervates muscle fibers

The time required for an impulse to traverse the synaptic cleft (100 to 200 angstroms across) is 0.1 to 0.3 ms. Therefore, the more synapses in a neural chain, the longer the travel time from receptor to target site.

Afferent neurons
neurons that carry sensory information to the brain and spinal cord

The postsynaptic neuron, when adequately stimulated, repeats the conduction and transmission of the impulse, chaining together the neurons. It may change the influence on the impulse, depending upon its transmitter type or the disposition of the next neuron.

Interneurons
neurons that synapse with alpha motor neurons and help to create opportunities for excitation or inhibition throughout the spinal cord

The last neuron in each chain is known as the efferent neuron or **motor neuron**. **Afferent neurons** or sensory neurons transmit impulses to the brain and spinal cord. **Interneurons** begin and end in the brain and spinal cord. A motor neuron releases its transmitter at the muscle fibers' neuroeffector junctions of its motor unit. The muscle then responds proportionately to the total number of fibers fired as well as the frequency of firing.

One of the most common transmitter substances is *acetylcholine* (Ach). Also stored in the vesicles, it significantly influences the fast-slow response characteristics of muscle fibers. Dopamine, a chemical transmitter found in the brain, has a clearly defined motor function. Individuals with Parkinson's disease, like Muhammad Ali, whose vignette was presented at the beginning of Section II, have benefited from the drug L-dopa. An amino acid precursor of dopamine, L-dopa supplies the chemical transmitter needed in receptor sites of the brain's basal ganglia to facilitate coordinated motor responses. Without the presence of dopamine, the individual exhibits tremors, rigidity, and delay in the initiation of movement (Nathanson & Greengard, 1977).

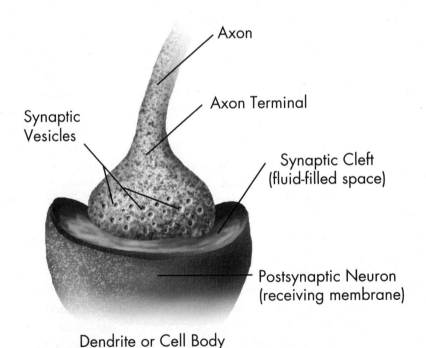

Synaptic Vesicles

Axon

Axon Terminal

Synaptic Cleft (fluid-filled space)

Postsynaptic Neuron (receiving membrane)

Dendrite or Cell Body

Synaptic transmission

5.3

FIGURE

NEUROMUSCULAR CONTROL

A seven-year-old girl fields a ground ball at her first tee-ball practice; a professional basketball player dishes the ball to another player for the dunk; an infant rolls onto her stomach for the first time. In these examples, how do neural chains at the cellular level "know" the target site for the transmission of impulses? These observable motor behaviors are combinations of communication and cooperation among the nervous system, the musculoskeletal system, and the sensory systems (somatosensory, visual, and auditory).

The intricate details of how this cooperation and integration are accomplished are not yet fully known. What *is* known, however, is that motor behavior is conducted through the brain and spinal cord, and that a series of feedback loops is created throughout the central nervous system to assist goal-directed behavior. The nervous system guides, oversees, and corrects; the musculoskeletal system performs movements and at the level of the central nervous system controls movements; and sensory systems provide information available to the central nervous system which, in turn, influences the musculoskeletal system and, ultimately, motor behavior.

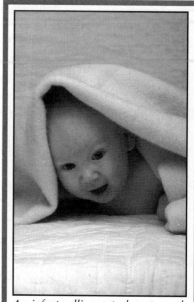

An infant rolling onto her stomach involves the use of neural chains.

To understand motor behavior from a motor control perspective, we must understand the neurological mechanisms involved in the guiding, oversight, and correction of goal-directed behavior. The central nervous system is at the center of this discussion, beginning with the brain.

THE BRAIN

Structurally, the brain is divided into three sections: **forebrain,** (cerebral hemisphere, basal ganglia, hypothalamus, thalamus); **midbrain** (superior colliculi, inferior colliculi); and **hindbrain** (pons; cerebellum; medulla) (Figure 5.4). Weighing approximately three pounds, it is encased in the skull and is one of the most sophisticated brains in any living creature.

The *brain stem,* referred to by anatomists as the hindbrain and midbrain, connects the brain to the spinal cord. The *medulla,* having ascending sensory-fiber tracts and descending motor tracts,

Forebrain
the part of the brain composed of cerebral hemisphere, basal ganglia, hypothalamus, and thalamus

Midbrain
the part of the brain consisting of superior colliculi, and inferior colliculi

Hindbrain
the part of the brain consisting of pons, cerebellum, and medulla

connects the brain to the spinal cord. This portion of the brain regulates respiration, heartbeat, and gastrointestinal function. Trauma to this area, such as a blow to the base of the skull, could be fatal.

The *pons*, located above the medulla, contains neurons that control movement. It connects the two hemispheres of the cerebellum and acts as a relay for the auditory system and movement, including eating and facial expression. The *cerebellum*, just above and behind the medulla, substantially contributes to the control of movement. It may provide a blueprint or a basic paradigm for movement. It may be that series of comparisons are made between sensory and motor neural pathways to rapidly adjust the paradigm with the goal and the environmental demands. The ability to provide a movement paradigm seems intimately connected with the cerebral cortex, the brain stem, and the spinal cord; they probably regulate the quality of movement and posture as well as coordinating adjustments in goal-directed movement. The cerebellum continuously orchestrates comparisons of movements performed with movements to be performed and movements to be performed with movements performed. In short, it detects and corrects errors in movement.

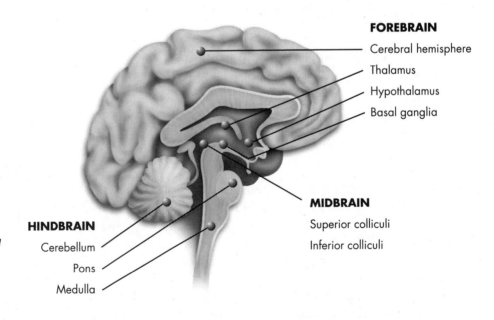

The brain divided into three subsections: forebrain, midbrain, and hindbrain

FOREBRAIN
Cerebral hemisphere
Thalamus
Hypothalamus
Basal ganglia

MIDBRAIN
Superior colliculi
Inferior colliculi

HINDBRAIN
Cerebellum
Pons
Medulla

5.4
FIGURE

The midbrain, located above the pons, contains the reticular formation. This structure plays major roles in arousal, consciousness, states of sleep, and relaxation. It also facilitates reflexes involving flexion and extension as well as responses from the motor cortex.

The remaining portion of the brain is the forebrain. Two cerebral hemispheres compose the **cerebral cortex.** The cortex accounts for nearly 80 percent of the weight of the brain. The *corpus callosum* divides the two hemispheres and functions as a pathway for nerves. Approximately three-fourths of all neurons in the nervous system are found within the cerebral cortex (Guyton, 1972). The cortex is composed of four basic lobes: the frontal, the parietal, the occipital, and the temporal (Figure 5.5). The *frontal lobe,* located toward the front of the cerebral cortex, contains the primary motor area or motor cortex. It has been found that the motor cortex is quite specialized and controls detailed movements (such as the fingers and hands of a concert cellist). The motor cortex has also been found to adjust muscular force during movement. In sustained movements (such as moving into and out of an arabesque on balance

Cerebral cortex
portion of the brain that contains two cerebral hemispheres and accounts for nearly 80% of the weight of the brain

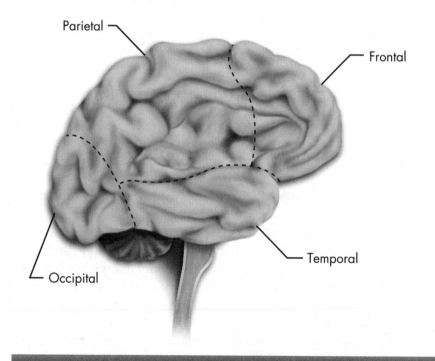

Parietal

Frontal

Occipital

Temporal

Cortex is composed of four basic lobes: Frontal lobe, parietal lobe, occipital lobe, and temporal lobe

5.5

FIGURE

beam or a cross on rings), this area contributes substantially, because these movements require repeated neural firing to initiate and continue the movement over time. The *parietal lobe,* adjacent to the frontal, contains the primary somatosensory projection area and the primary projection region for taste. The *occipital lobe,* located near the base of the skull, contains the primary visual projection area that guides movement. Finally, the *temporal lobe,* below the frontal, contains the primary auditory projection area as well as speech and smell.

Basal ganglia
an area of the brain, located near the center of the forebrain, that facilitates movement involving power, speed, direction, and amplitude in preparation for movement

Basal ganglia are located near the center of the forebrain. It is believed, through research conducted primarily on animals, that this area facilitates movement involving power, speed, direction, and amplitude in movement preparation. Because the basal ganglia seem to be involved in Parkinson's disease, their altered state contributes to the movement difficulty Muhammad Ali experienced when attempting to light the Olympic flame.

The *hypothalamus* is found adjacent to the brain stem. It functions to control body temperature and regulates the efficiency of fat and carbohydrate energy use. While the hypothalamus regulates bodily energy efficiency, the thalamus, directly above it, serves as a relay station for sensory and motor information. It transmits impulses from one cerebral hemisphere to the other and interconnects other subcortical areas.

A USEFUL MODEL OF MOTOR CONTROL

While the anatomical structure and functions of various parts of the nervous system are important, Brooks (1986) has devised a useful model involving motor control applications. He suggests studying the brain by its function during movement planning (Figure 5.6). He designates brain areas as the limbic system, the association cortex, the projection system, and the spinal system.

The *limbic system* includes parts of the brain that neurally connect to control behaviors involving emotion, motivation, and learning. This system's function provides the impetus for goal-directed behavior in environmental contexts. Parts of the thalamus, as well as the hypothalamus, amygdala, septal area, and hippocampus are included in the limbic system.

The second area in Brooks's neural model of goal-directed movement is the *association cortex.* It includes portions of the frontal, parietal, and temporal lobes of the brain. Receiving partially processed sensory information from other areas of the central nervous system, the association cortex identifies, chooses, and interconnects meaningful information for distribution to higher levels of the cortex. In principle, neural networks between the limbic system and the association cortex function cooperatively to generally guide goal-directed motor behavior. Information from sensory systems will also influence decisions made for motor behavior.

The *projection system* also plays an important role in goal-directed motor behavior. Previously it was mentioned that the limbic system and the association cortex provide general guidance, or the "what to do" for movement. The projection system seems to

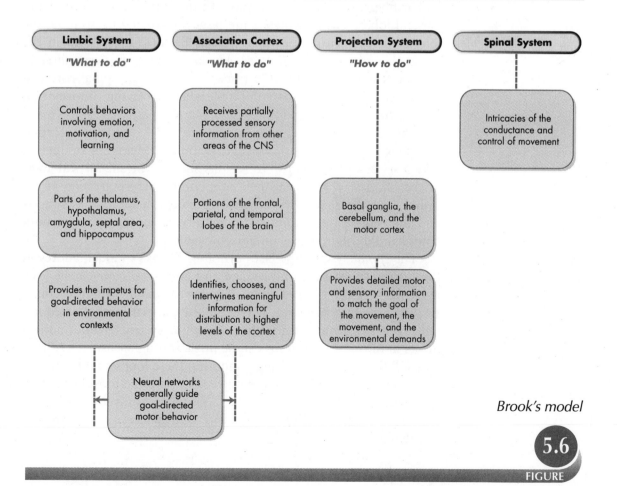

Brook's model

5.6

FIGURE

provide the specifics, or the "how to do" the movement. These neural networks provide detailed motor and sensory information to match the goal of the movement, the movement as specified by the limbic and association systems, and the environmental demands. The basal ganglia, the cerebellum, and the motor cortex are all part of this system.

A basic understanding of the mechanisms involved in transporting movement information is essential before the spinal system is presented. Two motor pathways are responsible for carrying movement information: the pyramidal and extrapyramidal systems. Once the impulses have arrived from the brain at these pathways, specialized neurons known as alpha motor neurons transmit the information to groups of muscles that will execute the movement. The pyramidal system consists of the corticospinal fibers and corticobulbar fibers. These fibers are axons in the cortex of the frontal and parietal lobes. Their diameters are large and their lengths long, the longest in the central nervous system. Because they begin in the cerebral cortex motor and sensory areas, they traverse directly down to the spinal cord. Motor neurons within the spinal cord can be selectively excited or inhibited when receiving information quickly for transmission.

The second pathway, the *extrapyramidal*, transports information much more slowly than the pyramidal. Messages frequently take a series of "side trips" to regions such as the subcortical areas of the brain so that signals can be modified before arriving at the spinal cord. These side trips increase the complexity of this system, and they create opportunities for modifying motor behavior both before and during the execution of movements.

The *spinal system,* the last portion of Brooks's model, addresses the intricacies of the conductance and control of movement. The muscular system is networked through neurons with the spinal system through a variety of nerve impulse patterns orchestrated initially, generally, and specifically by previous systems. Minor adjustments in movement patterns can be made through sensory feedback loops. By means of "sampling" impulses, these loops enable the system to compare the goal of the movement with the movement itself and with environmental demands. Coordinated movement, then, is the shared responsibility of the entire central nervous system, not just the brain.

- Skeletal muscles are controlled by the central nervous system.

- The central nervous system is composed of the brain and spinal cord, which work cooperatively to produce coordinated and skilled motor behavior.

- Feedback loops connect, consult, compare, adjust, correct, and fine-tune impulses throughout the nervous system.

- The nervous system is composed of two types of cells: neurons and neuroglia.

- The neuron receives and conducts impulses.

- It is composed of a receiving pole (dendrite), transmitting pole and conducting segment (axon), and cell body (soma).

- The axon is enclosed in a cellular sheath (myelin sheath).

- The primary function of a nerve cell is to transmit an impulse (or excitation) to other cells.

- Transmission of neural impulses from one cell to another to a target site requires an action potential to reach a junction (synapse).

- A synapse consists of an axon terminal button of the transmitting neuron (presynaptic neuron), a fluid-filled space (synaptic cleft), and a receiving membrane of a postsynaptic neuron. The last neuron in each neural chain is known as the efferent neuron (motor neuron).

- Afferent neurons or sensory neurons transmit impulses to the brain and spinal cord.

- Interneurons begin and end in the brain and spinal cord.

- Acetylcholine (Ach) is one of the most common transmitter substances.

- A series of feedback loops is created throughout the central nervous system to assist goal-directed behavior.

- The brain is divided into three sections: forebrain (cerebral hemisphere, basal ganglia, hypothalamus, thalamus), midbrain (superior colliculi, inferior colliculi), and hindbrain (pons, cerebellum, medulla).

- The brain stem connects the brain to the spinal cord and includes the hindbrain and midbrain.

- The medulla connects the brain to the spinal cord.

- The cerebellum, just above and behind the medulla, contributes to the control of movement.

- The midbrain is located above the pons.

- The forebrain has two central hemispheres composing the cerebral cortex.

- The cortex is composed of four basic lobes: frontal (containing the primary motor area); parietal (containing the primary somatosensory projection area and the primary projection region for taste); occipital (containing the primary visual projection area that guides movement); and temporal (containing the primary auditory projection area as well as speech and smell).

- Brooks's model involves motor control applications: the limbic system, the association cortex, the projection system, and the spinal system.

DISCUSSION QUESTIONS

1. What are the specific motor functions of the motor cortex in the control of human movement?

2. Describe how a neuron receives and conducts impulses.

3. What function does a synapse have in neuron transmission?

4. What is the role of transmitter substances in impulse conduction?

5. Describe the lobes of the brain and their function as they relate to motor behavior.

ADDITIONAL READINGS

Bennett, T. L. (1977). *Brain and behavior.* Monterey, CA: Brooks/Cole Publishing Company.

Brooks, V. B. (1986). *The neural basis of motor control.* New York: Oxford University Press.

Enoka, R. M. (1994). *Neuromechanical basis of kinesiology.* 2nd ed. Champaign, IL: Human Kinetics. (Chapters 6 and 7 refer to the spinal system and its responsibility for ongoing control and coordination.)

REFERENCES

Brooks, V. B. (1986). *The neural basis of motor control.* New York: Oxford University Press.

Guyton, A. C. (1972). *Structure and function of the nervous system.* Philadelphia: W.B. Saunders Company.

Nathanson, J. A. & Greengard, P. (1977). Second messengers in the brain. *Scientific American, 237*(2), 108.

Noback, C. R., and Demarest, R. J. (1972). *The nervous system: Introduction and review.* New York: McGraw-Hill Book Company.

Motor Neurons

CHAPTER FOCUS

- The central nervous system and motor behavior

- The central nervous system as it relates to motor behavior

- The structure and function of the brain as they relate to motor behavior

- Brooks's model of motor control as it relates to motor behavior perspectives

*T*he spinal system has the responsibility of providing the final details to the execution of continuous movements, which relates to the timing of motor patterns. The musculoskeletal system actually performs the movements. The interconnections of the central nervous system with the musculoskeletal system may appear to flow in only one direction, from the brain and spinal cord to the musculature, but this is hardly the case. The

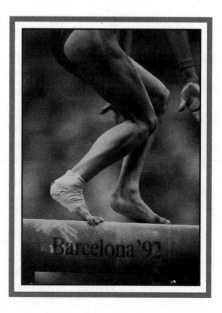

Barcelona'92

interconnections help the central nervous system to make comparisons in order to determine whether the planned action will meet the intended goal.

When you decide to kick a ball in a soccer game, the force needed to kick the ball with enough speed and accuracy to score a goal is determined by two factors (McCrea, 1992):

1. the total number of fibers needed to produce enough force to accomplish the goal; and

2. the type of joint that is involved with the action produced by the musculature crossing the joint.

The coordination and continuation of movement are the responsibility of the central nervous system and the musculoskeletal system. The spinal system contributes to the control and coordination of continuous voluntary movements. Other subsystems within the central nervous system play supporting roles at various times.

TYPES OF MOTOR NEURONS

To understand these roles, we must understand the function of motor neurons. Three types of motor neurons transmit impulses that relate to motor behavior. They are alpha motor neurons, gamma motor neurons, and interneurons.

The motor neurons that carry messages from the brain and spinal cord, forming a common final pathway to the appropriate musculature involved in the movement, are known as **alpha motor neurons.** These neurons are networked together to function in "teams" to innervate specific groups of skeletal muscles.

Gamma motor neurons carry their messages from the brain to muscle spindles. The neuromuscular spindles are highly specialized sensory organs that are located in the contractile fibers of skeletal muscles. The more spindles in the muscle, the more precisely can be the control of the muscle, because spindles provide necessary information for picking up movement errors and adjusting them to the goal and the environment.

Interneurons synapse with alpha motor neurons and, by doing so, help to create opportunities for excitation or inhibition throughout the spinal cord. They assist in what is referred to as reciprocal inhibition. For example, in order for a knee jerk reaction to occur, extensor muscles must contract while flexors must relax. Inhibitory

Alpha motor neuron
a nerve cell that innervates skeletal muscle

Gamma motor neuron
highly specialized neuron; located in contractile fibers of skeletal muscles, that carries messages to muscle

Interneuron
a neuron that synapses with alpha motor neurons and helps to create opportunities for excitation or inhibition throughout the spinal cord

interneurons whose axons reach the motor cells of the flexor muscles are relaxed, while alpha motor neurons provide impetus for the extensor muscles.

MOTOR NEURONS, MOTOR UNITS, MUSCLES, AND THE PRODUCTION OF FORCE

The journey of the nervous impulse that ultimately creates movement continues through the alpha motor neuron from the spinal cord to the skeletal muscles. Each axon divides into several branches after entering the muscle. Each branch forms a specialized ending called the motor end plate or **neuromuscular junction.** In this area, at the neuromuscular synapse, energy transmitted by the alpha motor neuron is changed to chemical energy, which is then infused into the muscle through membrane. This synaptic region has properties similar to those of excitation in the central nervous system. Acetylcholine, the neurotransmitter, sets the stage for the action potential threshold to be reached and creates opportunities for muscular contraction to occur when the proteins actin and myosin interact. This process, the conversion of electrical to chemical energy, followed by an action potential that sets up the opportunity for proteins to interact and create muscular force, is known as **excitation-contraction coupling.**

Neuromuscular junction
a motor end plate

Excitation-contraction coupling
the conversion of electrical to chemical energy, followed by an action potential that sets up the opportunity for proteins to interact and create muscular force

MOTOR UNIT, RECRUITMENT, AND RATE

A **motor unit** consists of one motor neuron, its axon branches, and all of the muscle fibers that it innervates. **Innervation** refers to the stimulation of a muscle by nerves. For example, each extrinsic eye muscle has a one-to-one (1:1) motor neuron–to–fiber innervation, creating velocities of 500 degrees of arc per second. There are 360 degrees in a circle. These velocities would mean that the impulse travels almost twice that distance in one second. The gastrocnemius muscle has an innervation of one to 1,700 (1:1700). Muscles that are used to generate force, like muscles in the legs and trunk, have large innervation ratios, while those used in fine or manipulative movements (e.g., hand, face, and eye) have small innervation ratios. Therefore, the smaller the innervation ratio, the more precise the motor control.

Motor unit
consists of one motor neuron, its axon branches, and all of the muscle fibers it innervates

Innervation
the stimulation of a muscle by nerves

Motor Units and Their Enlistment in Goal-Directed Motor Behavior

Concerning which motor units are enlisted to meet goal-directed motor behavior, there are three questions: (1) Which motor units are recruited? (2) How are they recruited? (3) At what rate are they recruited?

Motor units are recruited through their terminating points in specific muscles that are needed to execute a movement. For example, if the goal is to jog for one mile around the track, those motor units innervating the hamstring muscle group are called upon to extend the hip. The size of the motor unit innervating the muscle group will determine its activation longevity. In concept, the smallest motor neurons are recruited first and work the longest during muscular contraction. In other words, the larger the motor unit, the later it is recruited and the shorter is its firing duration. The smaller the motor unit, the sooner it is recruited and the longer is its firing duration. This concept is known as the **size principle.** As the electrical stimulus demand increases, larger motor units are recruited and activated until every motor unit available is firing.

The goal of the movement generally determines how many motor units will be used. People have particular sets of motor units that can be recruited. Each set is referred to as a **motor neuron pool.** As an increase in force is required, the orderly recruitment through each pool is increased. When the basketball player goes up for the rebound, when the figure skater executes a triple axel, when the gymnast travels across the mat in a roundoff, back handspring, back handspring, tuck double back somersault, each recruits all available units progressively. Force production has already been determined by the size principle, whereby motor units are recruited through the central nervous system. The complexity of the goal-directed motor behavior has already been somewhat simplified as a result of the size principle.

Additionally, the rate at which motor units are recruited completes the discussion of muscular force production. There are two types of motor units: *tonic* and *phasic*. **Tonic motor units,** having smaller fiber size and slower conduction velocities, have a high threshold to electrical stimuli. As a result, they create

Size principle
the concept holding that the size of the motor unit innervating the muscle group will determine its length of activation; the larger the motor unit, the shorter is its firing duration

Motor neuron pool
a set of motor units that is recruited for use in a voluntary movement

Tonic motor units
motor units that have smaller fiber size, slower conduction velocities, and a high threshold to electrical stimuli

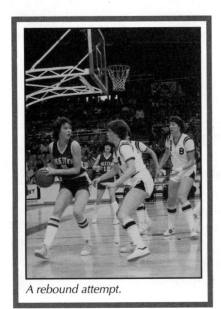

A rebound attempt.

smaller action potentials at a decreasing rate as muscular force is increased. **Phasic motor units,** having large fiber size, produce large action potentials with high conduction velocities. As a result, they create large action potentials with an increasing rate as muscular force increases.

As the rates are repeatedly coded through motor neuron size, the rate of firing can be manipulated to attempt to increase muscular force. As the time between firing becomes shorter, the muscular force created begins to "build up," thereby increasing the overall level of force.

The synchronization of motor unit firing may also lead to increased muscular force necessary for the completion of goal-directed motor behavior. Through strength training, it may be possible to synchronize motor unit firing, which will again increase the overall amount of force generated (Dawson, 1996; Bompa, 1996; Verkhoshansky, 1996).

The initial position of the body, including the limbs and each muscle's length, can add to or detract from the overall effectiveness and efficiency of the movement. For example, when a swimmer is waiting for the sound of the gun to start the 200 m freestyle race, a grab-start is usually used. The grab start elongates the limbs and muscles in the back and legs sufficiently to facilitate the production of force over a large range of motion, while sufficiently shortening important musculature in order to generate greater velocity through muscle length.

Skeletal muscles are attached to bones of the skeletal system, which is also comprised of joints. The types of joints and their corresponding muscles are factors in force production. Force production is not, however, solely based upon muscular contraction. The number of joints used in goal-directed movement will also help to determine the production of force. The more joints involved in the production of a movement, the more force that can be produced. The more joints involved, the more muscles involved, thereby connecting concepts of biomechanics with motor control. The baseball pitcher, when throwing the fastball, generates accelerating force by using joints in the hip, spinal column, feet and legs, arms and hand through the creation of torque in three-dimensional planes. Interestingly, the more joints involved in the movement, the more complicated the movement becomes to monitor, learn, and control.

Reflexes, responses that are mediated at the spinal cord level and require no conscious effort (rather than mediated at all levels of the central nervous system) — also play roles in motor control.

Phasic motor units
motor units of large fiber size that produce large action potentials with high conduction velocities

Reflexes
responses that are mediated at the spinal cord level and require no conscious effort

Several of these — the withdrawal reflex, the stretch reflex, and the gamma loop reflex — are worthy of explanation for better understanding of motor control.

Each of these reflexive movement patterns occurs in a coordinated combination of one to several joint movements, contractions of specific muscles, and relaxations of others. Reflexive movements are represented in the form of a circuit or loop. These circuits or loops can quickly provide necessary adjustments. The loops may be short or long in distance and duration, depending upon the type of adjustment necessary.

Stretch reflex
a short-loop reflex, involving a single synapse that adjusts the position of the skeleton continuously by contracting, through muscle spindles

The stretch reflex and the gamma loop reflex could be considered examples of short-loop reflexes. The **stretch reflex** involves a single synapse and is referred to as monosynaptic. The stretch reflex maintains upright posture by continuously adjusting the position of the skeleton. By contracting, through muscle spindles, the stretched muscles correct the displacement created by gravity. The stretch reflex is also used when there is a sudden increase in the force demands of a movement. For example, while conditioning, a tennis player performs a series of pushups. At the highest point of the pushup, a heavy dictionary is placed on the back. Alpha motor neurons fire in order to hold the high point of the pushup. Suddenly, the added weight causes the muscles to lengthen as the torso begins to drop. Muscle spindles within the muscles become stretched, firing increases, and the body in the highest pushup position is reestablished.

Alpha and gamma motor neurons constitute the two pathways to innervate specific groups of skeletal muscles. The gamma motor neuron carries its message to muscle spindles. This is particularly interesting, because as the alpha motor neuron innervates the extrafusal fibers to lengthen, the gamma motor neurons are sending messages back to contract, thereby making the intrafusal fibers more sensitive to miniscule adjustments that might be necessary.

Withdrawal reflex
a long-loop reflex which is a result of body parts being quickly withdrawn as a result of intensely painful stimuli

The **withdrawal reflex** is a result of body parts being quickly withdrawn as a result of intensely painful stimuli. For example, after frying chicken in a cast iron skillet on the stove, the cook barehandedly reaches to remove the skillet from the stove. Once in contact with the extremely hot handle, the cook instantaneously drops the skillet with the chicken to the floor. In this case, sensory neurons, through interneurons, connected with the spinal cord. The interneurons, in turn, inhibited flexors of the fingers and excited the extensors, thereby causing the fingers to open, causing the hot skillet to fall to the floor.

KEY
POINTS

- Three types of motor neurons transmit impulses that relate to motor behavior: alpha motor neurons, gamma motor neurons, and interneurons.

- Excitation-contraction coupling is a process that involves the conversion of electrical to chemical energy, followed by an action potential that sets up the opportunity for proteins to interact and create muscular force.

- Motor units are recruited in an orderly fashion on specific muscles that are needed to execute a movement.

- The two types of motor units are: tonic and phasic.

- The synchronization of motor unit firing may lead to increased muscular force necessary for the completion of goal-directed motor behavior.

- Force production is not solely based upon muscular contraction.

- The more joints involved in the production of a movement, the more force can be produced.

- Reflexes are responses that are mediated at the spinal cord level and require no conscious effort.

- The stretch reflex is monosynaptic.

DISCUSSION QUESTIONS

1. Describe the common pathway of motor neurons when messages are carried.

2. Determine the journey of a nervous impulse through the alpha motor neuron to the skeletal muscles.

3. Describe reflexes. What causes them to function? Why do we have them?

4. When an action occurs, which motor units are recruited? How are they recruited? At what rate are they recruited?

5. What role do muscles and joints play in motor skill performance?

ADDITIONAL READINGS

Brooks, V. B. (1986). *The neural basis of motor control.* New York: Oxford University Press.

Bloedle, J. R., Ebner, T. J., & Wise, S. P. (Eds.). (1996). *The acquisition of motor behavior in vertebrates.* Cambridge, MA: The MIT Press.

REFERENCES

Bompa, T. O. (1996). Variations of periodization of strength. *Strength and Conditioning Journal, 18(3),* 58–61.

Dawson, B. (1996). In Reaburn, P. & Jenkins, D. (Eds.), *Training for speed and endurance.* Sydney: Allen and Unwin, pp. 76–96.

McCrea, D. A. (1992). Can sense be made of spinal interneuron circuits? *Behavioral and Brain Sciences, 15(4),* 633–643.

Verkhoshansky, Y. V. (1996). Principles for a rational organization of the training process aimed at speed development. *New studies in athletics (Monaco), 11(2/3),* 155–160.

Learning Perspectives

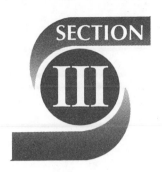

Known as the greatest female multi-event track and field athlete of all time, Jackie Joyner-Kersee has won three Olympic gold medals, one silver, and one bronze. She has competed in every Summer Olympic Games since 1984. She was the first woman to win a gold medal in the long jump, the first woman to earn more than 7,000 points in the heptathlon (seven events), the first athlete in sixty-four years to win gold medals in both multi-events and single events, and has held the world record in heptathlon since 1986. Born into poverty in East St. Louis, Illinois, Jackie could not afford sport activities that were not offered in school or through the community center. It was at the community center that she began to experience a wide variety of track and field events, basketball, and volleyball. Throughout high school, she was particularly interested in basketball, but she was also a good long jumper and 200-meter sprinter. Attending UCLA on a track scholarship, Jackie learned to run hurdles, throw the javelin, and put the shot. She competed in the heptathlon, the most grueling multi-event of track and field. What roles might the senses contribute to Jackie Joyner-Kersee's learning the "right stuff" to be the greatest woman multi-event athlete of all time?

Sensory Systems: Contributions to Motor Behavior

CHAPTER 7

CHAPTER FOCUS

- Sensory systems which are of particular relevance in motor behavior

- The structure and function of sensory systems as they relate to motor behavior

- The function of cutaneous and proprioceptors and motor behavior

- Sensory systems, their relationship, and motor behavior

- Feedback and motor behavior

You should now have an understanding of the basic motor behavior theories and a basic understanding of the physiological bases of motor control. The roles of sensory systems in motor behavior are also integral to the discussion. This section is devoted to the understanding of three sensory systems that are of particular relevance in motor behavior: the visual, auditory/vestibular, and somato-sensory systems. Because of the visual system's

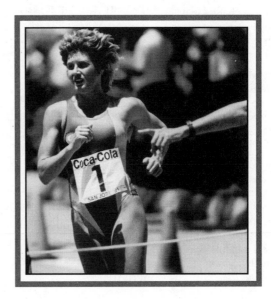

significant contribution to motor behavior, a separate chapter will be devoted to its structure, function, and influence at the end of the section.

Structurally and functionally each of these systems provides unique information, internally and externally, about the environment. Each system has specialized nerve cells that respond to certain changes in the individual or in the environment. These nerve cells, or **receptors**, transmit these responses to the nervous system. Each type of receptor cell is specialized to respond to a particular form of stimulus. Despite these uniquenesses, however, there are several core concepts that are common to the reception and transmission of information through these systems.

RECEPTORS AND THE TRANSDUCTION OF SENSORY INFORMATION

Information about the environment is received by sensory receptors. These receptors are located in the eyes (visual system), ears (auditory/vestibular system), and joints, muscles, and layers of skin (somatosensory system). Stimuli such as light waves, sound waves, and pressure can excite the specific receptor and, through a variety of processes, change the receptors' electrical characteristics. For example, receptors in the retina of the eye respond only to light with wavelengths between 400 and 800 nm (violet to red). Receptors of the ear are specialized to transduce fluctuations of air pressure (sound waves) with frequencies from 16 to 16,000 Hz (cycles per second). The electrical charges change firing patterns in the axons that lead into the central nervous system. This process is known as **sensory transduction**.

There are two basic types of receptor cells. One type has axons that communicate with other neurons by means of normal synaptic transmission. Known as **generator potential neurons**, they raise or lower the probability that a sensory neuron axon will fire. The other receptor type, having no axons, is referred to as **receptor potential neurons**. They transmit to other neurons having axons that are capable of producing action potentials. The receptor potential neurons alter firing rates. The difference between these two types is the presence or absence of axons. Figure 7.1 is a schematic diagram of how environmental stimuli are transduced into neural activity.

Receptors
specialized nerve cells in each sensory system that respond to certain changes in the individual or in its environment and transmit these responses to the nervous system

Sensory transduction
electrical charges that change firing patterns in axons that lead into the central nervous system

Generator potential neurons
receptor cells that raise or lower the probability that a sensory neuron axon will fire

Receptor potential neurons
a type of receptor, having no axon, transmitted to other neurons having axons that are capable of producing action potentials

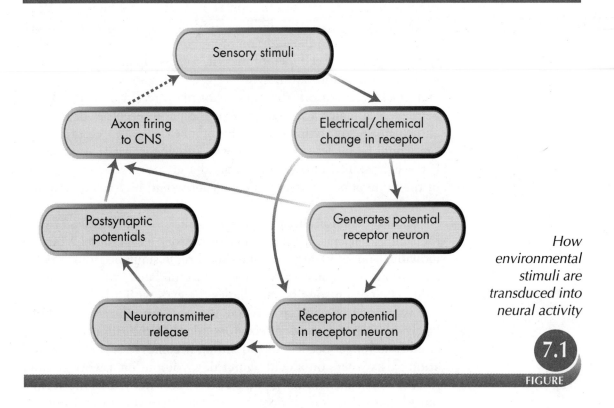

How environmental stimuli are transduced into neural activity

7.1 FIGURE

One of the common threads in all sensory transmission to the central nervous system is the announcement that something has occurred. This can be referred to as *sufficient* or **adequate stimulation**. Specific sensory receptors have specific thresholds for electrical energy conductance. Once this conductance happens, the central nervous system is informed. The meaning of this is quite clear when one considers light particles (photons) entering the eye. Without photons as stimuli, specific photoreceptive cells do not function.

Another common thread in all sensory transmission into the central nervous system is **coding.** Two types of coding exist: coding of **intensity** and coding of **frequency.** Referring again to the eye, the photon, a single unit of light, serves as the stimulus that excites retinal cells. Rods can detect light at brightness levels that are too dim for cones to respond. This addresses the issue of intensity. Frequency can be identified by the firing rate of each type of photoreceptor.

Within the concept of coding lies an additional concept that provides meaning to this thread. It involves temporal and spatial

Adequate (sufficient) stimulation
specific thresholds of specific sensory receptors for conductance of electrical energy

Coding
categorizing sensory transmission into the central nervous system, which can be designated through intensity or frequency

Coding intensity
the number of each type of photoreceptor for sensory transmission into the central nervous system

Coding frequency
the firing rate of each type of photoreceptor for sensory transmission into the central nervous system

summation. Temporal summation is a process by which the effects of closely spaced subthreshold excitations are cumulative. Spatial summation refers to the addition of potential changes from impulses to various parts of cell membranes. If, for example, a flashlight was suddenly shined into an individual's eyes while in a darkened room and quickly turned off, the number of photoreceptors firing would be huge; if a match was lighted near the photoreceptors of the eyes and then quickly extinguished, the number of photoreceptors that fire would be far less. This concept is known as **spatial summation**. If the light shined into the eyes caused a greater frequency of firing of the same photoreceptors, the concept would be termed **temporal summation**.

Spatial summation
a stimulus that causes the initial number of proprioceptors to fire

Temporal summation
a stimulus that causes more frequent firing of proprioceptors

Adaptation
sensory receptors changing to meet the needs of the stimulus

A third common thread involved in all sensory transmission into the central nervous system is that of sensory **adaptation**. When an individual initially steps out into the bright sunlight from a darkened room, the visual system becomes inundated with photons of light. The person squints and shades the eyes with a hand to block out some of the photons so that the photoreceptors can adjust. Fairly quickly, the sensory receptors adapt to the stimulus and the hand is no longer needed and squinting becomes less. A similar situation exists when, on a cold winter day, you put on a wool sweater for the first time. Initially, the sweater feels itchy, but the feeling quickly subsides. Soon it does not even feel like you are wearing the sweater.

GETTING SENSORY INFORMATION TOGETHER

Dorsal column route
one of two routes over which electrical impulses travel to the brain

Spinothalamic route
one of two paths over which electrical impulses travel to the brain

Orders of neurons
the first, second, and third orders of neurons in the dorsal column and spinothalamic route that facilitate input from receptors to the brain

With these common threads involved in sensory transmission, how does information get transmitted through the receptors to the cortex of the brain for further analysis, comparison, synthesis, and use? Part of the answer lies in the routes electrical impulses travel. Information generally travels to the brain using one of two routes: the **dorsal column route** or the **spinothalamic route** (Figure 7.2). Both of these routes have levels or **orders of neurons** (primary or first-order; secondary or second-order; third order) and synapses that facilitate input from receptors to the brain. Each of the receptors (vision, audition, and somatosensory) has structurally specialized and specific neural pathways which pass through the thalamus. First- and second-order neurons end in the thalamus, where their synapses connect and follow through to the somatosensory portions of the brain's cortex.

Dorsal Column Route (A)

touch, pressure, proprioception to the cerebral cortex

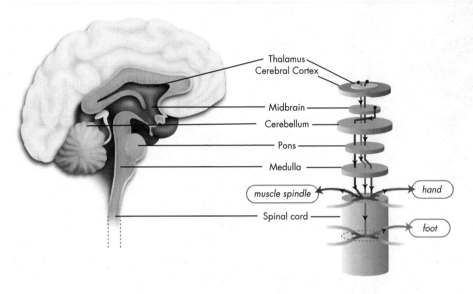

Spinothalamic Route (B)

pain and temperature to the cerebral cortex

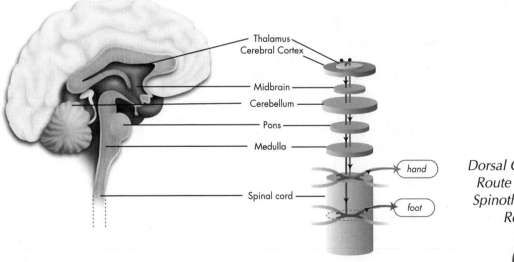

*Dorsal Column
Route (A) and
Spinothalamic
Route (B)*

7.2
FIGURE

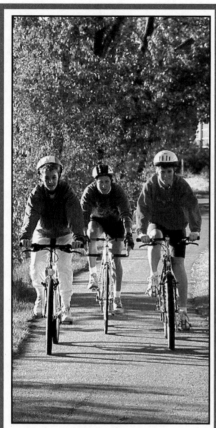

Cyclists, wearing protective helmets, are provided with protection from trauma to heads.

The thalamus (discussed in Section II) serves as a relay station for the sensory receptors of vision, audition, and somatosenses (pain). It allows information to flow to the part of the cortex that is relevant to the movement. Additionally, the thalamus, with its limbic system connections, induces emotional activity during sensory transmission. Ultimately, sensory receptor paths arrive at the cortex of the brain. Once the electrical impulses have arrived at the level of the cortex to the specific sensory area, the individual is able to receive and identify the stimulus. For example, visual information is routed to the occipital lobe, auditory information is channeled to the auditory cortex, while somatosensory information is sent to the parietal lobe. As a result, the individual can discriminate contrast, patterns, shapes, and shades of light; the individual can discern pitch (frequency) and intensity; and the individual can determine varying pressure on the skin and arm/leg position in three-dimensional space. The basal ganglia and motor tracts leaving the cortex, of course, are responsible for planning and recalling movement plans; therefore, the interconnectedness of the thalamus and limbic system provide multidimensional leveling of sensory transmission.

The ultimate integration of sensory transmission occurs in the association areas of the brain that are adjacent to the sensory areas. It is important for the cortex to be protected from trauma, as injury to any portion of it could result in a decrease in perceptual competence. It seems logical, then, as motor behavior professionals, to advocate for adequate head protection (particularly the cortex area) for people who participate in activities in which the head is vulnerable to trauma. The use of safety helmets while skateboarding, roller blading, bicycling, motorcycling, snow skiing, and batting is logical to provide protection from trauma.

The next section provides a detailed discussion of three systems that are primary contributors to learning and control in motor behavior. The somatosensory and auditory/vestibular systems will be discussed first, followed by a separate chapter on the visual system.

SOMATOSENSORY SYSTEM

The somatosenses provide information about pain, touch, warmth, cold, skin vibration, limb position, and movement. Their receptors are differentially referred to as **cutaneous receptors** and **proprioreceptors**.

Cutaneous Receptors

Cutaneous receptors can be specifically categorized as **thermoreceptors** (sensitive to temperature change), **mechanoreceptors** (sensitive to pressure changes through the mechanical deformation of the skin), and **pain receptors** (sensitivity to stimuli of a sufficient intensity to cause tissue damage).

The skin contains areas that are sensitive to stimuli. Generally, the closer cutaneous receptors are to each other, the better the individual can discern information. The lips, thumbs, and eyelids, for example, contain more cutaneous receptors than the arms, legs, or torso. Some areas of the body are particularly sensitive to cold, while others are particularly sensitive to heat. The skin participates in thermoregulation by producing sweat to cool the body or by restricting blood circulation to conserve heat through "goose bumps" (constricting of the skin, thereby leaving hair follicles protruded).

Cutaneous receptors
somatosensory mechanisms categorized in three areas: thermoreceptors, mechanoreceptors, and pain receptors

Proprioceptors
sensory receptors that provide information about the status of the body

Thermoreceptors
receptors that involve temperature

Mechanoreceptors
skin receptors that involve pressure-mechanical deformation of the skin

Pain receptors
receptors that determine intensity sufficient to cause tissue damage

LAB EXERCISE

SOMATOSENSORY (CUTANEOUS) RECEPTORS — PROPRIOCEPTION

Objective: To experience sensory awareness through tactile sensitivity

Equipment: One hairpin; partner; paper and pencil

Experience: Adjust the ends of a hairpin so that its points are 1½ inches apart. Partner A closes the eyes; Partner B places both points on the back of Partner A's forearm. What is the reaction to being able to feel one or two points? Adjust the hairpin so that the points are 1/8 inch apart. Partner B places both points on the index fingertip. What is the reaction to being able to feel one or two points?

Assignment: Select three additional body parts to assess. Chart the body's sensitivity, including the forearm and index finger points, for Partner A and Partner B.

Free nerve endings
the most widespread somatosensory receptors in the skin and through-out the body that can detect light touch and pressure

Meissner's corpuscles
cells in the fingertips, the lips, and other areas where distinguishing subtle differences in touch is important

Merkel's disks
the structural parts found near Meissner's corpuscles to transmit long-lasting signals that permit tolerance of constant contact with the skin

Pacinian corpuscles
cells that provide sensitivity to deep pressure sensations

Kinesthesis
movement sensation; the conscious appreciation and identification of movement and position of limbs

Organic sensitivity
receptivity to stimuli surrounding internal organs

Muscle spindles
body structures responsible for providing detailed information and having the ability to ascertain subtle and gross changes in muscle length; they stretch when the muscle lengthens and shortens when the muscle relaxes

Smooth skin contains **free nerve endings** and axons that terminate in specialized end organs. Free nerve endings (the most widespread somatosensory receptors found in the skin and throughout the body) can detect light touch and pressure. **Meissner's corpuscles** adapt rapidly to changes in pressure. They are found in the fingertips, the lips, and other areas where subtle differences in touch are important to distinguish. They assist in human communication through word pronunciation using the lips, "reading" Braille through the fingers, and "signing" through the hands and fingers. **Merkel's disks,** found near Meissner's corpuscles, though not as sensitive to pressure, probably transmit long-lasting signals that permit tolerance (or inability to tolerate) of constant contact with the skin (as in the case of wearing clothing). Ruffini endings, slow in their adaptation, detect and transmit information about continuous states of deformation of deeper tissue as well as deep, continuous pressure (sitting for hours in class). **Pacinian corpuscles,** rapid in their adaptation, provide sensitivity to deep pressure sensations (momentarily resting a weight on the chest during a bench press exercise) (Figure 7.3). All of these receptors, in varying ways, assist in the determination of pain.

Proprioceptors

Proprioceptors are sensory receptors that provide information about the status of the body. They allow a person to determine the position and movement of limbs in relation to the body, to determine where the body is located in space, and to determine when the bladder is full. **Kinesthesis** (from the Greek terms *kines* and *thesis* — movement sensation) refers to a conscious appreciation and identification of the movement and position of limbs. **Organic sensitivity** refers to stimuli surrounding internal organs. Because "kinesthetic sense" is an important contributor to motor behavior, specialized proprioceptors located in muscles, tendons, and joints will be discussed in detail.

Proprioceptors located within voluntary skeletal muscles provide information about the position and movement of limbs as well as details of movement. For example, when an individual kicks a football, under pressure from a defender, a distance of sixty meters, information about the stability of the plant foot and the speed and position of the kicking leg is attained through a variety of proprioceptors.

Muscle spindles, responsible for providing detailed information in this example, have the ability to ascertain both subtle and gross changes in muscle length. Intrafusal fibers are imbedded in the muscle and are parallel to the extrafusal muscle fibers, which attach to the sheath of the muscle. They are stretched when the muscle lengthens and shortened when the muscle relaxes.

The composition of the muscle spindle provides interesting information from both a sensory and a motor perspective. Each spindle contains two types of intrafusal fibers: **nuclear bag** and **nuclear chain**. Nuclear bag fibers are rather large and have many nuclei tightly packed together. The ends of the fibers are capable of contracting. Nuclear chain fibers are attached to the surface of nuclear bag fibers. Their ends are also capable of contracting. From a motor perspective, each muscle spindle has a 5:2 ratio of nuclear bag fibers to nuclear chain fibers: for every five nuclear bag fibers, there are two nuclear chain fibers. From a sensory perspective, each spindle is

Nuclear bag
one of two types of muscle spindles, having a 5:2 ratio with nuclear chains

Nuclear chain
one of two types of muscle spindles

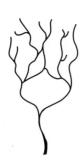

free nerve endings

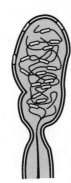

Meissner's corpuscles

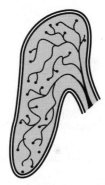

Ruffini endings

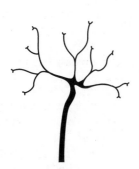

Merkel's discs

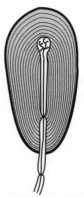

Pacinian corpuscle

Tactile Receptors

7.3

FIGURE

Primary neurons
rapid-firing neurons also
known as Group Ia

Secondary neurons
slow-firing neurons that
connect only to nuclear
chain fibers; also known
as Group II neurons

innervated with Group Ia and Group II afferents, which provide information about differences in extrafusal muscle length. Group Ia neurons, known as **primary**, rapid-firing neurons, are intertwined with the nuclear chain and bag fibers. **Secondary** (Group II) neurons, more slow-firing, connect only to nuclear chain fibers.

When any change in the muscle length is initiated, a similar change occurs in these mechanoreceptors. The change prompts the afferent neurons to fire, thereby sending sensory information to the spinal cord and central nervous system. Firing more rapidly than their secondary counterparts initially, the Ia afferent fibers seem to be in synchronization with the lower firing threshold of the nuclear bag fibers. It would seem logical, then, that if the nuclear bag fibers

LAB EXERCISE

SOMATOSENSORY RECEPTORS — WEIGHT DISCRIMINATION

Objective: To experience sensory awareness through discrimination of weighted objects

Equipment and Preparation: Eight weighted canisters; paper and pencil; stopwatch; partner. To make weighted canisters: Using a waterproof marker, label 8 empty canisters from 35 mm picture film on the bottoms with numbers 1 through 8. Place 20 BBs in the first canister; place 30 in the second, 40 in the third, and continue through canister 8, placing 90 in the last canister. Close each canister with the appropriate top.

Experience: Randomly place the canisters on a table in front of the partner. Using the preferred hand only, the canisters must be picked up one at a time and placed in a row so that the heaviest one is on the left, and the canisters become progressively lighter from left to right. The experience is timed so that the partner completes the task within one minute. After randomizing the canisters again, the other partner then completes the experience with the preferred hand. The first partner attempts the same task, this time using the other hand. The second partner then completes the task, using the other hand.

Assignment: To score each experience, determine the amount of error from correct placement and then total the numbers. For example, the correct progression from left to right should be: 1 2 3 4 5 6 7 8. A possible score might be: 2 3 5 7 4 1 6 8. The difference of 2 from position 1 is 1. The difference of 3 from 2 is 1. The difference of 5 from 3 is 2, etc. This individual's score would be: 1 + 1 + 2 + 3 + 1 + 5 + 1 + 0 = 11. Compare partner scores and time used; compare hands used. Explain the results.

have a lower firing rate threshold and are easily stretched, and Group Ia neurons are attached to nuclear bag fibers (while Group II are not), they would be the ones to fire during initial muscle length changes. The firing pattern of Group II, then, would be in synchronization with the more-resistant-to-stretch nuclear chain fibers. It also appears logical that Group II will fire once the length of the muscle begins its alteration. Finally, it would seem logical to conclude that the more manipulative the movement of a muscle or muscle group, the larger the number of muscle spindles found in the muscle. For example, many more muscle spindles are proportionately located in the extraocular muscle group controlling the eye than in the quadricep muscle group controlling the hip and knee.

Once the Group Ia and II afferents fire, information about muscle length travels through the sensory pathways to the spinal cord. Alpha motor neurons receive the transmission through synapses that provide detailed information about the stretched muscle so that

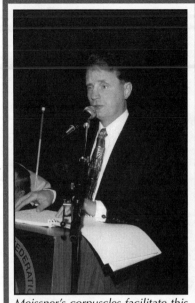

Meissner's corpuscles facilitate this man as he reads Braille.

the extrafusal muscle contracts, producing a shortening. The easiest way to demonstrate this activity is through the monosynaptic stretch reflex (Figure 7.4). The time interval between tapping the patellar tendon and the initiation of limb movement is approximately 50 ms (Bennett, 1977). This time period is too fast to allow the brain and the motor system to function full-circuit. The patellar reflex occurs in response to a brief, direct, and forceful stretch of the tendon.

The monosynaptic stretch reflex is important when initiating a movement to place a limb back into its original position. The brain assimilates the information from the muscle spindles to set a new firing level for the motor neurons, thereby keeping the limb in the appropriate position. For example, if a person placed a solid shot in the outstretched hand of a friend, that friend should be able to quickly adjust to the added weight and maintain the position. If, however, the afferent muscle spindle did not synapse with the alpha motor neuron, and the information was only sent to the brain, the lag time created by the increased weight and the initiation of muscle contraction would be too long, and the shot would be dropped. Conversely, if the shot were made hollow, its weight would be lighter than expected. The muscle would be prepared visually to be quickly contracted. In this case, the activity of the afferent muscle

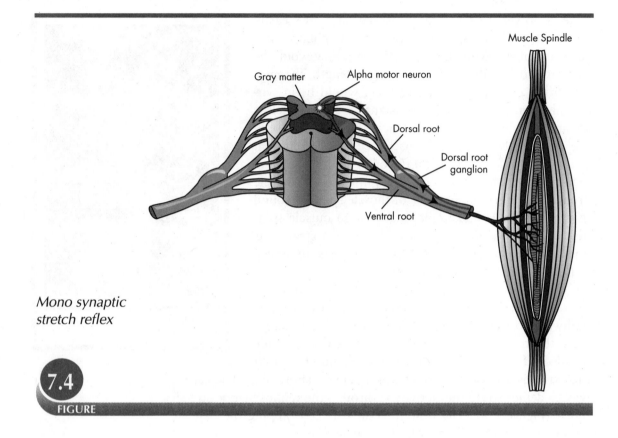

Muscle Spindle

Gray matter   Alpha motor neuron

Dorsal root

Dorsal root
ganglion

Ventral root

*Mono synaptic
stretch reflex*

7.4

FIGURE

spindle would be reduced, as would the rapid firing of the alpha motor neuron. Otherwise, the lightweight shot might be rapidly lifted into the air!

Stretch receptors are also located in the junctions between skeletal muscles and their tendons. They are referred to as **golgi tendon organs.** They contain Type Ib afferent fibers. There is a 10:1 ratio of extrafusal muscle fibers to golgi tendon organs in each skeletal muscle. In passive lengthening, these receptors assess the degree of stretch by their firing rates. They provide information on muscle tension and muscle relaxation. Their ability to assess tension rates indicates that they increase function during isometric muscular contractions, while muscle spindles decrease function during isometric contractions.

Voluntary muscular contractions (whether under isometric, isotonic, or isokinetic conditions) create different responsibilities for the organs and the muscle spindles. The tendon organs basically

Golgi tendon organs
stretch receptors located in the junction between skeletal muscles and their tendons

LAB EXERCISE

SOMATOSENSORY RECEPTORS — MONOSYNAPTIC STRETCH

Objective: To experience a simple functional neural pathway in the body.

Equipment: Adjustable stool, partner, paper, pencil

Experience: Partner A is seated on a stool high enough so that legs dangle in the air. Partner B lightly taps the patellar tendon of the right knee just below the patella. Partner B then lightly taps the patellar tendon of the left knee just below the patella. Change positions of partners and record again.

Assignment: Replicate the experience 5 times. Note any differences.

provide signals proportional to the contraction, while muscle spindle information becomes increasingly uneventful once muscular contraction is initiated.

Additionally, tendon organs, because of their ability to monitor intensity of contraction, protect muscles from overload. Interneurons, functioning as inhibitors, synapse with alpha motor neurons to stifle the firing of Ib afferent signals that travel through the spinal cord to reach alpha motor neuron synapses.

To summarize, muscle spindles are responsible for the assessment of muscle length changes; golgi tendon organs assess muscle tension changes. These proprioceptors provide varying responses from the spinal cord and brain, depending upon speed of response.

There has been increasing agreement about the contributions of muscle spindles to the positioning of joints (McCloskey, Cross, Honner, & Potter, 1983; Kelso, Tuller, Vatikoitis-Batesman, & Fowler, 1984). When researchers stretched muscle tendons surgically, subjects reported feelings of rotation in the joint involved. These findings changed the notion that when specific muscle tendons were stretched, feelings of muscle tension were also found. This raised questions about the individual's conscious ability to determine what is and what is not happening. A person may be unable to discern that a limb is not moving from the perception that it is (Brooks, 1986).

Another set of proprioceptors that provide information about movement and limb position is located in joint capsules and ligaments. These are called **joint receptors**. Neurophysiological investigations

Joint receptors
the parts of joint capsules and ligaments that provide information about movement and limb position

LAB EXERCISE

AUDITION

Objective: To experience the deception that the auditory system can display when using it exclusively for accurate information.

Equipment: Chair, partner (with the ability to snap the fingers), paper, pencil

Experience: Partner A, seated in the chair, focuses straight ahead. Partner B stands directly behind and facing the back of Partner A, 2 feet away.

Assignment: Snap the fingers a total of 20 times, randomly selecting quadrants of up/left, up/right, down/left, and down/right. Also include the cross area of the quadrants. Change positions of partners and record again.

(Clark & Burgess, 1975; Wetzel & Stuart, 1976) have revealed that joints, when placed in extreme positions of rotation, display inordinate amounts of joint receptor activity; the same joints, placed under middle-range rotation conditions, display little or no joint receptor activity. Based upon these findings, it is believed that joint receptors such as golgi tendon organ, Ruffini, and free nerve endings primarily assess distressful intensity of movement (pain receptors), whether they are static or dynamic, within the joint capsule and surrounding ligaments. Other proprioceptors function throughout movement to provide the individual with information about movement, joint, and limb position.

AUDITORY/VESTIBULAR SYSTEM

Yet another set of organs that provides sensory contributions in motor behavior is the vestibular/auditory system. This system and the visual system provide vast amounts of information from the environment. The type of information that is gleaned from the vestibular/auditory and visual systems can be termed **exteroceptive**, meaning information that is derived from outside the body. A discussion of their structure and function follows.

    In order for sound waves transmitted in the air to be heard, they must be converted to sound waves in liquid so that electrical impulses can be conducted, as was previously discussed in this section.

Exteroceptive information that is derived from outside the body

AUDITION/VESTIBULAR APPARATUS EXPERIENCE

Objective: To determine the effects of angular acceleration on semicircular canals

Equipment and Preparation: An unbreakable glass half full with water; record turntable

Experience: Place a glass of water on the exact center of a turntable. Start the turntable. After one minute, turn off the turntable.

Assignment: Describe what happens to the water in the glass.

The ears are sensory receptors and are divided into three: the *external*, the *middle*, and the *inner* ears. Sound waves travel through the external ear or *pinna* through the *external auditory canal* to the *tympanic membrane*, also known as the eardrum. The tympanic membrane, through vibration, converts sound waves from the air. The tensor tympani (muscle in the tympanic membrane) changes the tension in the membrane and controls the amount of sound entering the middle ear. The tympanic membrane transmits vibrations to the *ossicles*, the bones of the middle ear. The *malleus* (hammer), connected with the tympanic membrane, transmits vibrations through the *incus* (anvil) and the *stapes* (stirrup) to the inner ear (cochlea) (Figure 7.5).

The *cochlea*, with an oval window, is filled with fluid. The window is connected to the stapes. The ossicles, then, transmit vibrations to the membrane covering the oval window, creating waves in the cochlear fluid. The bones are mechanically efficient, causing sound waves to be directed from a relatively large tympanic membrane to a much smaller stapes and oval window.

A major proprioceptor, the inner ear functions much like an air traffic control center. It provides information about orientation, acceleration, and body position. It continuously monitors head position, constructs spatial relationships between body and environment, and details angular acceleration. Vestibular information is quite important, but it is not always readily noticed. It is, for example, quite evident when you ride the Tilt-A-Whirl at the amusement park. Before the ride begins, you have no difficulty with dynamic balance (balance used when in motion). At the end of the

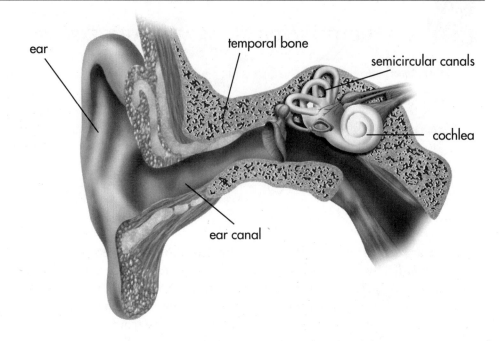

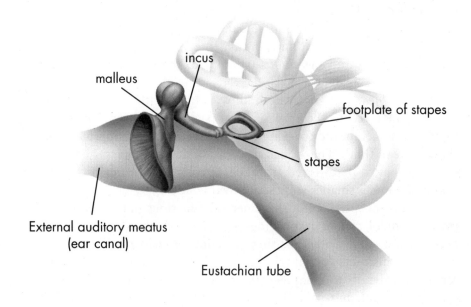

The ear and primary portions of the vestibular system

7.5

FIGURE

ride, dynamic balance is difficult to maintain. This set of receptors is constantly functioning, monitoring the dynamic positions of the head and body to maintain posture and movement. A little warm water in the ear can temporarily cause a state of **vertigo,** a severe disorientation in space, combined with nausea. Vertigo can also be caused by a virus lodging in the inner ear.

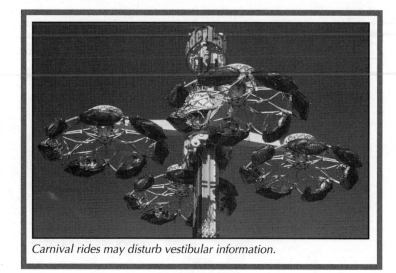

Carnival rides may disturb vestibular information.

Primary portions of the vestibular system include the utricles, saccules, and semicircular canals. These bony labrinths respond to differing stimuli (Figure 7.6). The canals represent the three major planes of movement: sagittal, transverse, and horizontal. As such, they assess angular velocities in their respective planes through hair cells. They also detect acute alterations in head rotation. The vestibular sacs (utricle and saccule) function differently. Having a patch of receptive tissue, the utricles and saccules assess gravitational orientation (e.g., linear acceleration of the head and static head position) through their hair cells. These hair cells, or cilia, contain crystals of calcium carbonate (otoconia), which shift in a gelatin-like substance. When head position changes, the movement produces a shearing effect on the cilia, thereby creating the perception of continued motion, even though the body and head have ceased moving.

Vertigo
severe disorientation combined with nausea

RELATIONSHIP OF SENSORY SYSTEMS TO EACH OTHER AND TO MOTOR BEHAVIOR

Some of the most interesting connections to the vestibular system are those that control the extraocular muscles. When an individual moves through space, the head also moves. The vestibular system directly influences the control of eye movement to compensate for sudden head movements. In this way a somewhat stable retinal or visual image is maintained. Distortions of the vestibular sacs through

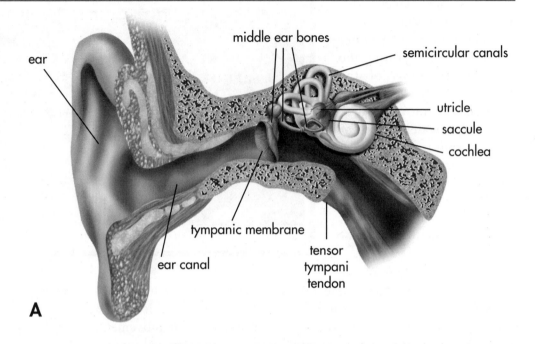

middle ear bones

semicircular canals

ear

utricle

saccule

cochlea

tympanic membrane

tensor tympani tendon

ear canal

A

Primary portions of the vestibular system (A), and orientation planes of the body (B)

7.6

FIGURE

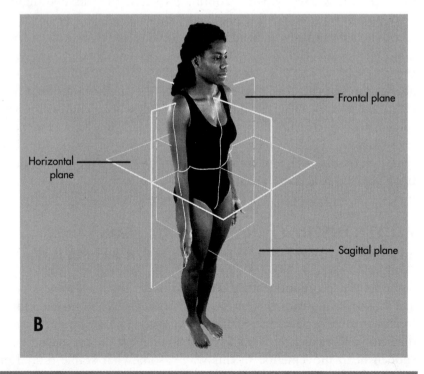

Frontal plane

Horizontal plane

Sagittal plane

B

low-frequency stimulation can produce nausea, and irregular stimulation of the semicircular canals can induce dizziness and nystagmus (eye movements that generally produce a lateral "shaking" motion of the iris).

The auditory/vestibular system, when functioning with other somatosensory systems, can provide accurate information in movement, such as providing static and dynamic balance. It can also contribute to sending conflicting sensory signals when vision has a substantial influence on movement information. For example, the inner ear can measure acceleration, but at constant speeds it provides no useful information. Vision must then become the primary influencer to assist in the determination of how fast the individual is moving. If vision is inhibited or not present, the individual is quite limited in the ability to determine rates of speed on the system.

When discussing the contributions of sensory systems to motor behavior, it is also important to mention the effect of changes that occur due to aging. During the aging process, many of the

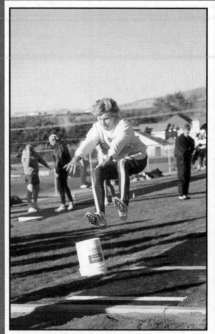

When performing the long jump, an individual utilizes information from the auditory/vestibular system.

somatosensory systems lose some of their adaptability, flexibility, and accuracy as sensory receptors. As dorsal column system pathways become affected, the ability to closely discern differences in touch or pressure decreases. For example, an individual can lose sensitivity to pressure in the feet. As a result, when a 70-year-old returns from a half-hour fitness walk and changes socks and shoes, she may find blisters on her foot that she did not feel. Sometimes the individual will also lose static and dynamic balance. At 75, an individual who is seated at a desk for an hour, may stand up, lose his balance, and fall. As spinothalamic system pathways become affected, temperature, pain, and touch information can be reduced. The 70-year-old woman who uses hot water for her bath and unknowingly scalds herself and the 78-year-old man who, while cooking, inadvertently touches the burner and unknowingly burns himself are examples of what can happen during the aging process. It is also possible for desensitization to occur in both the spinothalamic and dorsal column tracts as a result of scar tissue or lesions from trauma.

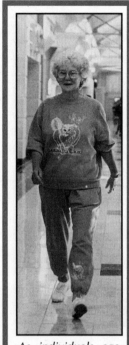

As individuals age, the ability to closely discern differences in pressure decreases.

Finally, many questions have arisen about sensory contributions to motor behavior and their role in performance enhancement. Motor behavior professionals have tried to augment proprioceptor information to enhance the learning process during practice. For example, parachutes have been attached to runners to create drag and have been used as training devices to heighten limb awareness. Vision occluders have been placed on basketball players to increase the necessity for tactile awareness and spatial orientation. Heavier bowling balls have been used by bowlers to augment limb awareness and speed of arm swing. Several investigations have proven these types of techniques to be effective in providing kinesthetic enhancement (Rothstein & Arnold, 1976; Laszlo & Bairstow, 1983; Winstein & Schmidt, 1988). In these studies, it has also been determined that kinesthesis improves as an individual ages to adulthood and that the motor behavior neural connections, once established, seem to be retained. For example, the phenomenon of riding a bicycle is an interesting one. A youngster learns to ride a bicycle around age 7. She continues to ride with frequency until the age of 11, but never rides between the ages of 11 and 32. At 32, she begins riding again with little or no difficulty, as if she had ridden only weeks before. It remains unclear why this phenomenon occurs and what role the senses play in performance success.

FEEDBACK PERSPECTIVES AND MOTOR BEHAVIOR

Feedback
sensory information obtained about movement

Because sensory systems provide information influencing motor behavior, sensory **feedback** (sensory information obtained about movement) is intimately woven into motor behavior. Feedback influences this tapestry in a variety of ways: in anticipation of or in preparation for and during movement (may also be considered feedforward, detailed in Chapter 8); about positions of the body in space prior to, during, and after movement; and in the initial learning of movement.

When one is preparing for a movement, information obtained beforehand — such as body posture — is important. It affects anticipation, the analysis of environmental demands, and the movement dimension selection. Once the movement has begun, discrete adjustments are possible if the movement is long enough, if new information from the dynamic environment is picked up, and if the adjustments are quick enough (milliseconds). For example, an individual playing badminton decides to overhead clear to the opponent's backhand from the opponent's overhead drop shot near the net. Once the clear has been executed, the player perceives that this has set up the opponent for a short and weak return shot. The shot is weakly returned by the opponent; the player, in the meantime, has moved in for the "kill" shot, the smash into the opponent's body. Without the benefit of proprioception, the player would have been unable to adequately prepare for the movement and be ready for discrete adjustments in shot selection (placing the smash in the line of the opponent's body movement, creating a collision of shuttle and body).

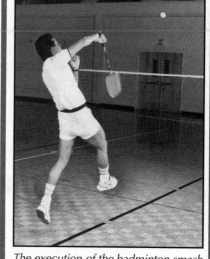

The execution of the badminton smash involves the use of proprioception.

As this example unfolds, the spatial body position of the player is important for success. The location of each body part in relation to the body's core (proprioceptive information) as well as the spatial location of the entire body (exteroceptive information) provides critical information for learning and performance success. Proprioceptive information about racket head position at contact with the shuttle during the smash and a sense of arm speed provide meaningful assessment information based upon outcome.

Future performances under similar environmental conditions can be enhanced. Through practice, sensory feedback enables the individual to rehearse this scenario, displaying similar sequences to learn new movements to accomplish the goal. The perspective of trial-and-success feedback also helps those who have injured a limb to learn to use that limb in order to play the piano, walk, or pick up and cuddle the dog.

Finally, signals from some exteroceptive sources can provide initially meaningful information, but ultimately alarming misinformation to the brain. For example, when someone approaches a viaduct through which an auto passes and the driver blows the horn, the other drivers have difficulty determining where the sound is coming from. The visual system provides meaningful information, but the auditory system provides misinformation to the brain.

In order to facilitate improved communication and ease of transmission, the quality of feedback also depends upon experience

parameters that closely resemble real-world environmental conditions. For example, using a spotting rig to learn a Tsukahara vault (roundoff/back somersault) in gymnastics; hand spotting a roundoff, back handspring, full twisting double back somersault in floor exercise; or using a mini tramp to improve timing on volleyball spiking may have a remarkable effect initially for a novice performer. Later, however, the change in sensory feedback can provide alarming results once the artificial enhancer is removed, which may inhibit the individual's learning.

KEY POINTS

- The visual system, the auditory/vestibular system, and the somatosensory system are sensory receptors that provide humans with information about the environment for movement.
- Two basic types of receptor cells are generator potentials and receptor potentials.
- Sufficient or adequate stimulation is a common feature of all sensory transduction.
- Coding of intensity, coding of frequency, spatial summation, and adaptation are also common to sensory receptors.
- Information generally travels to the brain by one of two routes: the dorsal column route or the spinothalamic route.
- The somatosenses provide information about pain, touch, warmth, cold, skin vibration, limb position, and movement. Their receptors are generally referred to as cutaneous receptors and proprioceptors.
- Cutaneous receptors are categorized into thermoreceptors, mechanoreceptors, and pain receptors.
- Ruffini endings, end bulbs of Krause, free nerve endings, Meissner's corpuscles, Merkel's disks, and Pacinian corpuscles are involved, in varying degrees, in the determination of pain.
- Kinesthesis refers to a conscious appreciation and identification of movement and limb position, while organic sensitivity refers to stimuli from internal organs.
- Muscle spindles and their components are responsible for providing detailed information about the position and movement of limbs.

- Stretch receptors are also located in the junctions between skeletal muscles and their tendons (golgi tendon organs).

- Structures in the ear include the pinna, external auditory canal, tympanic membrane, ossicles, malleus, incus, stapes, and cochlea.

- Primary portions of the vestibular system include the utricles, saccules, and semicircular canals.

- The aging process has an effect on the sensory systems and motor behavior.

- Feedback is intimately woven into the motor behavior tapestry.

- Signals from some exteroceptive sources can provide initially meaningful information, but ultimately alarming misinformation to the brain.

DISCUSSION QUESTIONS

1. Describe the structure of each of the following sensory systems: auditory/vestibular and somatosensory.

2. How are these systems alike in structure and function?

3. What does the word *kinesthesis* refer to? How does it contribute to motor behavior?

4. Describe the relationship of sensory systems to each other and to motor behavior.

5. How does feedback influence motor behavior?

ADDITIONAL READING

Houk, J. C., & Rymer, W. Z. (1981). Neural control of muscle length and tension. In V. B. Brooks (Ed.), *Handbook of physiology: Sec. 1: Vol. 2. Motor control* (pp. 257–323). Bethesda, MD: American Physiological Society.

REFERENCES

Bennett, T. L. (1977). *Brain and behavior.* Monterey, CA: Brooks/Cole Publishing Company.

Brooks, V. B. (1986). *The neural basis of motor control.* New York: Oxford University Press.

Clark, F. J., & Burgess, P. R. (1975). Slowly adapting receptors in the cat knee joint: Can they signal joint angle? *Journal of Neurophysiology, 38,* 1448–1463.

Kelso, J. A. S., Tuller, B., Vatikoitis-Batesman, E., & Fowler, C. A. (1984). Functionally specific articulatory cooperation following jaw perturbations during speech: Evidence for coordinative structures. *Journal of Experimental Psychology: Human Perception and Performance, 10,* 812–832.

Laszlo, J. I., & Bairstow, E. J. (1983). Kinesthesia: Its measurement, training, and relationship to motor control. *Quarterly Journal of Experimental Psychology, 35A,* 411–422.

McCloskey, D. I., Cross, M. J., Honner, R., & Potter, E. K. (1983). Sensory effects of pulling of vibrating exposed tendons in man. *Brain, 106,* 21–37.

Rothstein, A. L., & Arnold, R. K. (1976). Bridging the gap: Application of research on videotape feedback and bowling. *Motor Skills: Theory into Practice, 1,* 35–62.

Wetzel, M. C., & Stuart, D. G. (1976). Ensemble characteristics of cat locomotion and its neural control. *Progress in Neurobiology, 7,* 1–98.

Winstein, C. J., & Schmidt, R. A. (1988). Sensorimotor feedback. In D. H. Holding (Ed.), *Human skills* (2nd ed., pp. 17–47. New York: Wiley.

Vision: Its Contributions to Motor Behavior

*I*n Chapter 7, the auditory/vestibular and somatosensory systems were discussed in detail. The visual sensory system functions similarly to the other systems in its effect on motor behavior. Upon closer examination, however, the visual system is quite different than the others in its structure and function. We rely heavily on our visual system to provide information about the external environment. Visual information is then used to make decisions about movement that can be, at times, lifesaving. For example, to cross the

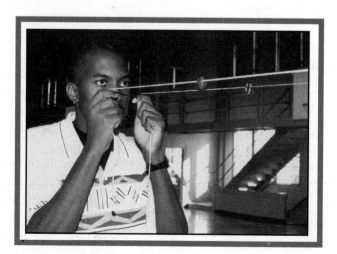

street, you rely upon visual information to determine the street's congestion, where autos, people, and curbs are located, the speed of autos, the flow of traffic, and the timing of the traffic lights. Based upon the visual information, you decide if and when it is appropriate to cross the street safely.

It has been estimated that about 85 percent of sensory information about the external environment is obtained through the visual system (Gavrisky, 1969). This important system provides at least three functions as it relates to motor behavior (Lee, 1978): proprioception, exteroception, and exproprioception. As was mentioned in Chapter 7, the visual system functions as one of the body's proprioceptors, at times in concert and at times at odds with the auditory/vestibular system. It also serves to provide information about the external environment, the spatial locations of objects, and the contours of the environment (**exteroception**). As a proprioceptor, it works in harmony with somatosensory systems to provide information about dynamic and static balance. Finally, the visual system provides information about body position in the environment, using the dimensions of time, force, and flow to influence movement (**exproprioception**). For example, it assists in coincidence anticipation (e.g., a center fielder moves to catch a ball hit between center and right fields). Before we examine the visual system's contributions to motor behavior, we should learn more about the structure and function of the system itself.

THE EYES AS SENSORY RECEPTORS

The **eyes** are sensory receptors that are sensitive to light waves of varying lengths and frequencies. These light waves, through transduction in the form of electromagnetic energy (discussed in an earlier chapter), comprise a narrow portion of the electromagnetic spectrum: 380 to 760 nm (nanometer — one-billionth of a meter) (Figure 8.1). Additionally, these light-sensitive receptors send 430 times more bits of information to the brain than do the ears (Seiderman & Marcus, 1989). The white opaque outer covering of the eye is called the **sclera**. Light waves enter the eye through the **cornea**, a fluid-filled nutrient chamber at the front of the eyeball. The fluid within the cornea is called the **aqueous humor**. The cornea impedes the light and bends or refracts it toward the center. The light reaches the **iris** (the portion that gives color to the eye), narrowing the dark hole in bright light and expanding the dark hole in dim light. The

Exteroception
information that is derived from outside the body

Exproprioception
the visual system providing information about body position in the environment, using the dimensions of time, force, and flow to influence movement

Eyes
sensory receptors sensitive to light waves of varying length and frequency

Sclera
white, opaque, outer covering of the eye

Cornea
a fluid-filled nutrient chamber at the front of the eyeball

Aqueous humor
a nutrient chamber at the front of the eyeball

Iris
the colored ring of the eye

Wavelengths in meters

Electromagnetic spectrum

8.1

FIGURE

dark hole, referred to as the **pupil**, regulates the amount of light that proceeds to the **retina** (a thin membrane of receptor cells located on the back of the eyeball) through the **lens. Pupillary size** is determined by sphincter and dilator muscles of the iris and depends on an individual's arousal level and the amount of light falling on the retina. The lens changes its shape by using **ciliary muscles** to focus light onto the retina. After leaving the lens, light travels through the main chamber of the eye, which contains **vitreous humor**, a pressurized fluid that maintains the shape of the eyeball. The **macula**, located near the center of the retina, is the area where greatest visual acuity

Pupil   the dark center of the eye that regulates the amount of light entering the retina

Retina   a thin membrane of receptor cells located on the back of the eyeball

Lens   a portion of the eye that allows light to enter and is refracted and focused onto the retina

Pupillary size   diameter of the pupil of the eye determined by sphincter and dilator muscles of the iris, dependent upon the individual's arousal level and the amount of light falling on the retina

Ciliary muscles   muscles that change the shape of the lens to focus light onto the retina

Vitreous humor   pressurized fluid in the main chamber of the eye through which light travels after leaving the lens; maintains the shape of the eyeball

Macula   the portion of the eye located near the center of the retina where vision is clearest

Fovea
the center of clearest visual acuity in the eye

Cones
color receptors in the eye that provide chronomatic vision and facilitate the highest acuity

Rods
long, slender cells located primarily in peripheral areas of the eye that are unable to detect color

Chromatic vision
sight in which the cones provide the highest acuity and color vision

Photopigments
chemicals of opsin and retinal used in the initial transduction of light in the eye

Trichromatic spectrum
the range of primary, secondary, and tertiary colors

occurs. The **fovea** (foveal pit) is the center of clearest visual acuity. When an individual focuses directly on an object, light falls directly onto the fovea. Figure 8.2 provides an illustration of the route light traverses to reach the retina.

Once light arrives at the retina, it encounters two types of photoreceptors: the **cones** and the **rods**. Cones are color receptors that provide **chromatic vision** and facilitate the highest acuity. They are densely packed at the back of the eye and thin out around the periphery. It should be no surprise that the fovea contains only cones. Cones are comprised of **photopigments** (chemicals of opsin and retinal used in the initial transduction of light) needed for the detection of object detail, hues (colors), saturation (richness of hue), and brightness (vividness of hue). The retina has three types of cones, each sensitive to a wavelength of light that corresponds to one of the primary colors in the **trichromatic spectrum**. Figure 8.3 displays a chart of primary, secondary, and tertiary colors. Since cone sensitivity is not exactly to red, blue, or green, overlap exists. Equal stimulation of all three types of cones is perceived as white light. Some people are unable to perceive correctly one or more of the primary colors (Gavrisky, 1969). This seems to be a sex-linked genetic trait in 8 to 10 percent of males compared to less than 0.5 percent of females. This

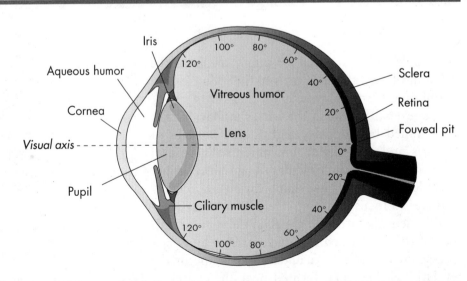

Route light traverses to reach the retina

8.2
FIGURE

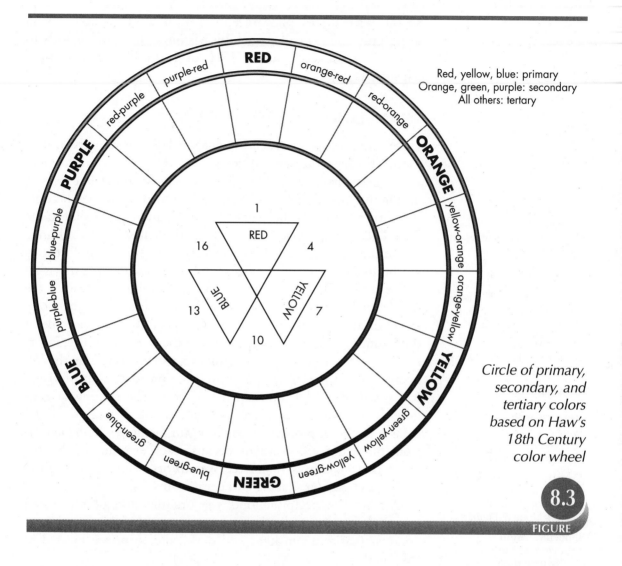

Red, yellow, blue: primary
Orange, green, purple: secondary
All others: tertiary

Circle of primary, secondary, and tertiary colors based on Haw's 18th Century color wheel

8.3
FIGURE

color deficiency (note the term *deficiency* rather than *blindness*) ranges from minor confusion of color hues to total lack of color identification. Total lack of color identification (color blindness) is quite unusual in humans. The most frequently reported deficiency occurs with red-green, because light having these specific wavelengths stimulates the same combination of cones.

Rods are long, slender cells located primarily in peripheral areas. They are unable to detect color — thereby providing only **monochromatic vision** — but are more light-sensitive than cones. Because rods function well in low levels of illumination, they serve

Color deficiency
a condition in which sensitivity of cones is not sufficient to stimulate color discrimination; generally, an inability to perceive correctly one or more of the primary colors

Monochromatic vision
eyesight that is unable to detect color, just blacks, whites, and shades of gray

Scotopic vision
night vision

Optic disk
the area in the eye where
no receptors are located

Optic tracts
optic nerves after entering
the brain and extending to
the lateral geniculate
nucleus of the thalamus

Lateral geniculate nucleus
portion of the brain where
the optic nerves enter and
become the optic tracts

Thalamus
portion of the brain involved
with visual perception

Optic radiations
a portion of the brain where
axons stemming from the
optic nerves run through to
the primary visual cortex in
the brain's occipital lobes

Primary visual cortex
main area of visual
perception, located in
occipital lobe of brain

Binocular vision
the eyes receiving
information from slightly
different angles, producing
two distinct images

Accessory optic nuclei
nuclei located in the brainstem that coordinate eye
movements that compensate
for head movements

Pretectum pathway
portion of the brain near
the superior colliculus that
assists in controlling size
of pupils of the eye

as the individual's photoreceptors at night (low-light vision using only rods is called **scotopic vision**). The ratio of rods to cones in each eye is roughly 17:1, or 120 million to 7 million (Anshel, 1990).

TRANSDUCTION TO THE BRAIN

Once visual impulses reach the deepest layer of the retina, they ascend through the **optic disk**, where no receptors are located, via the optic nerve and transmit the signals at speeds in excess of 420 mph (Anshel, 1990) to the brain. The optic nerves become the **optic tracts** once they enter the brain, and they extend to the **lateral geniculate nucleus** of the **thalamus**. These axons continue on through the **optic radiations** to the **primary visual cortex** in the brain's occipital lobe. Figure 8.4 details the route of visual image transmission through the brain. To reiterate some of the information, receptors stemming from one side of the body travel through pathways used to transmit to the opposite side of the brain. For example, when the eyes focus at a distance, information that is to the right of visual focus is detected by the left hemisphere of the brain, while information to the left of visual focus is detected by the right hemisphere. The routing of ganglion cells from the inner halves of the retina through the optic chiasm to the opposite side of the brain facilitates **binocular vision** (Binocular vision occurs because each eye, due to the distance that separates them, receives information from slightly different angles, producing two distinct images.)

Within the occipital lobe, the organization of the visual scene takes place. Cells that are specific to the identification of contrast (variances in light and dark) and form are located in this area.

Additionally, other pathways are taken by optic nerve fibers into the brain. Nuclei (**accessory optic nuclei**) located in the brain stem coordinate eye movements that compensate for head movements (Ito, 1977). The **pretectum pathway** is located near the superior colliculus and assists in the control of pupillary size (Sprague, Berlucchi, & Rizzolatti, 1973). The superior colliculus plays a role in attention to visual stimuli and control of eye movements. Here, vision is integrated with other sensory information from the somatosensory and auditory systems (Rodieck & Stone, 1965).

TWO VISUAL SYSTEMS AND MOTOR BEHAVIOR

It has been determined that there are two visual systems (Sanderson, 1972; Sanderson & Whiting, 1978), both of which contribute to human movement, but which differ in structure and function. These are the **focal** and **ambient** systems. Table 8.1 categorizes the characteristics of each system as it relates to human movement.

Focal vision
conscious and central eyesight used in identifying objects

Ambient vision
peripheral vision used in localizing objects, which is not central

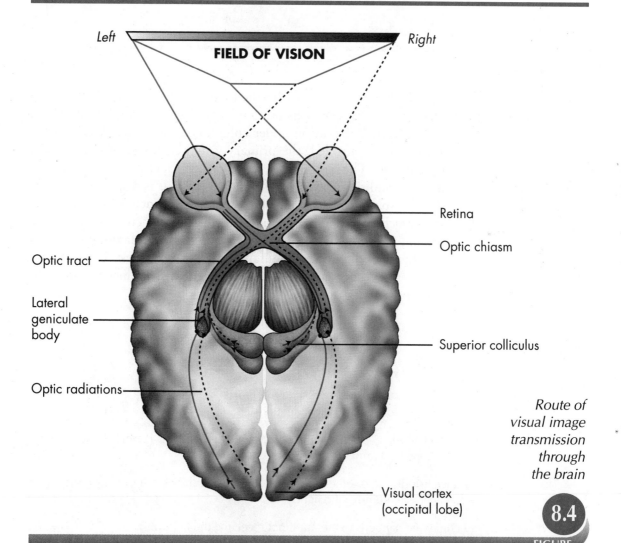

Route of visual image transmission through the brain

8.4
FIGURE

TABLE 8.1

Characteristics of Focal and Ambient Systems

Focal	*Ambient*
Conscious	Nonconscious
Central	Peripheral
High spatial frequencies	Low spatial frequencies
Identification	Localization
Body/photoreceptor	Body/spatial orientation
Gross movement control	Fine movement control
Bright light	Dim light

The focal system involves the fovea and is responsible for object identification. It performs best under well-lighted conditions and assesses detailed definition under voluntary control. Because it can be voluntarily controlled, the primary visual cortex serves as the area of control. The ambient system, which operates best in dimly lighted conditions, involves the entire retina. It is responsible for the general spatial location of objects. The ambient system must provide much of the information gleaned from the environment when driving at night, when playing a tennis game as dawn approaches, or when bicycling on a mountain roadway near dusk. When there is a decrease in focal sensitivity, there is generally an increase in ambient sensitivity.

LAB EXERCISE

PATHWAY OF THE VISUAL FIELDS

Objective: To determine how visual fields function.

Equipment and Preparation: 8" by 11" cardboard; partner; flashlight. Partner A places the divider between Partner B's eyes.

Experience: Partner B looks across the room while Partner A shines a flashlight indirectly into either eye. Remove the light.

Assignment: Record what happens to the pupil not receiving the light.

Another similar categorization is based upon cell structure and function. The **magno** system, designated by its large cells, is associated with peripheral vision, depth perception, movement identification, low luminance, high contrast sensitivity, rapid response, and low spatial frequency characteristics. The **parvo** system is associated with its central, texture, shape, color-sensitive, high luminance, low contrast sensitivity, high spatial frequency, and sustained response capacities (Bassi & Lehmkuhle, 1990).

These systems seem to be parallel processed, particularly during movement. Table 8.2 provides a perspective on these systems.

Magno system
a classification system identified by its peripheral, depth perception, movement identification, low luminance, high contrast sensitivity, rapid response, and low spatial frequency

Parvo system
a model characterized by central, texture, shape, color-sensitive, high luminance, low-contrast sensitivity, high spatial frequency, and sustained response

1. Peripheral vision	ambient/magno
2. Reaction time	ambient/magno
3. Brightness of objects	focal/parvo
4. Clarity of objects	focal/parvo
5. Ability to focus on an object	focal/parvo
6. Ability to shift focus from one object to another	focal/parvo
7. Ability to track an object	focal/parvo
8. Ability to fixate on an object in space	focal/parvo
9. Ability to locate object in space monocularly and binocularly	focal/parvo
10. Ability to concentrate visually with minimum tension	ambient/magno
11. Ability to concentrate visually without raising thresholds of other senses	ambient/magno
12. Ability to coordinate vision with other senses	ambient/magno
13. Ability to coordinate vision with other ANS functions	ambient/magno
14. Ability to coordinate vision with gross and fine motor systems	focal/parvo; ambient/magno
15. Ability to make texture judgment	focal/parvo
16. Ability to make fine depth judgments	focal/parvo
17. Ability to make gross depth judgments	ambient/magno

TABLE 8.2

Central/Peripheral Visual Mechanisms and the Focal/Ambient and Magno/Parvo Systems

THE BRAIN, PERCEPTION, AND MOTOR BEHAVIOR

Once the brain has received neural input from the eyes through visual pathways, the visual perception process unfolds. The processes that are involved and the models used to better understand these processes continue to be debated by the experts.

Visual perception theories continue to focus on two profoundly different tenets that: (1) visual perception is based upon one's understanding of the environment (**cognitive theories** of visual perception) through deductive internal processes; or (2) visual perception is taken directly from the environment through signals that function for us as a sort of detailed road map (**ecological theories** of visual perception). Cognitive theories stem from the notion that there is an additional step before information can be made meaningful to guide movement; ecological theories reflect the notion that environmental information can be meaningful and, therefore, directly used to guide behavior. It should be no surprise that the research designs used to attempt to prove the theories differ as well.

Published researchers of the cognitive approach (Sharp & Whiting, 1974; Sanderson & Whiting, 1978) used designs within controlled laboratory settings so that certain variables could be isolated to determine the effects. Those upholding the ecological approach (Gibson, 1979; Singer, Caraugh, Murphey, Chen & Lidor, 1991) have used real-time, real-event environments to determine the effects of environmental conditions.

The truth may lie somewhere in between. It may be that cognitive visual perception theory is at work when there is a dynamic environment, where decision-making is one of the major factors for performance success (Williams, Davids, Burwitz, & Williams, 1992). In racquetball, for example, complex decisions must be made about the angle of rebound from several potential surfaces. Other decisions involve force, spin, shot selection, and rules that govern the sport. In contrast, it may be that ecological visual perception theory is at work when the environment is stable, so that what is seen is what is known (Wieringen, 1988). When completing the last pass on balance beam, for example, the gymnast performs a front handspring punch front tuck somersault dismount. The **optic array** (the ambient light reflected from objects that present a unique texture to the brain at each point of observation) that is configured might be sufficient to guide the movement.

Cognitive theories
paradigms that explain that an additional step is present before information can be made meaningful to guide movement

Ecological theory
a paradigm explaining human movement, in which the individual interacts with the environment and interaction that is based upon the individual's perception

Optic array
ambient light reflected from objects, presenting a unique texture to the brain at each point of observation

What is currently known from the research provides conflicting pieces of information about visual perception and motor behavior. Real-time, real-event environments where detailed decisions must be made on the basis of advance visual cues, seem to provide a basic understanding about possible strategies to enhance learning and performance. It remains to be seen which approach will provide the most detailed information upon which to build effective strategies for performance success.

VISUAL/PERCEPTUAL SKILLS: THEIR ROLE IN INFLUENCING MOTOR BEHAVIOR

As an illustration of the complexity of vision in motor behavior, consider the following scenario from a basketball game: The player's attention is directed by the sound of the ball hitting the backboard (auditory system); she looks up and searches for the ball, locks onto it (using saccadic eye movements), and tracks its trajectory (using smooth pursuit eye movements) while positioning herself to intercept and catch it. Upon catching it, she dribbles repeatedly, sights the basket, and checks the position of opponents (using vergence eye movements). She aims before shooting the ball (maintaining balance through vestibular-ocular eye movements), and tracks its trajectory through the hoop (using vergence movements). In addition to the eye movements depicted in this scenario, other visual/perceptual skills are used to influence movement.

As a result of the increasing interest in the role that visual/perceptual skills play in motor performance, a relatively new, interdisciplinary area has evolved. Known as **sports vision**, it was initiated in the United States by optometrists and ophthalmologists in the 1960s who were interested in the topic from vision correction, vision enhancement, and ocular injury perspectives (Reichow, Coffey, Wacho, & Velnousky, 1981; Vinger, 1980; Gregg, 1987). Their emphasis emanated from the work of several behavioral optometrists (see Loran & MacEwen, 1995 for a detailed review in the Additional Readings for this chapter). With the works of early and contemporary researchers in the area of gaze behavior and sport success (Ludveigh & Miller, 1958; Hubbard & Seng, 1954; Bard & Fleury, 1981; Bahill & LaRitz, 1984; Vickers, 1996), dynamic visual acuity parameters (Burg, 1966; Trachtman, 1991; ten Napel, 1993), and contrast sensitivity function in sport (Ginsburg, 1983; Hoffman, Polan, & Powell, 1984; Kluka, Love, & Allen, 1989), there

Sports vision
an interdisciplinary area of sport science, initiated by optometrists, ophthalmologists, and sport science researchers who were interested in the relationship of vision to sport performance from perspectives of vision correction, vision enhancement, and ocular injury

has been substantial interdisciplinary collaboration, continued appeal in the area, and an explosion of information. Much, however, remains to be understood.

There seems to be a core of visual/perceptual abilities that influence motor skill acquisition: dynamic stereopsis, acuity (static/dynamic), accommodation, vergence (convergence/divergence), glare recovery, focal/peripheral vision, color perception, and contrast sensitivity function (Planer, 1994; Reichow, Coffey, Wacho, & Velnousky, 1981). An additional ability, **eye dominance** (ocular dominance), has received mixed reviews as to its importance in motor skill acquisition. Eye dominance can be divided into three types: sighting dominance, sensory dominance, and acuity dominance (Coren & Kaplan, 1973). **Sighting dominance** refers to the eye that is consistently used in aiming tasks — for example, the eye that is used to focus through a camera or the one that is tested with the hole-in-the-card test (Buxton & Crossland, 1937). **Sensory dominance** is indicated by the eye that holds monocular images longer (Porac & Coren, 1976). The third, **acuity dominance,** is found by determining which eye is more accurate on measures of static visual acuity. Generally, sighting dominance is used most frequently as the definition of eye dominance.

Eye dominance (sighting dominance; sensory dominance; acuity dominance)—the preferred eye; the eye that holds monocular images the longest; the eye that is more accurate on measures of static visual acuity

Sighting dominance the eye that is preferred through behavior

Sensory dominance refers to the eye that holds monocular images longer

Acuity dominance describes the eye that is more accurate on measures of static visual acuity

---

LAB EXERCISE

EYE (SIGHTING) DOMINANCE

Objective: To determine which eye is dominant at distance and near.

Equipment and Preparation: 4" by 6" card; two one-inch square colored papers; paper punch. Attach one square to the wall at eye level. Attach the other square to the top of a table. Punch a hole in the center of the card; partner; pencil and paper.

Experience: *(For distance)* — Standing 10 feet from a wall, hold the card by its sides with both hands. Extend the arms at the shoulders toward the wall. *(For near)* — Standing in front of the table, perform the same procedure, but hold the card as if reading from it. Look through the hole in the card and repeat the procedure.

Assignment: Look through the hole in the card with both eyes and focus on the square. Without moving the card, close the right eye; open it. Refocus on the square and close the left eye.

LAB EXERCISE

EYE MOVEMENTS AND PERCEPTUAL PROCESSING

Objective: To assess observational skill when viewing a scene.

Equipment and Preparation: Posterboard (18" by 22"); brightly colored marking pen; straightedge. Place a large triangle shape on the posterboard. Print the following words in the triangle in the following manner:

Shoot the ball
into the
the hoop

Experience: Partner A constructs the posterboard without letting Partner B see it before it is completed. Partner B is asked to read aloud what is on the posterboard. What is actually read? What is actually on the posterboard?

Assignment: Explain what the results might mean as they relate to the observation of motor behavior.

There seems to be a commonly held belief (Teig, 1980; Seiderman & Marcus, 1989) that in baseball and softball, players with cross-dominance (left-eye and right-handed batting dominance; right-eye and left-handed batting dominance) perform better at batting than those without (right-eye and right-handed batting dominance; left-eye and left-handed batting dominance). The idea is that in players with cross-dominance, the dominant eye has a better viewing angle of the pitch and can process information as much as 21 ms faster than the other eye (Teig, 1980). This belief has not been substantiated with research (Adams, 1965; Schrader, 1971; Ong & Rodman, 1972). The largest published investigation included over 200 NCAA Division I baseball players and over 120 youth players (Milne, Buckolz, & Cardenas, 1995). Using sighting dominance as their definition of eye dominance, researchers found no difference between cross-dominant and same-side-dominant batting performance or between eye dominance, hand dominance, batting side, or stance in collegiate and youth batters. A rather simple solution to the matter involves head placement. The axiom, "teach skills from the eyes down," is fully appropriate. By turning the head so that both eyes have an equal opportunity to view the approaching ball, dynamic stereopsis and other visual/perceptual skills can be more appropriately used.

Gauging the distance of objects appropriately (**dynamic stereopsis**) is one of the visual/perceptual skills that contributes to performance success. Because the eyes are separated (retinal disparity), they provide binocular cues for judging distance. The effectiveness of this separation, however, decreases with distance; therefore, the closer the object, the greater the stereo effect. For example, when a pitcher views the seams of a softball while holding it in her throwing hand as she prepares for the windup, the ball appears to be more rounded and three-dimensional. Once the ball has moved fifteen feet away, it loses some of its three-dimensionality. When the ball has reached the catcher's mitt, it appears to have little, if any, three-dimensionality. At that distance, the angle between the eyes and the object is rather small; therefore, the smaller the angle, the less the stereoscopic

Dynamic stereopsis
gauging the distance of objects in relative motion

LAB EXERCISE

DEPTH PERCEPTION (STEREOPSIS)

Objective: To determine the accuracy of depth perception.

Equipment and Preparation: Two one-half inch buttons of the same color; two screw eyes; 25 feet of heavy string; hammer; hand drill. Mount the two screw eyes on a wall at eye level so they are 6 inches apart horizontally. Thread the string through both screw eyes so the ends are even. Position one button 7 feet from the left end of the string (knot the string at both ends of the string after the buttons are placed on the string) and the other 5 feet from the right end; partner; paper and pencil.

Experience: Stand about 12 feet from the wall, holding one end of the string in each hand with hands extended straight ahead at eye level. With both eyes open, adjust the string until the buttons appear to be equidistant from the screw eyes. Release the string and measure the alignment of the buttons. If they are out of alignment by more than one inch, position the buttons so that they are directly across from one another, focus on the buttons, then change their positions so that they are 9 and 11 feet from the ends of the string and repeat the process.

Assignment: Attempt 10 trials, alternating the procedure so that the left button is closer than the right one for half the time. Record the distance of each trial and each button. Compare the results with a partner.

effect (or the flatter the object's appearance). Stereopsis is five times more sensitive at six feet than at 300 feet (Ogle, 1964).

Distance can also be estimated monocularly. This is particularly helpful when a person has only one eye or when the brain suppresses information in a binocular situation. Monocular cues depend upon the qualities of the objects themselves rather than upon any stereoscopic effect. The basic categories of stereopsis (House, Pansky, & Siegel, 1979) are linear and textural perspective, relative size of objects, aerial perspective, shadowing, interposition, movement parallax (or relative movement of objects), and upward dislocation.

For example, surface textures seem to become more dense with distance, thereby providing interesting perspectives of linearity and texture. Children often look for vacant lots to play pickup games of baseball or kickball. In the initial observation from the street, a lot may appear to have ground that is smooth enough to make a great field. Upon closer examination, however, the ground could have ruts big enough to make fielding the ball challenging.

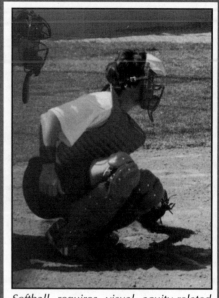

Softball requires visual acuity-related skills.

As was mentioned previously in this chapter, the ability to visually discern detail in objects is called **visual acuity**. Visual acuity can be divided into two parts: **static** (SVA) and **dynamic** (DVA). SVA is usually evaluated by the Snellen Eye Chart, where the smallest feature (usually letters) is distinguished in high-contrast conditions. DVA refers to visual clarity when there is relative motion (motion of an object, an individual, or an object and an individual). There are many factors that affect visual discrimination, including contrast, lighting, motion, time, color, age, and attentional demands. The most important factors appear to be contrast, lighting, and time and motion (McCormick & Sanders, 1982). If the contrast between object and background is low, the object needs to be larger to be as detectable as a smaller object with greater contrast. Greater illumination tends to improve acuity, but this effect tends to decrease over time (adaptation), and too much light may create glare that interferes with vision (McCormick & Sanders, 1982; Knudson & Kluka, 1997).

The time available to focus on an object also affects SVA. The time and motion factor distinguishes DVA from SVA. Because most

Visual acuity
(static; dynamic) the ability to visually discern detail of objects

Static visual acuity
clarity of features distinguished by the eyes under high-contrast conditions

Dynamic visual acuity
clarity of eyesight when there is relative motion

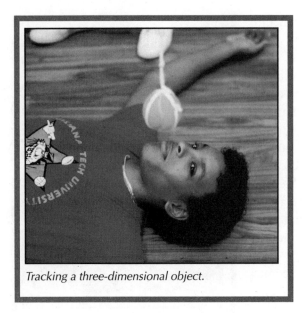
Tracking a three-dimensional object.

sports are dynamic, DVA may be an important variable in sport performance. SVA is weakly related to DVA at slow speeds but is not related to DVA at faster speeds (Morris, 1977). An individual's DVA decreases rapidly as eye angular velocities required to track an object exceed sixty to seventy degrees per second (Bahill & LaRitz, 1984; Burg, 1966). DVA improves from ages six to twenty, but begins to decline thereafter (Burg, 1966; Ishigaki & Miyao, 1994). Children under the age of ten may not, however, have DVA skills that have developed sufficiently to perform certain motor skills, because adult-like vision usually develops between the ages of ten and twelve (Schalen, 1980). Providing larger and less elastic balls, batting tees, and larger racket heads to learn basic motor patterns provides definite advantages for children. Additionally, researchers have shown improvement in DVA with training in adults (Schalen, 1980), but the exact length of time the improvement lasts is yet to be established. More research needs to be conducted in this area.

Accommodation
adjustment of the eye's lens to obtain clarity of an object, controlled by ciliary muscle contraction

Accommodation, the adjustment of the eye's lens to focus clearly on an object, is controlled by ciliary muscle contraction. It is of particular importance when an object is closer than twenty feet. As a person ages, accommodative function becomes less flexible. When a 57-year old recreational tennis player views the approaching ball from an opponent's backhand drive, he may experience difficulty focusing on the ball within fifteen feet of the racket. There has been little research to show improvements in accommodation in athletes. Efforts published to date have used research designs that involve relaxing accommodation through auditory and visual biofeedback (Trachtman, 1997; Trachtman & Venezia, 1994). Researchers have tried to test the notion that by relaxing accommodation, they can create an enhanced alpha brain wave state, thereby leading to improved athletic performance. An enhanced alpha brain state is one in which the individual is in a relaxed state that heightens awareness and sensitivity. Through several case studies, it was found that athletes were able to achieve substantial improvement in their abilities to participate in several simultaneous activities and to perceive objects in slow motion. Further research needs to be conducted in this area as well.

Vergence, the ability of the eyes to follow an object moving toward or away from the body, can be divided into convergence (eyes turning inward as an object approaches) and divergence (eyes returning to the neutral position) (Kluka, 1997). This visual/perceptual ability needs to be researched further to determine its precise role in motor skill acquisition.

Vergence (convergence; divergence) the ability of the eyes to follow an object moving toward or away from the body

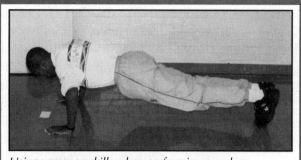

Using vergence skills when performing a pushup.

Glare recovery, the time it takes to redefine an object after bright light has bleached out the rods and cones, can be an important visual/perceptual ability. For example, when volleyball setters look up to see the ball and face the bright lights suspended from the ceiling, the ball is sometimes "lost" in the lights. Some sport facilities are constructed with built-in glare. The NFL's Cowboy Stadium in Dallas, Texas was designed with huge overhangs that cast shadows onto the field of play. When a late afternoon game is played, receivers are challenged by plays that take

Glare recovery the time required to redefine an object after bright light has bleached out the rods and cones of the eyes

LAB EXERCISE

VISUAL/PERCEPTUAL SKILLS — FUSION AND PERIPHERAL VISION

Objective: To experience the visual/perceptual skills of fusion and peripheral vision.

Equipment and Preparation: Poster (18" by 22" or larger) of someone performing a motor skill who is throwing a ball; posted on a wall so that the center of the poster is at eye level.

Experience: Stand at least 10 feet away from the wall and the poster. Place the tips of both index fingers together, extending both arms out to three inches in front of the eyes. Look at the throwing hand of the picture displayed on the wall. Separate the finger tips 1/2 inch. What happens to the appearance of the fingers? Then wiggle both fingers simultaneously. Still focusing on the throwing arm on the poster, what happens to the appearance of the fingers?

Assignment: Explain the phenomenon that has occurred. How does this phenomenon relate to motor performance?

them into the shadows to catch the ball. Part of their success may depend upon how quickly they can recover from glare. There has been little research into this particular visual/perceptual ability and its contributions to performance. It is unclear whether or not glare recovery can be improved and if its improvement is beneficial to successful motor performance.

Yet another visual/perceptual ability that influences motor behavior success is **contrast sensitivity function** (CSF). CSF is the ability to process or filter spatial and temporal information about objects and their backgrounds under varying lighting conditions. It is determined by measuring the least amount of contrast required to detect a visual stimulus. CSF can be represented by graphing an individual's sensitivity relative to spatial frequency. Grating patterns that vary in width and brightness have been used to determine contrast sensitivity threshold in athletes. Spatial frequency is designated by the reciprocal of the visual angle displayed by a light and dark bar pair (Figure 8.5).

Contrast sensitivity function
the ability to process or filter spatial and temporal information about objects and their backgrounds under varying lighting conditions

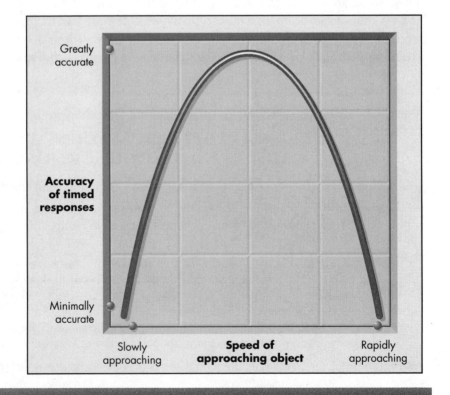

Inverted-U relationship between speed of the approaching object of interest and accuracy of timed responses

8.5 FIGURE

It has been theorized (Ginsburg, 1983) that CSF decreases as an object's velocity increases. In principle, the higher the individual's CSF profile and the higher the individual's CSF profile across frequencies, the more likely the individual is to discriminate an object as its velocity increases. A model of visual abilities and characteristics of the magno and parvo systems for optimal athletic performance has been developed (Trachtman & Kluka, 1993) and shown in Table 8.2. Note the role contrast sensitivity plays in characterizing each of the systems.

Several investigations have been published about the role of CSF and vision in sport performance. The progression of research focus can be summarized as follows: (1) the status of CSF in athletes through CSF performance profiles and types of instruments used for assessment, (2) the effects of physiological fatigue on CSF, and (3) the effects of sports vision enhancement programs on CSF.

The earliest published investigations to determine the status of male athlete CSF (Hoffman, Polan, & Powell, 1984) hypothesized that male collegiate athletes achieved better CSF performance scores than a sedentary population. The results supported this hypothesis. Collegiate female athlete CSF scores were also found to be significantly higher than accepted sedentary female population norms (Kluka, Love, & Allen, 1989). Extensive profiling of athletes by sport and by ability level was also conducted (Kluka, Love, Sanet, Hillier, Stroops, & Schneider, 1995). Olympic (volleyball and softball) and professional (ice hockey and football) athletes were comparable in their profiles. Within each sport (volleyball, softball, football, basketball, ice hockey) , the higher the performance level (beginner to professional/elite), the higher the CSF profile. The CSF profile difference may distinguish the expert from the novice. It is yet to be determined whether this ability is learned or inherent.

To determine the effects of physiological fatigue on CSF, researchers (Love, Kluka, & Cobb, 1996) investigated the effect of blood glucose levels on CSF in female athletes. The longer the athlete aerobically exercised, the less sensitive was the athlete's central vision to changes in contrast; blood glucose levels were unaffected. These findings help to substantiate the notion that when aerobically based activity is engaged in, an athlete's central (focal) vision is affected first.

Enhancing CSF through sports vision training programs was investigated by several researchers. CSF within central vision was improved as a result of relaxation of accommodation through biofeedback training, while CSF within central and peripheral vision was improved as a result of sport-specific vision training (Kluka, Love, Kuhlman, Hammack, & Wesson, 1996). Further investigations need to be conducted in real-time, real-environmental conditions in order to more fully determine the short-term and longitudinal effects of such programs on motor performance improvement.

FEEDFORWARD AND FEEDBACK PERSPECTIVES

Vision is used in a variety of situations to assist in the determination of static and dynamic human movement. Proprioceptors, as was indicated in Chapter 7, provide sufficient information for adults to maintain erect posture. For example, those who lose their sight during adulthood can readily maintain erect posture and continue to move by relying on sufficient information from proprioceptors. Children who are sighted at birth, however, seem to rely more heavily on the visual system to guide behavior; there is evidence that other proprioceptive information may not be well integrated until between the ages of one and three for postural and movement success (Sigelman & Shaffer, 1995). Those born without sight move adequately through intersensory perception involving the recognition of postural and dynamic movements from one sense (touch or audition) by what has been learned through another sense (proprioception).

Feedforward
the process of launching signals prior to movement that gives meaning to information as a result of movement

Vision has also been found to be useful in providing **feedforward** information. Feedforward refers to the process of launching signals prior to movement so that information stemming from movement has meaning. It serves as a precursor to determining the dimensions of objects in the environment, the terrain of the environment, and time and space in the environment. Christa McAuliffe (the first teacher to be enrolled in the NASA space program), while experiencing weightlessness for the first time, relied heavily upon vision to serve a feedforward movement prediction function. When she was learning to move from one side of the simulated space shuttle to another, the information gained ahead of time about object location and the presence of walls, floors, ceilings, and instrumentation was invaluable. The primary challenge in weightlessness is to utilize feedforward information quickly to perform a movement in opposition to what would be done in a weighted state to get the desired result!

Feedforward is also used in situations where foot or body placement influences performance success. Infants as young as seven months were found to be already using feedforward information about terrain in crawling success (Gibson & Walk, 1960; Campos, Langer, & Krowitz, 1970). When placed in situations where terrain was level and where dropoffs were created, infants avoided the dropoffs and remained on level ground when attempting to reach their mothers, positioned several feet away. It was also determined that when the surface remained smooth, crawling patterns were generally controlled by the spinal system, with limited feedforward information needed from vision.

For adults, foot placement is also critical when running cross country. Whether jogging for health or racing competitively, vision used as a feedforward mechanism provides important cues for a successful experience. For example, when one sees the hill ahead with no trees or stumps to impede progress, information is forwarded in advance to the brain to facilitate adjustments in stride length, body lean, and arm position to "charge" up the hill. Conversely, at the top of the hill, vision assists in the assessment of bushes and small trees for the descent. Misjudging a dip in the terrain cannot only be unexpected but can also be painful. Kicking into a tree root because ground distance was misjudged or not seen

LAB EXERCISE

BALANCE (STATIC AND DYNAMIC)

Objective: To experience variations in static and dynamic balance.

Equipment and Preparation: Balance boards, bean bags, 4" ball, 8" ball, 4" in diameter PVC pipe, cut in 12" sections; 24" by 12" balance boards cut out of 3/4" plywood; target, similar to that used in archery to be placed on a wall, eye height when on balance board.

Experience: Attempt the following balances using the balance board constructed:

(a) Balance as long as possible.

(b) Balance with eyes on center of target for as long as possible.

(c) Balance while bouncing the 8" ball for as long as possible.

(d) Balance while tossing the 4" ball overhead from hand to hand for as long as possible.

Assignment: Record the results of each of the above experiences and compare with others in the class. How do the results compare? Why?

is an example of the feedforward mechanism failing to appropriately communicate.

Foot placement can also be critical in sports that have spatial and temporal components that require takeoffs and landings, such as track and field high jump, long jump, triple jump; gymnastics vaulting, balance beam, parallel and uneven bar mounts using propulsion boards; and diving. For a handspring vault, a key to successful takeoff is the placement of the plant foot and the position of the body's mass prior to the jump onto the board. The objective of the vault is to convert horizontal motion to sufficient vertical motion, using an optimum angle of trajectory to propel the body, through the hands, off the horse to a controlled landing on the other side. Using an approach run of sixty feet, the gymnast can make adjustments, using feedforward mechanisms, in stride length, speed, and foot plant prior to the vault action (Meeuwsen & Magill, 1987).

When one is landing from heights, vision plays an interesting feedforward role as well. While jumping from three different heights (0.72 m, 1.04 m, 1.59 m) onto a force plate, subjects were asked to visually focus on the plate throughout each jump. The researchers (Sidaway, McNitt-Gray, & Davis, 1989) recorded EMG activity of the rectus femoris muscle to determine if individuals used *optical tau* (developed by Lee, 1978, 1980) regardless of the jump heights, to trigger muscular contraction. It was determined that tau was used to estimate time-to-contact.

The ability to change body position in space and intercept objects that are moving depends upon many variables during the early part of execution. The processing of visual information has been thought to be attained from the changing visual display or optic array. These theorists contend that a single optic variable provides enough information to estimate time to contact. This optic variable, known as **optical tau** is the ratio at any moment of the distance of point from the center of an expanding optical pattern to its velocity away from the center (Bruce, Green, & Georgeson, 1997). More simply stated, tau is the inverse of the time it takes to dilate the image on the retina. Tau supplies the time to contact with a surface rather than a specific distance. By determining the speed at which an approaching object fills the visual field, one can interpret when action should be initiated. Ice hockey goalies can determine how quickly the puck approaches using tau. As the puck approaches, the goalie's visual field fills. The faster it fills, the faster the speed of the puck. It was found that optical tau was used as the triggering

Optical tau
a mathematical formula that details the time an object travels to contact a given point in space

mechanism to activate muscle contraction at different times, corresponding with varying jump heights. This important role is noticeable in parachute jump landing, plyometric landing and takeoff, landing from a high bar, and ski jump landing.

Biofeedback — also referred to as augmented sensory physiological feedback — has been used to facilitate feedforward information. Through the use of biofeedback, researchers have begun to argue that parallel processing and slow motion perception occur during enhanced alpha brain wave states with the eyes open (Trachtman & Venezia, 1994; Boer, 1986; Griffin & McBride, 1986). They contend that athletes who function in an enhanced alpha state utilize visual feedforward information more rapidly, thereby producing improved reaction times. Much of the work has been conducted on jet fighter pilots. These pilots are required to do complex tasks involving analog and digital visual displays, auditory information, target location and fixation, and approaching enemy aircraft. In addition, they also endure tremendous rates of speed (1,000 to 2,000 feet per second), low oxygen, high g-forces, and the stress of combat (Crowley, 1989). As a result, eye movement latency (approximately 200 ms) contributes to the loss of a clear image for 200 to 400 feet; accommodation latency (approximately 250 ms) contributes to a loss for 250 to 500 feet (Trachtman, 1997). The use of feedforward information for those involved in multitask, high-velocity activities seems extremely important.

Biofeedback
the immediate display of an individual's biological signals through specialized electronic equipment

VISION AS THE DOMINANT SENSE

Vision has been found to serve as the dominant sensory system used to provide feedback. Several researchers (Reeve, Mackey, & Fober, 1986) determined that when vision was available, individuals relied on it as the primary source of information, even though it might provide inaccurate information that led to a lack of performance success.

Information provided by the eyes in terms of feedforward or feedback information is not always exact and uncomplicated. Every visual cue that involves spatial and temporal decision-making has the potential for misinterpretation. When uncertainty exists, it is known as an **illusion**. It is also used in information theory terms to indicate a lack of information rather than misinformation.

Visual illusions can be complicated. There are several basic assumptions about the phenomenon of visual illusion (Tolansky,

Illusion
a visual cue involving spatial and temporal decision making that is uncertain and subject to misinterpretation

VESTIBULAR/OCULAR SENSORY SYSTEM

Objective: To determine what happens when the systems interact.

Equipment and Preparation: Jump rope and sports scene picture on a wall; metronome.

Experience: Place a picture of a sports scene on the wall, at least ten feet away. Facing the wall, jump rope under the following conditions:

    (a) at 30 bpm on two feet; then changing feet; then on one foot

    (b) at 60 bpm on two feet; then changing feet; then on one foot

    (c) at 90 bpm on two feet; then changing feet; then on one foot

Assignment: Determine which is the most difficult condition in which to keep the scene appearing steady. Why?

1964): (1) Circles tend to be underestimated in size. (2) Straight lines are generally overestimated in length. (3) Acute angles are overestimated, (4) while obtuse ones are underestimated. (5) A square appears to be taller than it is wide, and (6) the perceived size of a square depends upon where it is standing (e.g., in a corner or on one side).

One illusion worth mentioning in this chapter that relates to motor behavior is that of **apparent motion.** This illusion is the perception of motion that results from viewing appropriately timed sequences of stationary stimuli. One of the most familiar scenes to illustrate this is Christmas lights — when they blink sequentially across the rooftop of a house, they can create the illusion of motion. The notion of apparent motion (phi phenomenon) plays a role in anticipation, prediction, and timing. The Bassin timer is also based on the construct of apparent motion.

Apparent motion
an illusion that perceives motion as the result of viewing appropriately timed sequences of stationary stimuli

ANTICIPATION, PREDICTION, AND TIMING

Anticipation in skilled motor behavior involves the ability to know or predict a series of events that coincide with an external environmental demand (Tyldesley, 1981). Decisions in anticipation must be made that involve visual search about what to do and when to do it. Decisions must also be made in timing to control movement. For example, anticipation, prediction, and timing are critical to the success of a corner hit in field hockey. After all players remain stationary, the ball is hit into play by the offense. The defending team must predict where the ball will be hit, who will receive it, where it might be passed, and who will ultimately shoot for goal. The goalkeeper must determine this information by a visual search of the approaching players, from body position prior to ball contact, and as the ball is contacted in order to begin movement to a position where the ball might be hit to within the goal area. As the ball is hit, the goalkeeper must move her body to a line that will cut off the

LAB EXERCISE

ANTICIPATION

Objective: To successfully catch as many balls as possible.

Equipment and Preparation: Partner; tennis ball; area of at least twenty feet, unobstructed.

Experience: Standing with a partner twenty feet away,

1. Toss the tennis ball to each other ten times, using any type of throw that will cover the distance without the ball bouncing. Upon completion, one partner turns his or her back to the other. The other partner, with the ball (thrower), says "now" and throws the ball as before.

2. When the partner (catcher) hears the "now," (s)he turns around to catch the ball.

3. This time, the thrower and catcher face one another. The thrower releases the ball at a 45-degree angle so that the catcher must move to catch the ball five times. Then the catcher turns his or her back to the thrower. The thrower informs the catcher that the ball will be thrown just as before to the same side at a 45-degree angle. When the catcher hears the "now," (s)he turns around to catch the ball.

4. Finally, the thrower makes the choice of randomly throwing the ball five times at a 45-degree angle to the left or to the right as both partners face one another. Then the catcher turns his or her back to the thrower. The thrower informs the catcher that the ball will be thrown to either side, randomly. When the catcher hears the "now," (s)he turns around to catch the ball.

Assignment: Observe the behavior when the partner turns around to catch the ball in each of the above situations. Determine what happened in each situation. Did performance remain the same, improve, or get worse? What role did coincidence anticipation play in each? What cues were important for appropriate anticipation?

impending shot on goal. The body is stopped and planted; the hips, knees, and ankles prepare to flex in anticipation of the ball's arrival so that the ball gets cushioned by the body upon contact.

Despite its importance in performance success, anticipation still remains one of the least investigated areas in visual/perceptual perspectives of motor behavior (Adams, 1966; Schmidt, 1975; Graydon, Bawden, Holder, Dyson, & Hurrion, 1996). Part of the challenge lies with designing the research and using valid instrumentation to appropriately and succinctly measure the variables involved in visual interception and to adequately answer the questions posed (von Hofsten, 1987; Whiting, Savelsbergh, & Faber, 1988). The concept of anticipation has been categorized as either receptor anticipation or perceptual anticipation (Poulton, 1957). Sometimes, predictions must be made on the basis of pieces of information and past experiences. This is the case in **receptor anticipation.** The use of this type of anticipation results when the individual is unable to constantly see the approaching object of interest. Cues that might provide lead-time information (advance cues) are not available. Temporal uncertainty may play a role in this form of anticipation. For example, one modification for dribbling a basketball is to wear "flippers" (a device similar to spectacles worn over the eyes to block one's vision of the ball). The dribbler must learn to rely on other proprioceptors to provide meaningful information for anticipating, predicting, and timing the ball-to-hand contact.

Perceptual anticipation results when the individual can see the approaching object of interest consistently. Temporal uncertainty is reduced. Spatial uncertainty may play a role in creating a need for anticipation. Baseball or softball catchers have the opportunity to know what pitches are being thrown ahead of time. Based upon that knowledge, they can anticipate, predict, and time their behaviors. Sometimes, however, the anticipated drop ball actually rises instead. Experienced catchers can anticipate, predict, and time alternative behaviors in such cases to make the necessary adjustment. Consistency of viewing may provide enough cues to facilitate the adjustment.

Anticipation involves prediction and timing. When anticipation timing is investigated, a popular instrument used to measure error is the Bassin Anticipation Timer or some variation of it. The instrument is based on the concept of apparent motion. As a stimulus appears, subjects are asked to view a set of light-emitting diodes (LEDs) on a runway. By pressing a button or making some type of

Receptor anticipation expectation based on when the individual is unable to constantly see the approaching object of interest, based on pieces of information and past experiences

Perceptual anticipation the point at which the individual is able to see the approaching object of interest consistently

movement to break the plane of a photoelectric cell when they think the final light on the runway will illuminate, they stop the timer. The time recorded is the difference between the time the timer was stopped and the time the last light was displayed. Through the use of this device and others in laboratory settings, researchers (Christina, 1977; Wrisberg, Hardy, & Beitel, 1982; Kluka, 1985) have revealed several important generalizations about the predictability of objects of interest:

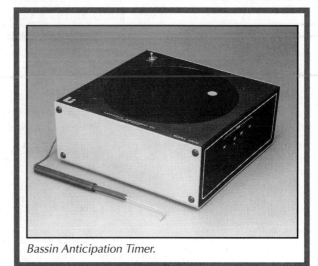

Bassin Anticipation Timer.

1. The more predictable the approaching object of interest is, the easier it is to make an accurate movement. For example, in indoor volleyball, once the ball has left the setter's hands for a high-outside left-front attack, it follows a predictable flight path until it reaches the attacker's hand. This consistency of trajectory (spatial consistency) and speed (temporal consistency) of the typical high-outside set attack provides the attacker and defense little variation to deal with. When the setter learns a variety of sets for a left-front attack (first and second tempo), spatial and temporal consistency diminish (introducing stimulus consistency or temporal and spatial uncertainty). This forces the receivers to make individual judgments about every play.

2. The faster the speed of the approaching object of interest, the more accurate the response, to a point. There seems to be an inverted-U relationship (Figure 8.5) between the speed of the approaching object of interest and the accuracy of timed responses (Magill, 1993). Slowly moving objects are more difficult to accurately respond to than faster ones. Accuracy seems to improve as the speed of the object of interest increases, to a point. The point at which the object moves too fast appears to be related to the visual system's ability to continuously track the object (Wrisberg, Hardy, & Beitel, 1982). When playing slow-pitch softball, batters seem to experience more success in hitting balls that approach more rapidly and have a flatter flight path than those that have lofty flight

paths and less velocity. When playing fast-pitch softball, batters experience a point at which the pitcher's fastest fastball completely eludes them. This produces a decline in batting speed and performance accuracy.

3. Practice improves timing accuracy whether the object of interest moves at the same speed or at different speeds. Again, focusing upon baseball and softball, batters working in a batting cage with a pitching machine are provided with literally hundreds of pitches at varying speeds and elevations. By practicing the timed events, batters improve regardless of the type of the ball delivery.

From a reality-based perspective, it is also important to discuss the relevance of tau when catching and hitting objects. The research has established that (1) if the object, once airborne, remains in a predictable flight path, it is important that the individual initially view its release for approximately 300 ms (0.3 s) in order to successfully catch it (Whiting, Gill, & Stephenson, 1970). From a cognitive visual perception perspective, information that is received in the first few moments of the object's flight path provides enough details to time a movement for the catch. (2) If the flight path remains constant, continuously tracking the object is not important for success

LAB EXERCISE

OCCLUSION OF VISION AND APPARENT MOTION

Objective: To observe variations in occlusion of vision and apparent motion.

Equipment and Preparation: Electric fan; scissors; inexpensive 8" paper plate; straight pin; pencil with new eraser. Cut 8 narrow, evenly spaced slots around the rim of an inexpensive paper plate. Place a pin through the center; stick the pin into an eraser of a pencil so that the plate can be spun.

Experience: Spin the plate in front of one eye. Focus on the electric fan. Spin the plate so that it revolves slowly. Spin the plate so that it revolves increasingly faster.

Assignment: Explain what happens when the plate is moving slowly; when it is moving at an intermediate speed; when it is moving at a high rate of speed. What causes this apparent motion? How can this concept be used during practice in ball sports?

(Whiting, Gill, & Stephenson, 1970). (3) It is important that the hands are viewed just prior to catching the object (200 to 350 ms) (Smythe & Marriott, 1982). The hands, during this time, should be in their final position to make the catch (Sharp & Whiting, 1975). The fingers are positioned to grasp the object within the last 32 to 50 ms of flight (Alderson, Sully, & Sully, 1974). After the object contacts the hand, it is easier to understand how vision can serve in a feedforward capacity rather than a feedback capacity.

As early as 1608, researchers were comparing the eye to a darkened chamber, or camera, focusing an image on its posterior surface. Eye movements could be taken into account in one of two ways. *Outflow* theorists suggested that motor commands sent to eye muscles were used in interpreting image movement. *Inflow* theorists proposed that sensory signals from the eye muscles were taken into account when movement in the retinal image was interpreted. These theories formed the basis for the investigation of eye movements to determine their contribution to the gaining of information about the environment.

Early studies of eye movements dealt with the classification and measurement of the basic types of ocular behavior. The eyes performed several definite types of movements instead of moving in a steady sweep from one fixation point to another. Four basic types of movements were identified (Bahill & LaRitz, 1984): saccadic, vestibulo-ocular, vergence, and smooth pursuit. The role of saccades is to direct the gaze to different points of the optic array, or peripheral field, so that the high acuity of the fovea can be used to gather information of interest clearly. Smooth pursuit movements assist in locking the gaze onto specific objects for continuous tracking. Vergence movements — convergence and divergence — are used when the distance of an object from the observer changes. If an object comes within a few centimeters of the face, it is impossible to display convergence, so the object becomes blurred. Vestibulo-ocular movements are used to maintain relative balance when the scene or the observer is moving.

Also known from the research:

1. Continuous tracking (using smooth pursuit eye movements) of a fast-moving object (greater than 70 degrees/s) to contact is physiologically impossible (Bahill & LaRitz, 1984; Adolphe, Vickers & Laplante, 1997). The adage of "keeping your eyes on the ball to contact" is technically impossible; however, it

has some practical value in teaching, because it focuses the individual's attention on the object for as long as possible.

2. Movement adjustments before contact generally occur within the first few hundred ms that the object is observed (up to 500 ms) (Hubbard & Seng, 1954). Movement must be co-ordinated to coincide with the object's release.

3. The more highly skilled the performer, the longer the individual tracks the object before contact (Bahill & LaRitz, 1984; Adolphe, Vickers, & Laplante, 1997). It is still unclear if it is essential to view the actual contact by highly skilled performers if they track the object longer.

4. When time to contact is shorter, more force is applied to the swing to quicken its speed (Bootsma & van Wieringen, 1990; Graydon, Bawden, Holder, Dyson, & Hurrion, 1996). The adage "swing faster" provides redirection of proprioceptor information to feel the swing through contact as well as modifying the time it takes them to swing. A faster swing also provides a few ms more to track.

5. Visual/perceptual information serves as a catalyst for swing initiation; it also provides guidance for subtle minute adjustments during the swing (Bahill & LaRitz, 1984; West & Bressan, 1996). Because it is possible to subtly adjust the swing just prior to contact, using saccadic eye movements that "jump" focus from the object to contact point is important.

PERFORMANCE MEASUREMENT OF VISION IN MOTOR BEHAVIOR

Researchers have been interested in measuring various aspects of this important sensory mechanism and its role in perception and cognition as it relates to the performance of motor skills. Several techniques have been developed to assist in the assessment of visual abilities and the interrelatedness of the eye, brain, and body in human movement. Notably, characteristics of the visual/perceptual system used in sport have been proposed (Trachtman & Kluka, 1993; Schalen, 1980) in which the focal, ambient, magno, and parvo systems are all involved in human movement control. The status of visual/perceptual systems in athletes has been determined (Coffey & Reichow, 1989; Kluka, Love, Sanet, Hillier, Stroops, &

Schneider, 1995), and sport-specific enhancement programs have been devised (Kluka, Love, Kuhlman, Hammack, & Wesson, 1996; MacLeod, 1991; Long, 1994) and tested. Additionally, expert-novice paradigms (Bard & Fleury, 1981; Allard & Starkes, 1980; Abernethy & Russell, 1984; 1987) have been characterized and developed. Varying parts of the visual display (visual occlusion) have also been investigated (Abernethy & Russell, 1987; Starkes & Deakin, 1984; Starkes, Edwards, Dissanayake & Dunn, 1995). Instrumentation used in the recording of eye movements (Kluka & Love, 1990; Dell'osso & Daroff, 1988) has been documented. The manner in which the eyes are used to gain information has also been detailed (Bard & Fluery, 1981; Abernethy & Russell, 1987; Vickers & Adolphe, 1997). These investigations have begun to determine visual/perceptual performance, but none have investigated the contribution of vision in the motor learning process.

Assessing the status of visual/perceptual abilities in tandem with human motor performance is important when discussing learning and performance. The debate in the expert/novice literature is whether the differences are learned or are innate. Such things as strategy and pattern recognition can be learned, but there is still much debate about whether or not some visual abilities can be learned. Visual/perceptual abilities for sport have been assessed through sophisticated instrumentation devised primarily by the optometric and ophthalmologic communities (e.g., Stereo Optical Company, Wayne Engineering, Inc., Lafayette Instrument Company, AcuVision International). These abilities include static visual acuity (SVA), dynamic visual acuity (DVA), ocular motility, eye/body coordination, eye dominance, color perception, binocularity/stereopsis, accommodation and vergence facility, peripheral vision, visual reaction time, visual adjustability, and contrast sensitivity function (Coffey & Reichow, 1990; Planer, 1994). Each of these abilities can be assessed by a variety of instruments that have been validated with athletic populations, such as the Stereo Optical Vision Tester 2500, Saccadic Fixator, Reaction Plus, Tachistoscope, Cover Test, Vectograms, Accommodative Rock, and Bassin Anticipation Timer. Many have standardized norm-referenced profiles specifically developed for those populations.

Once the status of visual abilities has been determined, the visual system should be corrected to its "best fit" through correction using spectacles, contact lenses, or refractive surgery (such as radial keratotomy) in order to provide accurate measurements statically and dynamically. Whether visual abilities are learned or capable of enhancement has been debated for several decades (Wold, Pierce, & Keddington, 1978; Vinger, 1980; Zinn & Solomon, 1985). Several researchers have contributed data to the debate by creating sport-specific visual skill enhancement programs. Using pre- and post-tests and stationwork approaches in experimental designs, some visual skills significantly improved in those sports investigated (e.g., volleyball, soccer, and baseball). Researchers have emphasized that the programs must be sport-specific and based on real-time experiential conditions in order to be effective.

Questions have been raised about the use of static tests (Burg, 1966; Trachtman & Kluka, 1993) when attempting to extrapolate meaningful information about visual/perceptual abilities and the environment for human movement. The need to conduct research using real-time measurements is paramount in order to draw insightful conclusions about visual/perceptual abilities and their contributions to motor behavior.

A straightforward method of determining the status of visual/perceptual abilities relating to motor performance compares the

LAB EXERCISE

SPAN OF RECOGNITION

Objective: To successfully hit the ball and the wall 10 of 10 times.

Equipment and Preparation: A wall; a rolling pin; six different colored pieces of tape (red, green, blue, black, orange, yellow); old tennis ball; 15' of heavy string; partner. Place the string through the tennis ball. Suspend the ball and string from the ceiling at eye level. Place two different colored pieces of tape at opposite ends around the rolling pin. Place the same two different colored pieces on the wall so that they have the same pattern as on the pin and are two feet apart. Stand two feet from the wall, holding the rolling pin at the ends in both hands.

Experience: Hit the ball with the color on the pin called by the partner to the corresponding color on the wall. Increase the span of choices progressively to 6 on the wall and on the rolling pin. Hit to a different color on the wall, depending upon the partner's call.

Assignment: Determine the time it takes to get 10 out of 10. Compare results with 10 others in class.

performances of experts and novices. In this **expert-novice paradigm,** researchers assess the characteristics of elite athletes and their novice counterparts in visual search patterns, speed of visual search, how rapidly relevant information is extracted from the environment, and the length and position of gaze (Vickers & Adolphe, 1997). The paradigm establishes "profiles" of novice visual/perceptual behaviors and expert behaviors. For example, it has been determined that experts scan the visual environment more rapidly and extract meaningful information more succinctly. Experts also access the information more easily in later situations once the information is coded, stored, and learned (Vickers & Adolphe, 1997; Abernethy, 1991). It has also been found that expert coaches visually search in a different manner than novice coaches when watching skill performance (Bard & Fleury, 1980; Bard & Fleury, 1976). Expert coaches generally focus on core body movements, while novice coaches focus on appendage movement.

A technique used to assess visual/perceptual skills is *visual occlusion.* By using this technique, researchers have been able to "profile" experts and novices and their skills to predict the results of movements. For example, the coach who can determine the success of a roundoff, back handspring, back somersault combination in floor exercise based upon viewing hand position on the roundoff can provide meaningful information to the gymnast in less time.

Techniques have been devised to limit or filter parts of the visual display from the performer's vision. One such technique is videotape occlusion. The researcher videotapes a specific skilled performance and then blocks out or occludes portions of the video so that the individual viewing the tape cannot see the movement's outcome. Using this traditional technique, several researchers (Abernethy & Russell, 1987; Starkes & Deakin, 1984) found that skilled observers accurately determined the results of movements without viewing the total movement sequence. Specifically, expert badminton players were able to identify where the bird landed by only viewing the shuttle until milliseconds before racket contact; novice players viewed the shuttle for a longer period of time. Specific body parts (hips and legs, nonracket arm, racket arm, and head) were also occluded to determine which segments were used as cues to gain advanced information about the movement outcome.

This technique has its challenges. It is time-consuming to first video and then occlude segments of the tape to be viewed. It has

Expert-novice paradigm a model by which researchers assess characteristics of elite athletes and their novice counterparts

also been difficult to provide adequate viewing perspectives of the skill (shown from the front, the back, the side, or above).

The most recent improvement in technology has involved the use of liquid crystal spectacles (Milgram, 1987). For example, the StrobeSpex – Model 1000 allows the researcher to adjust the amount of vision available through a series of electrical impulses delivered through the lenses. The lenses can produce a flickering effect (similar to strobe lights) or can occlude vision for one or more seconds. This type of technology should provide much greater mobility for investigations under actual practice conditions.

EYE MOVEMENT MEASURES

The earliest method of measuring eye movements was known as the *simple inspection technique* of gross eye movement. No quantitative assessment was possible using this procedure. Researchers (Javal, 1879) simply qualitatively described the type of eye movement and reported the number of pauses made.

Instrumentation that facilitated observations of eye movement made greater accuracy possible in collecting data. The *afterimage technique*, used for the assessment of saccadic eye movements, was one such improvement (Landolt, 1891). The subject fixated on one end of a line. When a lamp was turned on, the subject quickly focused the eyes on the other end of the line. The individual then closed his eyes and reported the afterimage.

Saccadic eye movements became the interest of many early researchers. They devised several instruments to assess those movements: a tube resembling a telescope with a twenty-diopter convex lens at the end (Javal, 1879; Newhall, 1928); the corneal cup method, a plaster of paris cup fitted over the eye, with one end of a thread attached to the cup and the other attached to a recording lever (Delabarre, 1898; Huey, 1898); and the Dodge and Chicago apparatus, and Stanford modification (Dodge, 1907; Gillian, 1921; Miles & Shen, 1925), in which the sclera, iris, and pupil were photographed while a swinging pendulum time line and a falling plate were viewed in the background. Another technique of recording eye movements, the photokymographic technique, used a strip of light-sensitive paper that moved while a beam of light was projected through a small slit in another piece of paper. This exposed the sensitive paper and made a mark that could be measured (Wendt & Dodge, 1938).

With the advent of more sophisticated technology, eye movements could be measured using electromyography (Shackel, 1967) by attaching electrodes to skin areas over selected extraocular muscle bellies. This, however, has not proven to be the most effective method of measurement, as the most accurate determination of muscular activity in extraocular muscles requires the use of indwelling electrodes. Placing needle electrodes into the bellies of muscles surrounding the eye is extremely difficult.

Currently, the most reliable method of eye movement recording is the *corneal reflection technique*, devised by Stratton (1906). Others (Tinker, 1931; Brandt, 1937; Mott, 1954) further enhanced the technique. The NAC Eye Mark and ASL System Recorders have been used in many of the contemporary investigations (Bard & Fleury, 1981; Goulet, Bard, & Fleury, 1989; Vickers & Adolphe, 1997). The devices measure the pupil and corneal reflex monocularly by placing a small light source on the corneal surface to determine the line of gaze (focus).

The use of present technology to record eye movements is not without difficulties. The camera that films the eye is generally mounted on top of a helmet worn by the subject. A reflective visor is also present to provide magnification of the eye. An infrared light source is retro-reflected off the retina. Video imaging is processed by a digital computer. Another camera, used to film the environment, displays the individual's field of view. This configuration makes it challenging for the equipment to be used easily in field-based research settings. Calibration of the instrument is rather laborious as well.

Two other concerns have been expressed (Adams, 1966; Trachtman & Kluka, 1993; Rose, 1997). Researchers assume that eye movements and fixations reflect what the individual attends to and actually views and processes. If this is not a valid assumption, data collected and interpreted has substantially less meaning. Additionally, present-day instruments cannot assess peripheral vision and focal vision simultaneously. Both focal and ambient vision provide information in motor behavior. As improvements in technology continue, researchers will be able to address these concerns. All psychological and physiological assessments relating to motor behavior will be enhanced as technology improves.

Recently, Conrad, Westenberg, Smith, Korf, and Hartfel (Spence, 1997), have devised a system that uses the concept of **video overlay** to monitor and assess the motor behavior of elite athletes. Video

Video overlay technique which produces live video images shown on a screen with various measurements specific to a sport

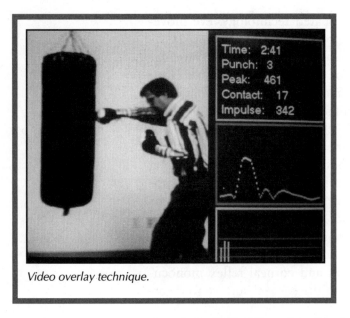
Time: 2:41
Punch: 3
Peak: 461
Contact: 17
Impulse: 342

Video overlay technique.

overlay produces live video images that are shown on a screen with various measurements specific to a sport. For example, in shooting a basketball free throw, a laser beam is projected from the shooter's hand to the hoop that indicates the exact trajectory the ball should travel to create the swish. This is displayed on one of two screens. On another screen, a live picture of the shooter is shown, including hand placement on the ball, eye blinks, and eye movements. At the bottom of the screen are the shooter's heart rate and breathing rate and the velocity of the ball. When the shot is taken, the aim can be seen on one side of the screen, the shooter's mechanics on another, as well as heart rate, breathing rate, eye blinks, eye movements, and ball velocity. Through this technology, the shooter can get immediate external feedback before, during, and after the movement. Because this technology is in its infancy, it is premature to estimate its overall impact on motor behavior. It is, however, worth mentioning, as performance enhancement and technology developed for its assessment are important to motor behavior professionals.

A PERFECT SYSTEM?

The visual/perceptual system is not without its limitations. A newborn cannot effectively see further than the width of a basketball (eight to ten inches) and is unable to coordinate the eyes. The eyes are coordinated through six extraocular muscles that work in contractile opposition. Most information from the external environment is synthesized through touch (tactile sense) and somatosensory input. From birth, the infant begins to explore the environment, first with the hands, then with the eyes. As the child develops, vision plays an increasingly important role. By age six months, the youngster begins to coordinate eye movements with arm movements and is comfortable within a radius of two feet. Attention can be shifted from nearby to a distance. This is particularly significant, as the eyes begin to team together to gain understanding of time and space. Depth perception, however, is in its beginning stages (Sigelman & Shaffer, 1995).

By the age of one year, the eyes focus within a radius of three feet and comfortable space is extended to ten feet. Objects are scanned for meaning and information is discriminatingly perceived. By age two, the child begins to integrate vision, language, and movement. The eyes and head begin to lead movement without turning the body, and vision begins to become the dominant sense. Binocular vision extends to three feet, but is quite immature (Seiderman & Marcus, 1989).

Between the ages of three and four, eye-hand movements are refined enough to color and paint with relative precision, and binocular vision extends to around ten feet. The child begins attending to objects out to sixteen feet, and begins to be able to successfully coordinate eye-body actions to catch and throw objects, follow objects with the eyes when they are airborne, and run with agility. Visual information, however, is still rather inaccurate until the ages of seven to eight (Williams, 1983).

During these formative years, visual disorders may begin to emerge. Only 1 to 2 percent of newborns have **myopia** (nearsightedness) (Seiderman & Marcus, 1989). The myopic child may avoid physical activity or be easily surprised because objects in the environment are not clearly defined. Generally, myopia can be resolved with glasses or contact lenses.

Myopia
nearsightedness

Another condition, **strabismus**, may be observed as early as eighteen months of age and is found in 2 to 4 percent of the population (Seiderman & Marcus, 1989). One eye is turned in or out, preventing binocular vision because the brain receives two differing images. The child's ability to judge distances and anticipate approaching objects can be affected. The condition can be improved by surgery or vision therapy.

Strabismus
a condition in which one eye is turned in or out, preventing binocular vision

The visual system does not become adultlike until the ages of ten to twelve. Through the age of twelve, the child becomes increasingly reliant upon the visual/perceptual system as a basis for controlling motor behavior. The system remains stable through the third decade. During this time period, the system acquires improved discriminatory abilities as they relate to decision-making, motor selection, and movement control.

By the time the individual reaches his or her mid-forties, the system begins to lose flexibility. Most notably, near focus becomes increasingly difficult because the lens loses some flexibility (**hyper-opia**). Typically, bifocals or "reading" glasses provide assistance in viewing clearly what is within three feet of the eyes.

By ages sixty-five to eighty-five, individuals may develop cataracts. Cataracts diminish the amount of light available to the eye, thereby creating "haze" or "fog" when looking at objects in the environment. Frequently, surgery for cataract removal provides substantially improved sight.

Occasionally, visual deficits occur from trauma to the head, tumors in visual pathway areas of the brain, or stroke. These deficits can include complete, partial, or temporary blindness. Because these deficits are caused by trauma, a physician should be consulted as soon as possible after the head trauma has occurred.

Hyperopia
increasing difficulty of the lens of the eye to focus on near objects as a result of diminishing flexibility as the individual ages

KEY POINTS

- Approximately 85 percent of sensory information about the external environment is obtained through the visual system.

- The visual system provides at least three functions as they relate to motor behavior: proprioception, exteroception, and exproprioception.

- The eyes serve as sensory receptors sensitive to light waves of varying lengths and frequencies.

- The cornea impedes the light and bends or refracts it toward the center.

- The macula is the area where greatest visual acuity occurs.

- The fovea is the center of the macula where clearest visual acuity occurs.

- Two types of photoreceptors are the cones and the rods.

- The ratio of rods to cones in each eye is roughly 17:1.

- Color deficiency ranges from minor confusion of color hues to total lack of color identification.

- Color blindness — total lack of color identification — is quite unusual in humans.

- Receptors stemming from one side of the body traverse through pathways specifically used to transmit to the opposite side of the brain.

- The organization of the visual scene takes place within the occipital lobe.

- In the superior colliculus, vision is integrated with other sensory information from the somatosensory and auditory systems to create a multisensory experience.

- The focal system involves the fovea and the specifics of object identification.

- The ambient system involves the entire retina and assesses the general spatial location of objects.

- The magno and parvo systems seem to be parallel processed, particularly during movement.

- Visual perception theories continue to be based on two profoundly different tenets.

- Eye dominance can be divided into three types: sighting dominance, sensory dominance, and acuity dominance.

- Because the eyes are separated, they provide binocular cues for judging distance.

- Stereopsis is five times more sensitive at six feet than at 300 feet.

- Monocular cues depend upon the qualities of the objects themselves rather than stereoscopic effect.

- Visual acuity can be divided into two parts: static and dynamic.

- If the contrast between object and background is low, the object needs to be larger to have visual detectability comparable to that of a smaller object with great contrast.

- It has been theorized that contrast sensitivity function decreases as an object's velocity increases. This is important in motor behavior, because the clarity of moving objects can be important in decision-making.

- Feedforward in the visual system helps one to determine the dimensions of objects in the environment, the terrain of the environment, and time and space within the environment.

- Vision is the dominant sensory system used to provide feedback.

- Apparent motion is the illusion of motion that results from viewing appropriately timed sequences of stationary stimuli.

- The concept of anticipation has been divided into two basic forms: receptor anticipation and perceptual anticipation.

- Characteristics of the visual/perceptual system used in sport have been proposed.

- The status of visual/perceptual systems in athletes has been determined.

- Sport-specific enhancement programs have been devised.

- Expert-novice paradigms have been characterized and developed.

- Varying parts of the visual display have been investigated.

- Instrumentation used in the recording of eye movements has been documented, and as the manner in which the eyes are used to gain information has been detailed.

- A wide variety of instrumentation has been developed to assess the contribution of vision to motor behavior.

- Continuous tracking of a fast-moving object to contact is physiologically impossible.

- Movement adjustments before object contact generally occur within the first few milliseconds that the object is observed.

- The more highly skilled the performer, the longer the performer can track the object before contact.

- When time to contact is shorter, more force is applied to the swing to quicken its speed.

- Visual/perceptual information serves as a catalyst for swing initiation; it also provides guidance for minute adjustments during the swing.

- Myopia, strabismus, and hyperopia are disorders associated with the visual system.

DISCUSSION QUESTIONS

1. Compare/contrast the functions of proprioception, exteroception, and exproprioception of the visual system in reference to motor behavior.

2. Describe the transduction of light through the eye to the brain, describing parts of the eyes and their functions.

3. Determine the characteristics of the two visual systems that contribute to human movement. Then, integrate the characteristics of the magno/parvo systems with the characteristics you have described.

4. Compare the cognitive and ecological theories of visual perception. Provide one example of each theory in a motor behavior situation.

5. Discuss the different types of visual/perceptual skills and their role in influencing motor behavior.

6. Determine the visual system's role in feedforward and feedback in movement.

7. Describe the concept of optical tau and its importance to anticipation and prediction of movement.

8. Determine the role of apparent motion in anticipation timing.

9. Discuss visual/perceptual system limitations and some of the visual disorders that may occur throughout the life span. Determine ways in which the system might be enhanced.

ADDITIONAL READINGS

Gibson, J. J. (1979). *The ecological approach to visual perception*. London: Houghton Mifflin.

Lee, D. N. (1980). Visuo-motor coordination in space-time. In G. E. Stelmach & J. Requin (Eds.), *Tutorials in motor behavior* (pp. 281–295). Amsterdam: North Holland.

Loran, D. F. C., & MacEwen, C. J. (1995). *Sports Vision*. Oxford, UK: Butterworth-Heinemann, Ltd.

Posner, M. I., Nissen, M. J., & Klein, R. (1976). Visual dominance: An information processing account of its origins and significance. *Psychological Review, 83,* 157–171.

Williams, A. M., Davids, K., & Williams, J. G. (1999). *Visual perception and action in sport*. London, UK: E + FN Spon, Routledge.

REFERENCES

Abernethy, B. (1991). Visual search strategies and decision making in sport. *International Journal of Sport Psychology, 22,* 189–210.

Abernethy, B., & Russell, D. G. (1984). Advance cue utilization by skilled cricket batsmen. *The Australian Journal of Science and Medicine in Sport, 16,* 2, 2–10.

Abernethy, B., & Russell, D. G. (1987). The relationship between expertise and visual search strategy in a racquet sport. *Human Movement Science, 6,* 283–319.

Adams, G. L. (1965). Effect of eye dominance on baseball batting. *Research Quarterly, 36*(2), 3–9.

Adams, J. A. (1966). Some mechanisms of motor responding: An examination of attention. In E. A. Bilodeau (Ed.), *Acquisition of skill* (pp. 169–200). New York: Academic Press.

Adolphe, R. M., Vickers, J. N., & Laplante, G. (1997). The effects of training visual attention on gaze behaviour and accuracy: A pilot study. *International Journal of Sports Vision, 4*(1), 28–33.

Alderson, G. J. K., Sully, D., & Sully, H. G. (1974). An operational analysis of a one-handed catching task using high speed photography. *Journal of Motor Behavior, 6,* 217–226.

Allard, F., & Starkes, J. L. (1980). Perception in sport: Volleyball. *Journal of Sport Psychology, 2,* 22–33.

Anshel, J. (1990). *Healthy eyes, better vision*. Los Angeles: The Body Press.

Bahill, A. T., & LaRitz, T. (1984). Why can't batters keep their eyes on the ball? *American Scientist, 72,* 239–243.

Bard, C., & Fleury, M. (1976). Analysis of visual search activity during sport problem situations. *Journal of Human Movement Studies, 3,* 214–222.

Bard, C., & Fleury, M. (1980). Analysis of gymnastics judges' visual search. *Research Quarterly, 51,* 267–273.

Bard, C., & Fleury, M. (1981). Considering eye movement as a prediction of attainment. In I. M. Cockerill and W. W. MacGillivray (Eds.), *Vision and sport* (pp. 28–41). Cheltenham, UK: Stanley Thornes Publishers.

Bassi, C. J., & Lehmkuhle, S. (1990). Clinical implications of parallel visual pathways. *Journal of the American Optometric Association, 61*(2), 98–110.

Boer, L. C. (1986). Attention tasks and their relation to aging and flight experience. *National Technical Information Service*, Report S2421.

Bootsma, R. J., & van Wieringen, P. C. W. (1990). Timing an attacking forehand drive in table tennis. *Journal of Experimental Psychology: Human Perception and Performance, 16,* 21–29.

Brandt, H. F. (1937). A bidimensional eye movement camera. *Journal of American Psychology, 49,* 666–670.

Bruce, V., Green, P. R., & Georgeson, M. A. (1997). *Visual perception: Physiology, psychology, and ecology* (3rd ed.). East Sussex, UK: Psychology Press.

Burg, A. (1966). Visual acuity as measured by dynamic and static tests: A comparative evaluation. *Journal of Applied Psychology, 50*(6), 460–466.

Buxton, C. E., & Crossland, H. R. (1937). The concept of "eye-preference." *American Journal of Psychology, 49,* 458–461.

Campos, J. J., Langer, A., & Krowitz, A. (1970). Cardiac responses on the visual difference in pre-locomotor human infants. *Science, 170,* 196–197.

Christina, R. W. (1977). Skilled motor performance: Anticipatory timing. In B. R. Wolman (Ed.), *International encyclopedia of psychiatry, psychology, psychoanalysis, and neurology* (Vol. 10, pp. 241–245). New York: Van Nostrand Reinhold.

Coffey, B. & Reichow, A. (1989). Athletes vs. non-athletes: Static visual acuity, contrast sensitivity, dynamic visual acuity. *Investigative Ophthalmology and Vision Science, 30,* suppl 517.

Coffey, B., & Reichow, A. (1990). Optometric evaluation of the elite athlete: The Pacific Sports Visual Performance Profile. *Problems in Optometry, 1, 2,* 32–58.

Coren, S., & Kaplan, C. P. (1973). Patterns of ocular dominance. *American Journal of Optometry, 50,* 283–292.

Crowley, J. S. (1989). Cerebral laterality and handedness in aviation: Performance and selection implications. *National Technical Information Service,* Technical Paper U8915.

Delabarre, E. B. (1898). A method of recording eye movements. *American Journal of Psychology, 9,* 572–574.

Dell'osso, L. F., & Daroff, R. B. (1988). Eye movement characteristics and recording techniques. *Clinical Ophthalmology, 2,* 1–15.

Dodge, R. (1907). An experimental study of visual fixation. *Psychological Review, 7,* 454–465.

Gavrisky, P. (1969). The colors and color vision in sport. *Journal of Sports Medicine and Physical Fitness, 9*(1), 43–53.

Gibson, E. J., & Walk, R. D. (1960). The "visual cliff." *Scientific American, 202,* 64–71.

Gibson, J. J. (1979). *The ecological approach to visual perception.* Boston: Houghton Mifflin.

Gillian, A. R. (1921). Photographic methods for studying reading. *Visual Education, 2,* 21–26.

Ginsburg, A. (1983). Contrast sensitivity: Relating visual capability to performance. *Medical Service Digest, 34*(3), 15–19.

Goulet, C., Bard, C., & Fleury, M. (1989). Expertise differences in preparing to return a tennis serve: A visual information processing approach. *Journal of Sport Psychology, 11,* 382–398.

Graydon, J., Bawden, M., Holder, T., Dyson, R., & Hurrion, P. (1996). The effects of binocular and monocular vision on a table tennis striking task under conditions of spatio-temporal uncertainty. *International Journal of Sports Vision, 3*(1), 35–40.

Gregg, J. R. (1987). *Vision and sports: An introduction.* Boston: Butterworth.

Griffin, G. R., & McBride, D. K. (1986). Multitask performance: Predicting success in Naval aviation primary flight training. *National Technical Information Service,* Report U8619.

Hoffman, L. G., Polan, G., & Powell, J. (1984). The relationship of contrast sensitivity function to sports vision. *Journal American Optometric Association, 55*(10), 747–752.

House, E. L., Pansky, B., & Siegel, A. (1979). *A systematic approach to neuroscience.* New York: McGraw-Hill.

Hubbard, A. W., & Seng, C. N. (1954). *Research Quarterly, 25,* 42–57.

Huey, E. B. (1898). Preliminary experiments in the physiology and psychology of reading. *American Journal of Psychology, 79,* 575–586.

Ishigaki, H., & Miyao, M. (1994). Implications for dynamic visual acuity with changes in age and sex. *Perceptual and Motor Skills, 4,* 231–235.

Ito, M. (1977). Neuronal events in the cerebellar flocculus associated with an adaptive modification of the vestibulo-ocular reflex of the rabbit. In *Control of gaze by brain stem neurons: Developments in neuroscience.* Amsterdam: Elsevier.

Javal, E. (1879). *Anales d'Oculistique, 79,* 197–240.

Kluka, D. (1985). *Coincidence anticipation accuracy in light- and dark-eyed adult females as measured by a microcomputer program.* Unpublished doctoral dissertation, Texas Woman's University.

Kluka, D. (1997). The eye-brain-body connection. *FIVB: The Coach, 4,* 8–12.

Kluka, D., & Love, P. (1990). The study of eye movements related to sport: A review of the literature. *Sportsvision, 6, 1,* 23–29.

Kluka, D., Love, P., & Allen, S. (1989). Contrast sensitivity function of selected female athletes. *Sports Vision, 5,* 18–24.

Kluka, D., Love, P., Kuhlman, J., Hammack, G., & Wesson, M. (1996). The effects of a visual skills training program on selected intercollegiate volleyball athletes. *International Journal of Sports Vision, 3*(1), 23–34.

Kluka, D., Love, P., Sanet, R., Hillier, C., Stroops, S., & Schneider, H. (1995). Contrast sensitivity function profiling by sport and physical ability level. *International Journal of Sports Vision, 2*, 1, 5–16.

Knudson, D., & Kluka, D. (1997). The impact of vision and vision training on sport performance. *JOPERD, 68*(4), 17–24.

Landolt, A. (1891). Novelles Recherches sur las physiologie des mouvements des veus. *Archives d'Optamologie, 11*, 385–395.

Lee, D. N. (1978). A theory of visual control of braking based on information about time-to-collision. *Perception, 5*, 437–459.

Lee, D. N. (1980). Visuo-motor coordination in space-time. In G. E. Stelmach and J. Requin (Eds.), *Tutorials in motor behavior* (pp. 291–295). Amsterdam: North-Holland.

Long, G. M. (1994). Exercises for training vision and dynamic visual acuity among college students. *Perceptual and Motor Skills, 78*, 1049–1050.

Loran, D. F. C., & MacEwen, C. J. (1995). *Sports Vision.* Oxford, UK: Butterworth-Heinemann, Ltd.

Love, P., Kluka, D., & Cobb, T. (1996). The effect of blood glucose levels on contrast sensitivity function in female athletes. *International Journal of Sports Vision, 3*(1), 5–17.

Ludveigh, E. J., & Miller, J. W. (1958). Study of visual acuity during the ocular pursuit of moving test objects. *Journal of Optical Society, 48*, (4), 799–802.

MacLeod, B. (1991). Effects of Eyerobics visual skills training on selected performance measures of female varsity soccer players. *Perceptual and Motor Skills, 72*, 863–866.

Magill, R. (1993). *Motor learning: Concepts and applications* (4th ed.). Madison, WI: Brown & Benchmark Publishers.

McCormick, E. J., & Sanders, M. S. (1982). *Human factors in engineering and design* (5th ed.). New York: McGraw-Hill.

Meeuwsen, H., & Magill, R. A. (1987). The role of vision in gait control during gymnastics vaulting. In T. B. Hoshizaki, J. Salmela, and B. Petiot (Eds.), *Diagnostics, treatment, and analysis of gymnastic talent* (pp. 137–155). Montreal: Sport Psyche Editions.

Miles, W. R., & Shen, E. (1925). Photographic recording of eye movements in the reading of Chinese in vertical and horizontal axes: Methods and preliminary results. *Journal of Excremental Psychology, 8*, 344–362.

Milgram, P. (1987). A spectacle-mounted liquid-crystal tachistoscope. *Behavior, Research Methods, Instruments and Computers, 19*, 449–456.

Milne, C., Buckolz, E., & Cardenas, M. (1995). Relationship of eye dominance and batting performance in baseball players. *International Journal of Sports Vision, 2*(1), 17–21.

Morris, G. S. D. (1977). Dynamic visual acuity: Implications for the physical educator and coach. *Motor Skills: Theory with Practice, 2*, 15–20.

Mott, J. (1954). Eye movements during initial learning of motor skills. Doctoral dissertation: University of Southern California at Los Angeles.

Newhall, S. M. (1928). Instrument for observing ocular movements. *American Journal of Psychology, 40*, 628–629.

Ogle, K. N. (1964). *Research in binocular vision.* New York: Hafner.

Ong, J., & Rodman, T. (1972). Sex and eye-hand preference difference in star-tracing performance. *American Journal of Optometry and the Archives of the Academy of Optometry, 49*, 436–438.

Planer, P. J. (1994). *Sports vision manual.* Harrisburg, PA: International Academy of Sports Vision.

Porac, C., & Coren, S. (1976). The dominant eye. *Psychological Bulletin, 83*(5), 880–897.

Poulton, E. C. (1957). On prediction in skilled movements. *Psychological Bulletin, 54*, 467–478.

Reeve, T. G., Mackey, L. J., & Fober, G. W. (1986). Visual dominance in the cross-modal kinesthetic to kinesthetic plus visual feedback condition. *Perceptual and Motor Skills, 62*, 243–252.

Reichow, A., Coffey, B., Wacho, C., & Velnousky, D. (1981). Visual evaluation of the elite athlete: Optometric visual profiling. *American Journal of Optometry and Physiological Optics, 63*, 80.

Rodieck, R.W., & Stone, J. (1965). Response of cat retinal ganglion cells to moving visual patterns. *Journal of Neurophysiology, 28*, 819–832.

Rose D. J. (1997). *Multilevel approach to the study of motor control and learning.* Boston, MA: Allyn and Bacon.

Sanderson, F. H. (1972). Visual acuity and sporting performance. In H.T.A. Whiting (Ed.), *Readings in sports psychology.* London: Kimpton.

Sanderson, F. H., & Whiting, H. T. A. (1978). Dynamic visual acuity: A possible factor in catching performance. *Journal of Motor Behavior, 10*(7), 14.

Schalen, P. (1980). A developmental model of the visual system. *Journal of the American Medical Association, 80,* 762–766.

Schmidt, R. A. (1975). *Motor skills.* New York: Harper & Row.

Schrader, C. W. (1971). The effect of visual differences on hand-eye coordinated performance. *Western Carolina University Journal of Education, 2,* 28–33.

Seiderman, A. S., & Marcus, S. E. (1989). *20/20 is not enough: The new world of vision.* New York: Alfred A. Knopf.

Shackel, B. (1967). Eye movement recording by electrooculography. *A manual of psycho-physiological methods.* In P. H. Venables & I. Martin (Eds.). Amsterdam: North Holland.

Sharp, R. H., & Whiting, H.T.A. (1975). Information processing and eye movement behavior in a ball catching skill. *Journal of Human Movement Studies, 1,* 124–131.

Sharp, R. H., & Whiting, H. T. A. (1975). Information processing and eye movement behavior in a ball catching skill. *Journal of Human Movement Studies, 1,* 124–131.

Sidaway, B., McNitt-Gray, J., & Davis, G. (1989). Visual timing of muscle preactivation in preparation for landing. *Ecological Psychology, 1,* 253–264.

Sigelman, C. K., & Shaffer, D. R. (1995). *Life-span human development* (2nd ed.). Belmont, CA: Brooks/Cole.

Singer, R. N., Caraugh, J. H., Murphey, M., Chen, D., & Lidor, R. (1991). Attentional control, distractors, and motor performance. *Human Performance, 4,* 55–69.

Smythe, M. M., & Marriott, A. M. (1982). Vision and proprioception in simple catching. *Journal of Motor Behavior, 14,* 143–152.

Spence, M. C. (1997). Video overlay and sport science. *The Olympian,* 22–24.

Sprague, J. M., Berlucchi, G., & Rizzolatti, G., (1973). The role of the superior colliculus and pretectum in vision and visually guided behavior. In *Handbook of sensory physiology, central processing of visual information, part B.* Berlin: Springer.

Starkes, J., & Deakin, J. M. (1984). Perception in sport: A cognitive approach to skilled performance. In W. F. Straub and J. M. Williams (Eds.), *Cognitive Sport Psychology* (pp. 115–228). Lansing, NY: Sport Science Associates.

Starkes, J., Edwards, P., Dissanayake, P., & Dunn, T. (1995). A new technology and field test of advance cue usage in volleyball. *Research Quarterly for Exercise and Sport, 66,* 2, 162–167.

Stratton, G. M. (1906). Symmetry, linear illusion, and the movements of the eye. *Psychological Review, 13,* 82–96.

Teig, D. S. (1980). Sports vision care: The eyes have it. *Journal of the American Optometric Association, 51*(7), 671–674.

ten Napel, J. A. (1993). Eye injuries in sports. *Klinika Oczna, 92*(3), 48–49.

Tinker, M. A. (1931). Apparatus for recording eye movements. *American Journal of Psychology, 43,* 115–118.

Tolansky, S. (1964). *Optical illusions.* Berkeley, CA: University of California Press.

Trachtman, J. (1991). Visual demands of minor league baseball players. *Sports Vision, 7,* 8–11.

Trachtman, J. (1997). Finding the zone: Case studies of parallel processing and electroencephalogram training. *International Journal of Sports Vision, 4*(1), 6–11.

Trachtman, J., & Kluka, D. (1993). Future trends in vision as they relate to peak sport performance. *International Journal of Sports Vision, 1*(1), 1–7.

Trachtman, J., & Venezia, C. M. (1994). Central information processing and beta brain waves. *Proceedings of the 1994 Association for Applied Psychophysiology and Biofeedback* (pp. 172–175). Wheat Ridge, CO: Association for Applied Psychophysiology and Biofeedback.

Tyldesley, D. A. (1981). Motion prediction and movement control in fast ball games. In I. M. Cockerill & W. W. MacGillivary (Eds.), *Vision and sport* (pp. 91–115). Cheltenham, UK: Stanley Thornes Publishers, Ltd.

Vickers, J. N. (1996). Location of fixation, landing position of the ball, and spatial visual attention during free throw shooting. *International Journal of Sports Vision, 3*(1), 1–10.

Vickers, J. N., & Adolphe, R. M. (1997). Gaze behavior during a ball tracking and aiming skill. *International Journal of Sports Vision, 4,* 1, 19–28.

Vinger, P. (1980). Sports-related eye injury. A preventable problem. In M. L. Rubin (Ed.), *Perspectives in refraction.* New York: Survey of Ophthalmology.

von Hofsten, C. (1987). Catching. In H. Heuer & A. F. Sanders (Eds.), *Perspectives on perception and action* (pp. 33–46). Hillsdale, NJ: Erlbaum.

Wendt, G. R., & Dodge, R. (1938). Practical directions for stimulating and for photographically recording eye movements of animals. *Journal of Comparative Psychology, 25,* 9–49.

West, K. L., & Bressan, E. S. (1996). The effects of a general vs. specific visual skills training program on accuracy in judging length-of-ball in cricket. *International Journal of Sports Vision, 3*(1), 41–45.

Whiting, H. T. A., Gill, E. B., & Stephenson, J. M. (1970). Critical time intervals for taking in-flight information in a ball-catching task. *Ergonomics, 13,* 265–272.

Whiting, H. T. A., Savelsbergh, G. J. P., & Faber, C. M. (1988). Catch questions and incomplete answers. In A. M. Colley and J. R. Beech (Eds.), *Cognition and action in skilled behaviour* (pp. 257–271). Amsterdam: North-Holland.

Wieringen, P. Van. (1988). Discussion: Self-organization or representation? Let's have both! In A. M. Colley and J. R. Beech (Eds.), *Cognition and action in skilled behaviour.* Amsterdam: North-Holland.

Williams, A. M., Davids, K., Burwitz, L., & Williams, J. (1992). Perception and action in sport: A review. *Journal of Human Movement Studies, 22,* 147–204.

Williams, H. G. (1983). *Perceptual and motor development.* Englewood Cliffs, NJ: Prentice-Hall.

Wold, R. M., Pierce, J. R., & Keddington, J. (1978). Effectiveness of optometric vision therapy. *Journal of the American Optometric Association, 49,* 9, 1047–1054.

Wrisberg, C. A., Hardy, C. J., & Beitel, P. A. (1982). Stimulus velocity and movement distance as determiners of movement velocity and coincident timing accuracy. *Human Factors, 24,* 599–608.

Zinn, W. J., & Solomon, H. (1985). A comparison of static and dynamic stereoacuity. *Journal of the American Optometric Association, 56,* 9, 712–715.

Memory: Contributions to Motor Behavior

CHAPTER FOCUS

- Contribution of memory to perception
- Theories of memory and their role in learning
- Types of memory
- Types of knowledge base memory
- Concept of the engram
- Principle of equipotentiality
- Types of amnesia and their causes
- Concept of forgetting
- Memory strategies

*The use of sensory information, which has been discussed in the previous chapters of this section, involves a myriad of structures and functions within the human body. **Perception**, the application and interpretation of sensory-stored information (Thomas, Thomas, & Gallagher, 1993), shifts throughout the life span. In very young children, tactile and somatosensory information predominates;*

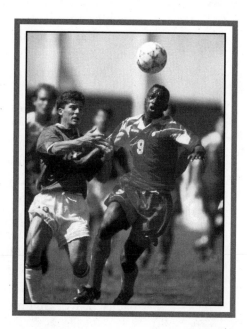

Perception
the application and interpretation of sensory-stored information

Memory
(sensory; short-term; working) a component of information processing that stores information for retrieval

Sensory memory
brief holding of sensory information before it is processed into short-term memory

Short-term memory
a passive rehearsal buffer for information

Working memory
the active part of long-term memory that can temporarily hold small bits or chunks of information

later, information gleaned from the visual system dominates. As the information is perceived, it is processed into movement selection and response. **Memory**, a part of information processing that stores information for retrieval, is also involved in perception. Memory has been called a capacity for benefiting from previous experiences (Tulving, 1985).

MEMORY TYPES

Memory is typically divided into three types: sensory, short-term, and long-term. **Sensory memory** briefly holds sensory information just prior to its being processed into short-term memory. **Short-term memory** is defined as a passive rehearsal buffer for information (Atkinson & Shiffrin, 1968). A more contemporary perspective of the same concept is that of **working memory** (Baddeley & Hitch, 1974), which can be described as the active part of long-term memory. It incorporates sensory, perceptual, attentional, and short-term memory components that are involved with information processing. Working memory can temporarily hold between five to nine items of information (Miller, 1956) so that comparisons can be made between information newly presented and information that has been stored in long-term memory. For example, when you hear a para-diddle produced by a drummer for the cadence of a marching band, you can temporarily hold the rhythm in working memory. You can quickly tap out its rhythm as the marching band fades from sight. As another band approaches with a different cadence, you can no longer remember the initial cadence.

The functions of working memory involve making decisions, solving problems, producing and evaluating movement, and creating long-term memory. It is a place where many functions can interact with each other to produce the necessary behavior, which is especially important for the mixing of long-term memory with information in working memory.

Early investigations involving movement information and its duration in working memory (Peterson & Peterson, 1959; Adams & Dijkstra, 1966) supported the premise that information in working memory remains there for twenty to thirty seconds. Information that is not additionally processed is lost.

The amount of information that can be retained in working memory is also a concern. Originally, it was proposed that the capacity of working memory is five to nine items (Miller, 1956). More information can be retained if pieces of information are grouped into chunks. Chunking enables individuals to retrieve substantially more information.

From a motor behavior viewpoint, it is difficult to determine the size of the chunk of an item necessary for retention. When an *item* referred to an appendage movement through space, working memory capacity was similar to the five to nine items as in verbal working memory capacity (Wilberg & Salmela, 1973). Interestingly, young novice and skilled ballet dancers were presented with typically sequenced ballet movements and unrelated ballet movements. Up to eight movements could be recalled by the skilled ballet dancers if the movements were in typical ballet sequence. If the dance movements were unrelated, only half of them were recalled. The novice dancers

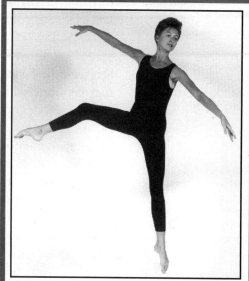

Skilled ballet dancers chunk information into memory through practice.

recalled the unrelated movements better than the skilled dancers (Starkes, Deakin, Lindley, & Crisp, 1987). This information supports the notion of chunking (Miller, 1956), whereby grouping pieces of information into memory through practice facilitates recall. The skilled ballet dancers effectively chunked the eight sequenced movements into one, while the novice dancers recalled unrelated movements in isolation. Chunking seems to be used in the context of the situation.

Long-term memory, having unlimited capacity (Chase and Ericsson, 1982), stores information somewhat permanently. It contains information about specific events in the past as well as general information about the environment. **Rehearsal** is one of the memory strategies that seems to transfer information from working memory to long-term. By repeating the paradiddle over and over, an individual can successfully transfer it to relatively permanent recall.

Within the last decade and a half, researchers have referred to long-term memory as **knowledge base memory** (Tulving, 1985; Thomas, Thomas, & Gallagher, 1993). They divided memory into three basic categories, based upon knowledge: declarative, procedural, and strategic. **Declarative knowledge** refers to an understanding of factual information and what to do. This idea is also connected with Gentile's model of learning (1972). The first stage of

Long-term memory
the type of memory that stores information rather permanently

Rehearsal
performing a movement repeatedly

Knowledge base memory
long-term memory

Declarative knowledge
an understanding of factual information and what to do with it

Procedural knowledge
an understanding of how to do something

Strategic knowledge
an understanding of the general principles that facilitate what to do and how to do it

learning involves "getting the idea of the movement." **Procedural knowledge** involves an understanding of how to do something. This again follows Gentile's model, whereby the individual moves to Stage Two in which the individual achieves performance of the skill. **Strategic knowledge** is an understanding of the general principles that facilitate what to do and how to do it.

These categories are based upon the work of Tulving (1985) and others (Thomas, Thomas, & Gallagher, 1993). Tulving's model of long-term memory is the standard model used when discussing long-term memory. Three systems are present in this model: procedural, episodic, and semantic memory. The **procedural memory system** stores information about motor skills. This system utilizes the information of *how* to do something. Procedural memory facilitates the exhibition of specific behaviors that accomplish specific goals, based upon learned responses.

Procedural memory system
information storage about motor skills that pertains to how to do something

Episodic memory system
a system of storing an individual's events with time relevance

Stored in the **episodic memory system** are specific events that have been experienced by the individual with time relevance. Important moments in life might include graduation day, the birth of a baby, the Challenger explosion, the assassination of President Kennedy, or the accomplishment of a tuck back somersault for the first time. Episodic memory can be expressed verbally, emotionally, and motor behaviorally.

Semantic memory system
storage of information about the general environment that has developed over time

The **semantic memory system** stores information about the general environment that has developed over time. For example, the knowledge that 0 degree Celsius equals 32 degrees Fahrenheit, that water boils at 100 degrees Celsius or 212 degrees Fahrenheit, that a German shepherd, a Westhighland terrier, and a Siberian husky are dogs, and that fear, anger, love, joy, and grief are emotions are represented in semantic memory. These examples are indicative of no specific way in which semantic memory is exhibited. With this information as a backdrop, theories of memory become important to gain more understanding of memory.

THEORIES OF MEMORY

It is important to understand relevant theories that have been proposed by researchers to explain that which is still somewhat inexplicable. Three theories have been of particular interest to researchers over the past two generations. The first, a multiple memory theory; the second, a levels of processing theory; and the third, a neurobiological theory, all attempt to explain the nature of memory. One is based on a structural perspective, another on a functional one, and still another on a combination of the two.

During the 1960s, there was substantive growth in the area of computer development and use. Models were constructed likening the brain to a computer in order to explain cognitive behavior. It should be no surprise that researchers (Atkinson & Shiffrin, 1968; Shiffrin & Schneider, 1977) developed models that simulated computers to explain human thinking involving memory. Of particular interest was the **multistore model** (Atkinson & Shiffrin, 1968). Researchers hypothesized that computer hardware was analogous to memory structure and that "software," under an individual's control, facilitated the flow (processing) of information stored and retrieved. This model (Figure 9.1), depicting a structural perspective, registers sensory information (in sensory store or in a sensory register) for brief amounts of time. That which is determined to be relevant by attention is briefly registered. What is irrelevant is released. Memory represents data, while store represents a structural component. Shapes, contrast in lighting, object and terrain texture, and environmental sounds might be included in the "byte" of information registered. Sensory information is initially held in short-term store. Short-term stores are designed for temporarily holding limited

Multistore model
a paradigm of memory structure using a computer hardware and software analogy as under an individual's control, facilitating the flow of information stored and retrieved

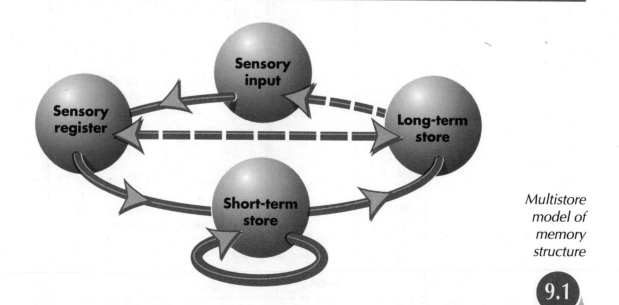

Multistore model of memory structure

9.1
FIGURE

amounts of relevant information before it is involved in the decision-making process for movement strategies. The longer the information remains in short-term memory, the greater the likelihood it will be transferred to long-term memory. Correct attention to sensory cues facilitates the encoding of information through processing into short-term, followed by long-term stores. Rehearsal and organization facilitate the transfer of information from short- to long-term storage.

With an unlimited storage area, the long-term store structure is fairly permanent. What is stored includes concepts, procedures, and details as well as images that are continuously compared to incoming stimuli. Figure 9.2 graphically depicts the exchange of information made continually between long-term store information, sensory input, and sensory register areas.

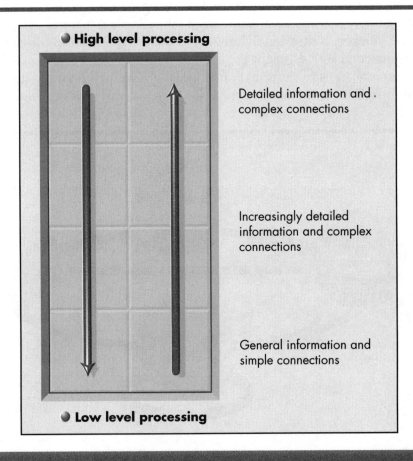

The continuous exchange of information between long-term store information, sensory input, and sensory register areas

9.2
FIGURE

Researchers who developed the **levels of processing theory** (Craik & Lockhart, 1972) attempted to explain *how* information is encoded (or categorized) and remembered. The determination of how information was processed was quite a different approach than how memory was structured.

Two basic premises exist in this theory: (1) there is a limited amount of information an individual can process at any moment, and (2) the nature of the stimulus depends upon the time available for processing. Because the nature of the word *process* implies dynamic or ever-changing, incoming information could be controlled by the individual through attention. That which received priority in processing was referred to as primary memory; that which was not processed was referred to as secondary memory. The individual, through attentional control, could determine the depth of processing by determining its significance and linking it to previously remembered information.

The significance of this theory centers around the notion that how the individual prioritizes the information is vital to remembering. How deeply information is processed into memory depends upon the initial level of attention, the attempt made to understand meaning, and the interpretation of usefulness.

The third and final theory of memory is referred to as the **dual systems theory.** Some researchers (Petri & Mishkin, 1994) believe that there are essentially two systems responsible for learning and

Levels of processing theory
a paradigm explaining that the individual, through attentional control, determines the depth of processing by determining its significance and linking it to previously remembered information

Dual-systems theory
a paradigm that explains the two systems responsible for learning and memory: cognitive memory and habit memory

LAB EXERCISE

MEMORY AND RETENTION

Objective: To determine the importance of information presentation.

Equipment and Preparation: Ten people; knowledge of the Highland Fling. Randomly divide the ten people into two groups.

Experience: Demonstrate the first section of the Highland Fling without music to one of the groups. Send this group to another room to practice for five minutes after the demonstration. To the other group, demonstrate the same section; add word cues describing the pattern and in the rhythm of the pattern. For example, "1, 2, 3, 4, 5, 6, 7, apart, together, break right." Ask this group to repeat the rhythm and the word cues to themselves as they are practicing. At the end of the practice session, each group presents what it has accomplished.

Assignment: Record the results of what is observed from each group. What can be attributed to what has been observed?

memory. Like the magno and parvo systems within the visual/perceptual system, they are quite unique in their structure and function and traverse different neural networks, packaging information for storage differently and storing portions of experiences in different places. **Cognitive memory** is responsible for the storage of neural images that will link individual memory experiences together. **Habit memory** facilitates skilled behaviors that appear automatic, such as the individual performing a full twisting double back somersault with seeming effortlessness. Additional research is vital for the further substantiation of this, and the other models, presented.

The development of a *parallel distributed processing model* (Rumelhart & McClelland, 1986) offers a computational point of view based on the complex networking of simple processing units rather than fixed capacities and limitations for memory, knowledge, and attention. This model does not describe the characteristics of units, structures, or resources. It describes performance as being composed of an entire network of integrated operations. This model attempts to bring together the neurophysiological with the psychological to explain memory. Perhaps a short discussion of memory from a neurobiological perspective will provide additional understanding.

MEMORY AND NEUROBIOLOGY

Researchers continue to try to determine the locations and structures of the brain directly responsible for memory. Early researchers wondered where memories were stored. The search for the **engram** (memory trace) was begun at the neocortex for several reasons: (1) it was the most easily accessible portion of the brain; (2) it was the most sophisticated portion of the human brain in terms of higher-order functioning; (3) it controlled complex behavior, which requires a high degree of memory process; and (4) it contained a myriad of interconnections that would be required by trillions of pieces of information (Hebb, 1949; Konorski, 1948). In searching for the engram, a researcher (Lashley, 1950) used rats and monkeys to determine that well-defined, conditioned stimulus-response reflex paths did not exist as originally thought (Pavlov, 1927), and that the motor cortex was unnecessary for the retention of sensory-motor associations or skilled manipulative patterns of responding. It was also determined that memory was not located in any one region of the cortex. This finding was particularly significant for motor behavior. Known as the **equipotentiality principle**, this idea holds that

Cognitive memory
memory responsible for storing neural images that link individual memory experiences

Habit memory
memory that facilitates skilled behaviors that appear automatic

Engram
a memory trace

Equipotentiality principle
the concept that certain tasks related to a sensory system are stored in a sensory region of the brain rather than at a specific location; hence, the region has an equal potential for storing memory

certain tasks related to a sensory system are stored in a sensory region of the brain rather than at a specific location. The region, then, has an equal potential for storing memory.

Most researchers now believe that the limbic system (hippocampus and amygdala), thalamus, temporal and frontal lobes, motor cortex, association cortex, and basal ganglia seem to possess memory functions (Dudai, 1989; Bennett, 1979). From research conducted on individuals and monkeys with damaged hippocampal structures (O'Keefe & Nadel, 1978; Mishkin, 1982), it was found that the hippocampus plays a role in cognitive map storage. **Anterograde amnesia,** the inability to remember events that transpire after an injury to the brain, is also associated with hippocampal damage from brain trauma. (**Retrograde amnesia** is the inability to remember events that transpire prior to the brain injury.) This would suggest that the hippocampus is involved in the creation of new memories involving places, how to find things, and where things are located in space (Zola-Morgan, Squire, & Amarai, 1986). When the thalamus and frontal lobe of the brain become injured in monkeys (Aggleton & Mishkin, 1983), anterograde amnesia again results, intimating the role they play in memory creation and retention.

Anterograde amnesia inability to remember events that transpire after an injury to the brain

Retrograde amnesia inability to remember events that transpired prior to brain injury

The temporal lobe association areas have also been shown to be repositories for memory (Penfield, 1959). By electrically stimulating the temporal lobes in humans, complex and forgotten memories have been enunciated.

Additionally, neural pathways have been found to connect the basal ganglia with the sensory, association, and motor cortexes. They seem to provide interneural networks, substantiating the rationale used by early researchers to investigate the neocortex as part of the memory storage mechanism (Cook & Kesner, 1984). These neural network pathways may be responsible for the encoding of information, information retrieval, and coordinating new sensory input with previously stored information. By investigating these neural pathways, researchers have begun to better understand that new connections between neurons represent the underpinnings of long-term memory.

FORGETTING

As detailed as the memory theories appear to be, the issue of the inability to remember or retrieve information is one that must also be discussed. There seem to be two basic theories of forgetting: trace decay theory and interference theory (Shea, Shebilske, & Worchel, 1993). Forgetting can occur when the neural connections involved in memory are not strong enough. This idea is referred to as the **trace decay theory**, and it holds that this "decaying" of the connection occurs over time. The second theory, the **interference theory**, supports the notion that forgetting occurs because other memories preclude or interfere with memory that one is trying to locate.

Specific to interference theory, there are two types of interference: proactive and retroactive inhibition. When something new is presented, old memories interfere with learning the new. This can be attributed to **proactive inhibition**. For example, an individual has learned to deliver a straight ball in bowling. In order for the individual to ultimately throw a perfect game (300), a hook ball must be learned. The hook ball is presented, but because of the similarity of the straight ball in much of its rhythm and pattern, the memory of the straight ball serves to proactively inhibit the learning of the hook.

In **retroactive inhibition**, new learning interferes with already established memories. An individual has already learned to throw the straight ball and is having difficulty learning the hook, so she decides to return to throwing the straight ball. To her surprise, she now has difficulty throwing the straight ball.

MEMORY STRATEGIES

In order to overcome the forgetting phenomenon, it is important to understand the effectiveness of strategies utilized in memory development. There has been much discussion by researchers (Bjorkland & Buchanan, 1989; Ornstein, Baker-Ward, & Naus, 1988) about what strategies are most effective.

The following memory strategies (**mnemonics**) have been found to be effective when working with children and adults: labeling, rehearsal, and organization (Thomas, Thomas, & Gallagher, 1993). They will be discussed in greater detail in Section IV.

Labeling, providing a short, meaningful image to a movement through verbalization, can assist performance. Using the verbal cue of "explode like a missile" to describe the body's appearance when driving the feet into the floor exercise mat after a back handspring to set up for a layout back stepout somersault provides the individual with a vivid visual and kinesthetic image. Understanding the what, why, how, appearance, and feel of the movement provides solid strategies for memory development.

Trace decay theory
the notion that a person can forget when the neural connections involved in memory are not strong enough and "decaying" of the connection occurs over time

Interference theory
paradigm supporting the notion that people forget because other memories preclude or interfere with memory

Proactive inhibition
interference of new learning by old memories

Retroactive inhibition
interference of new learning with already established memories

Mnemonics
memory strategies

Labeling
providing a short, meaningful image to a movement through verbalization

Rehearsal, or actively performing a movement, has great benefit to memory development because it combines practice with experience. When practicing a song on the piano (physical), singing the melody (verbally) and seeing the fingers hitting the appropriate keys (mentally) can help one to develop an integrated memory experience for future comparisons.

Organization strategy is used to combine information meaningfully in order to reduce cognitive demands. Another term for this strategy is **chunking**. By grouping and coding information into manageable bits, the individual can readily grasp and remember sequences and concepts. For example, a rather detailed folk dance, the Highland Fling, is more easily learned in strains and break steps. Once the break step is learned, it is easily inserted after each strain is learned. Chunking up the dance into smaller meaningful bits reduces the cognitive complexity of the performance.

Rehearsal
active performance of a movement

Chunking
grouping meaningful information into manageable bits

KEY POINTS

- Perception shifts throughout the life span from tactile and somatosensory to visual.

- Memory is a part of the perceptual process, involving sensory, short-term, and long-term memory.

- Short-term memory is also referred to as working memory; long-term memory is also known as knowledge base memory.

- Declarative knowledge is an understanding of factual information; procedural knowledge involves an understanding of how to do something; strategic knowledge is an understanding of general principles associated with ways to enhance memory.

- The theory of multiple memory is based upon a computer model, with hardware and software analogies.

- The levels of processing theory details how information is encoded and remembered.

- The dual-systems theory states that there are essentially two systems responsible for learning and memory: cognitive and habit memory.

- An engram was originally believed to be begun at the neocortex level.

- The principle of equipotentiality is particularly significant for motor behavior.

- Cases of retrograde and anterograde amnesia have helped researchers to determine the function of various brain structures relative to memory.

- There are two basic theories related to forgetting: trace decay and interference.

- Specific to interference theory, proactive and retroactive inhibition describe reasons for forgetting.

- Labeling, rehearsal, and organization are memory strategies that are effective in enhancing memory retention.

DISCUSSION QUESTIONS

1. Compare and contrast the types of memory.

2. Describe the three theories of memory and provide examples of each as it relates to actual motor behavior.

3. Describe the principle of equipotentiality and its impact on motor behavior.

4. How do proactive and retroactive inhibition affect memory?

5. Discuss three memory strategies that could be used to enhance memory development. Provide two examples of each.

ADDITIONAL READINGS

Christina, R. W., & Bjork, R. A. (1991). Optimizing long-term retention and transfer. In D. Druckman & R. Bjork (Eds.), *In the mind's eye: Enhancing human performance* (pp. 23–56). Washington, DC: National Academy Press.

Magill, R. A. (1984). Influences on remembering movement information. In W. F. Straub & J. M. Williams (Eds.), *Cognitive sport psychology* (pp. 175–188). Lansing, NY: Sport Science Associates.

Mishkin, M. (1982). A memory system in the monkey. *Philosophical Transactions of the Royal Society of London, 298*, 85–95.

Tulving, E. (1985). How many systems of memory are there? *American Psychologist, 40*, 385–398.

REFERENCES

Adams, J. A., & Dijkstra, S. J. (1966). Short-term memory for motor responses. *Journal of Experimental Psychology, 71*, 314–318.

Aggleton, J. P., & Mishkin, M. (1983). Memory impairments following restricted medial thalamic lesions in monkeys. *Experimental Brain Research, 52*, 199–209.

Atkinson, R. C., & Shiffrin, R. M. (1968). Human memory: A proposed system and its control processes. In K. W. Spence and J. T. Spence (Eds.), *The psychology of learning and motivation: Advances in research and theory* (Vol. 2, pp. 89–197). New York: Academic Press.

Baddeley, A. D. & Hitch, G. (1974). Working memory. In G. H. Bower (Ed.), *The psychology of learning and motivation: Advances in research and theory* (vol. 8, pp. 47–89). New York: Academic Press.

Bennett, T. L. (1979). A gating function for the hippocampus in working memory. *The Brain and Behavioral Sciences, 2*, 322–323.

Bjorklund, D. F., & Buchanan, J. J. (1989). Developmental and knowledge base differences in the acquisition and extension of a memory strategy. *Journal of Experimental Child Psychology. 48*, 451–471.

Chase, W. G., & Ericsson, K. A. (1982). Skill and working memory. In G. H. Bower (Ed.), *The psychology of learning and motivation* (vol.16., pp. 1–58). New York: Academic Press.

Cook, D. G., & Kesner, R. P. (1984). Memory for egocentric spatial localization in an animal model of advanced Huntington's disease. *Neuroscience Abstracts, 10*, 133.

Craik, F. I. M., & Lockhart, R. (1972). Levels of processing: a framework for memory research. *Journal of Verbal Learning and Verbal Behavior, 11*, 671–676.

Dudai, Y. (1989). *The neurobiology of memory: Concepts, findings, trends.* Oxford: Oxford University Press.

Gentile, A. M. (1972). A working model of skill acquisition with application to teaching. *Quest,* Monograph XVII, 3–23.

Hebb, D. O. (1949). *The organization of behavior: A neuropsychological theory.* New York: Wiley.

Konorski, J. (1948). *Conditioned reflexes and neuron organization.* London: Cambridge University Press.

Lashley, K. S. (1950). In search of the engram. *Society for Experimental Biology,* Symposium 4, 454–482.

Miller, G. A. (1956). The magical number seven, plus or minus two: Some limits on our capacity for processing information. *Psychological Review, 63*, 81–97.

Mishkin, M. (1982). A memory system in the monkey. *Philosophical Transactions of the Royal Society of London, 298*, 85–95.

O'Keefe, J., & Nadel, L. (1978). *The hippocampus as a cognitive map.* Oxford: Oxford University Press.

Ornstein, P. A., Baker-Ward, L., & Naus, M. J. (1988). The development of mnemonic skill. In F. E. Weinert & M. Perlmutter (Eds.). *Memory development: Universal changes and individual differences* (pp. 31–50). Hillsdale, NJ: Erlbaum.

Pavlov, I. (1927). *Conditioned reflexes: An investigation of the physiological activity of the cerebral cortex.* New York: Oxford University Press.

Penfield, W. (1959). The interpretative cortex. *Science, 129,* 1719–1725.

Peterson, L. R., & Peterson, M. J. (1959). Short term retention of individual verbal items. *Journal of Experimental Psychology, 58,* 193–198.

Petri, H. L., & Mishkin, M. (1994). Behaviorism, cognitivism and the neuropsychology of memory. *American Scientist, 82,* 30–37.

Rumelhart, D. E., & McClelland, J. L. (1986). *Parallel distributed processing: Explorations in the Microstructure of cognition* (Vol. 1). Cambridge, MA: M.I.T. Press.

Shea, C. H., Shebilske, W. L., & Worchel, S. (1993). *Motor learning and control.* Englewood Cliffs, NJ: Prentice-Hall.

Shiffrin, R. M., & Schneider, W. (1977). Controlled and automatic human information processing: II. Perceptual learning, automatic attending, and a general theory. *Psychological Review, 84,* 127–190.

Starkes, J. L., Deakin, J. M., Lindley, S., & Crisp, F. (1987). Motor versus verbal recall of ballet sequences by young expert dancers. *Journal of Sport Psychology, 9,* 222–230.

Thomas, J. R., Thomas, K. T., & Gallagher, J. D. (1993). Developmental considerations in skill acquisition. In R. N. Singer, M. Murphey, & L. K. Tennant (eds.), *Handbook of research on sport psychology* (pp. 73–105). New York: MacMillan.

Tulving, E. (1985). How many memory systems are there? *American Psychologist, 40,* 385–398.

Wilberg, R. B., & Salmela, J. (1973). Information load and response consistency in sequential short-term motor memory. *Perceptual and Motor Skills, 37,* 23–29.

Zola-Morgan, S., Squire, L. R., & Amarai, D. G. (1986). Human amnesia and the medial temporal region: Enduring memory impairment following a bilateral lesion limited to field CA1 of the hippocampus. *Journal of Neuroscience, 6,* 2950–2967.

Multidimensional Learning

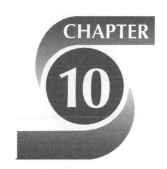

*M*otor skill acquisition and the performance of those motor skills must continuously be viewed from a multidimensional perspective. Each of the topics included in this chapter provides an additional twist of the kaleidoscope that displays a slightly different picture. Twisting the kaleidoscope provides unique previews of an individual's sphere of focus (the self), sphere of influence (interaction with others in social contexts), and sphere of concern (interaction with the self, with others in social contexts,

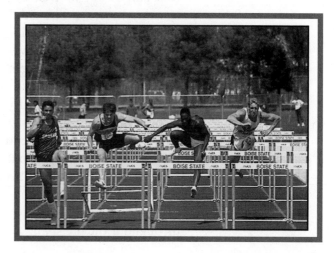

and with the environment). This chapter's theme, an individual's sphere of focus, involves the characteristics of the learner.

CHARACTERISTICS OF THE LEARNER

The following learner characteristics have multidimensional implications: sex, age, experience level, capability, and style of learning. The extent to which each influences multidimensional learning and motor behavior will be briefly discussed.

Sex: There is some support for the idea that females continue to have, on average, fewer motoric experiences than males throughout their formative years (Shapiro & Schmidt, 1982). With the passage of Title IX in 1972, however, opportunities to participate in sport for females have become increasing prevalent. Many investigations were conducted in the early 1980s involving females and sport participation (Del Rey, Whitehurst, & Wood, 1983, Del Rey, Wughalter, & Whitehurst, 1982). Since that time, literally millions more girls have participated in sport. Investigations that include the variables of sex and experience are necessary to more completely understand the role of these characteristics in multidimensional learning and motor behavior. There is also some support for the notion that because of differences in capabilities related to muscular strength, skeletal size, body composition, and cardiorespiratory function, women and men will be limited in their capabilities by sex (Pearl, 1993).

Age: It has been argued (Shapiro & Schmidt, 1982; van Rossum, 1987) that chronological age plays an important role in learning motor skills. Adults supposedly can be expected to have previously learned behaviors for tasks that are used to assess performance. Children, however, can be expected to have relatively limited experiences, thereby limiting the availability of previously learned behaviors used to assess performance. Physiological and cognitive readiness to learn also become variables in the equation. Generally, children, by virtue of physical and physiological parameters, do not possess the detailed neuroanatomical circuitry of adults. Similarities in the motor patterns of children and inexperienced and experienced adults have been noted (van Rossum, 1987). The assessment of motor behavior patterns such as basic throwing, striking, and kicking provide legitimacy in experiencing movement throughout the life span.

Experience level: In Section I of this text, several stages of learning were discussed. In the initial stage, regardless of what model is used (Gentile, Fitts, Bernstein, or Schmidt), theorists explain that learners try to get the general notion of the movement. At the next level, they try to determine and perform what it takes to integrate cognitive with motoric efforts into coordinated, purposeful movement. At the third level, learners try to refine that purposeful movement into action that is repeatable, flexible, and automatic. In several different investigations (Del Rey, 1989; Goode & Wei, 1988; Del Rey, Whitehurst & Wood, 1983), it was determined that learners, in order to learn most efficiently, must possess enough experiences to have an understanding of the parameters of specific skills.

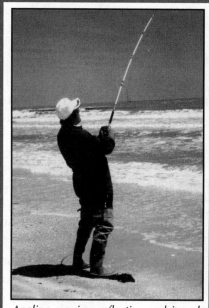

Angling requires reflective and impulsive learning styles.

Individual capability: Physical and physiological characteristics of the individual, including skeletal size, weight, muscular power, strength and endurance, agility, flexibility, and cardiovascular and muscular endurance contribute to the learner's characteristics and readiness to learn motorically. For example, the average size for quarterbacks in the National Football League is approximately 6 feet 2 inches (about two meters) tall, 215 pounds (about 97.5 kilograms); outstanding running backs complete the 40-yard sprint in less than five seconds (Clark, 1997); and professional male volleyball athletes routinely record vertical jumps of 36 inches (Briner, 1998). People's abilities may be limited to the parameters that have been genetically determined.

Style of learning: Learning styles have also been found to influence motor behavior. It was determined (Jelsma & Pieters, 1989; Jelsma & Van Merrienboer, 1989) that an individual's reflective or impulsive cognitive learning style influences the performance of motor skills. Those who display a **reflective learning style** (one that reflects proactivity rather than reactivity to the environment), when confronted with activities that involve speed and accuracy, choose to perform with greater accuracy than those who display an impulsive learning style. Self-paced activities display reflective learning styles; externally paced activities display **impulsive learning styles**. An illustration of self-paced learning style will be shared a little later in this chapter.

Reflective learning style the propensity to react to the environment proactively rather than reactively (self-paced activities)

Impulsive learning style a way of learning that reflects reactivity rather than proactivity to the environment (externally paced activities)

Learning style has also been referred to as *perceptual style*, or that which integrates the individual and the environment. Perception, as has been previously stated, not only involves the dimension of reasoning, but also adds the process of interpretation. Previous experiences, including positive response experiences, combine with age, sex, and neuroanatomical and structural characteristics to provide relevance to information from the environment.

Related to characteristics of the learner and one of the most visible factors contributing to the learning process is that of concentration. **Concentration,** focusing and maintaining attention on relevant environmental cues, is central to the discussion from a multi-dimensional learning perspective. **Relevant cues** are meaningful to and are interpreted by the performer. In tennis, when an individual serves, focusing on the seam of the ball during the toss provides a relevant cue to assist in the determination of direction and force. Relevance can also be established by the use of a key word or **trigger word** that centralizes attention. Using tennis again, the individual, just before the opponent serves, announces to herself "focus" in order to key in to the server's toss of the ball to contact point with the racket. Irrelevant cues, or **distractors**, might include spectators standing at the fence or the individual's desire to show off for a friend. Maintaining concentration is characterized by duration and intensity. **Duration,** or how long an individual remains focused, and **intensity,** the quality of attentional focus, provide interesting dimensions.

Discerning an object of interest is dependent upon two conditions: (1) the number of objects in the environment, and (2) how similar the object is to others in that environment. Generally, the more objects, the longer it takes to discern that which is important (Carter, 1982; Farmer & Taylor, 1980). Additionally, when the environment includes objects that are familiar or obvious, the time it takes to discriminate remains almost the same (Jonides & Gleitman, 1972).

ATTENTION

Although there has been an attempt to adequately define the word **attention** (Stelmach & Hughes, 1983), there has not been a clearly understood meaning for the word. Generally, it is defined as an individual's capacity to process information (Schmidt, 1991; Magill, 1993). It has also been explained by its features (Schmidt, 1991): (1) attention can be dynamic, changing initiation and duration

Concentration
focusing attention on relevant environmental cues and maintaining that focus

Relevant cues
pieces of information that are meaningful to the individual

Trigger words
key terms that centralize attention

Distractor
an irrelevant cue or a cue that takes attentional focus away from object of interest

Duration
how long something occurs

Intensity
the depth to which something occurs

Attention
processing information by focusing on relevant stimuli; alertness; selectivity

throughout time; (2) attention has limited capacity; (3) attention requires effort and is a component of arousal; and (4) attention limits the individual's capacity to combine actions.

Attention can be dynamic, in that it moves focus from one task, item, or thought to another rather rapidly. Attention can be directed to external events, such as a player passing the ball to another in soccer; attention can be directed internally so that the individual feels the aching of the hamstring muscles while sprinting for the finish line; or attention may be directed internally to recall a play that should be run during the current offensive drive in American football.

Attention has limited capacity in that it becomes difficult for a person to attend to more than two tasks at a time, especially if the tasks are complex. When the main task is fairly simple and does not require much attention, the person can perform a secondary task as well. It is likely that an experienced sports journalist can successfully conduct a telephone interview (main task) with Jackie Joyner-Kersee while typing the story on the computer (secondary task). A novice sports journalist, however, may find the main task too complex to be able to show good secondary performance results, because the main task requires more attention.

The challenge lies with adjusting to a potential overload of information, particularly in environments where high-level skill performance is necessary and information is abundant. It is important to learn what relevant information to attend to, when to attend to it, when to make adjustments in action, and how to anticipate future actions for performance success.

The notion of attention has also been appropriately divided along three dimensions (Posner & Boies, 1971). Attention may be viewed (1) as alertness; (2) as a limited capacity or resource; and (3) as selectivity. Each of these categories will be discussed separately.

Alertness refers to the state of mental preparation an individual can activate (intensity) and sustain (duration) prior to performance. Several researchers (Bertelson, 1967; Bertelson & Tisseyre, 1968) have determined that the presentation of a piece of meaningful information (stimulus) prior to performance can alter, even facilitate, the performance. Typically, reaction time measurements (Borwinick & Thompson, 1966) are used to show that reaction time slows dramatically when the time between the warning signal and the stimulus is in excess of four seconds. Alertness, then, is dynamic and is limited by an individual's ability to sustain attention. It is dependent upon an individual's state of arousal.

Alertness
the state of mental preparation at which an individual can activate and sustain discrete performance

Arousal
a state of internal excitement or alertness

Arousal reflects a physiological and psychological state of energy that is activated at a particular moment in time. The autonomic nervous system communicates the arousal level, using sympathetic and parasympathetic neural conductance involving the reticular formation and the hypothalamus. The pupils of the eyes become dilated, heart rate increases, blood pressure and respiration elevate, and sweating increases. Psychological states of arousal are often referred to as *anxiety*. Anxiety represents a high level of arousal that generally resembles fear or apprehension. Arousal levels may flow back and forth on a continuum, ranging from comatose to frenzy (Figure 10.1).

Inverted-U hypothesis
a paradigm that attempts to explain the relationship between arousal levels and performance

Yerkes-Dodson Law
the relationship between performance and arousal. When graphed, is displayed as an inverted-U

The relationship between arousal levels and performance is depicted as the **inverted-U hypothesis** (Duffy, 1962) or as the **Yerkes-Dodson law** (1908). Whether using reaction time laboratory tasks (Lansing, Schwartz, & Lindsley, 1956) or ecologically based movement skills (Weinberg & Ragan, 1978), there seems to be a specific level of arousal at which performance is maximized (optimal level of arousal). Above or below that optimal level, performance will be less than maximum. The optimal level of arousal depends upon the complexity of the task. Those movements that require fine motor skills (e.g., pistol shooting, dart throwing, golf putting) are performed better during lower levels of arousal. Those movements that require power and strength (e.g., powerlifting, hammer throw, shot put) are performed better during higher levels of arousal. In movements that combine fine and gross motor skills (e.g., biathlon, fencing, gymnastics/balance beam), arousal levels will fluctuate situationally for optimal performance.

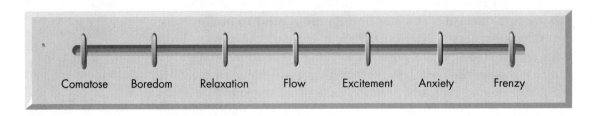

Comatose   Boredom   Relaxation   Flow   Excitement   Anxiety   Frenzy

10.1 *Arousal levels*

FIGURE

INFORMATION PROCESSING

Information processing can occur in parallel or in serial. Parallel processing occurs when two or more sets of information enter the individual simultaneously and are processed together with no interference. Processing in its peripheral sensory stages can be parallel. The **Stroop phenomenon** provides a rationale for this type of logic. In an experiment conducted by Stroop (1935), individuals were asked to respond as quickly as possible to the color red or black by depressing one key for red and another for black. The colors were represented by symbols or words for red and black. The word *red* was printed in black, while the word *black* was printed in red. The fact that the words were depicted in opposite colors produced longer reaction times. The two stimuli, the word and the color, are parallel processed. Interference occurs when the response required is different. Figure 10.2 provides a depiction of the phenomenon.

Stroop phenomenon
the depiction of objects in opposites, which produces longer reaction times, thereby displaying parallel processing

Additionally, events that require response selection are characterized by **controlled processing**. Controlled processing is a method of information processing that is marked by the following features: (1) It is serial. It occurs before or after other task processing. (2) It is slow, as evidenced by the Stroop phenomenon. (3) It is under voluntary control and can be initiated, stopped, or redirected. (4) It requires attention; competing processing interferes with it. A bowler, just prior to initiating his approach, is asked a question by another bowler on his team. He rolls a gutter ball and is unable to answer the question posed to him. These two tasks are in competition with one another. Both are performed, in this case, poorly.

Controlled processing
a method of information gathering marked by serial processing, which is slow, is under voluntary control, and requires attention

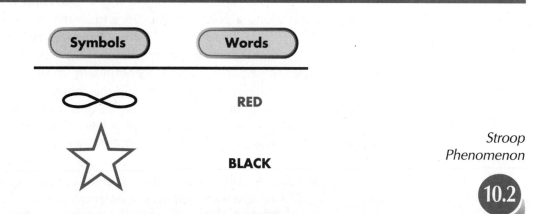

Stroop Phenomenon

10.2
FIGURE

Those who are highly skilled perhaps have learned to process information differently. They have developed **automatic processing**: (1) It is fast. (2) It requires little attention. (3) It is parallel. (4) It is involuntary. This type of processing may be the result of tremendous amounts of practice. Jackie Joyner Kersee, when performing the high jump, seems to perform effortlessly and automatically. During the jump, Kersee is able to focus on the specifics of the jump, such as the placement of the takeoff leg or hip height at the apex of the jump.

Automatic processing
a method of information that requires little attention and is fast, parallel, and involuntary

ATTENTIONAL FOCUS

Another construct is that of **attentional focus**. This refers to a state of focus in which irrelevant stimuli are extinguished and relevant ones are enhanced. A small attentional field with vivid details is referred to as **focal attention**. A wider span of the attentional field with less vivid details is referred to as **diffuse attention**. In activities such as boxing and fencing, it has been found that the person's attention is drawn to an intermediate area between the opponent's body and the glove or foil tip in an attempt to determine as many relevant cues as possible (Ripoll, 1988). This ability to adjust attentional focus leads us into a discussion of attentional styles.

Attentional focus
a state of focus in which irrelevant stimuli are removed and relevant ones are enhanced

Focal attention
attending to a small field with vivid details

Diffuse attention
a wider span of the attentional field with less vivid details

ATTENTIONAL STYLES

One of the most useful descriptions of attentional styles was developed from a theoretical perspective (Nideffer, 1976; 1979). Attentional focus can be viewed along two dimensions: direction (internal/external) and breadth (broad/narrow) of focus. *Direction* refers to the orientation along a continuum from within the individual to outside the individual. *Breadth*, on the other hand, refers to the orientation along a continuum of the environment from broad to narrow. The styles of attention used are continually changing within the individual over time, in tasks, or within the context of the situation. By placing these dimensions on continuums and intersecting them, four categories emerge: broad/external; broad/internal; narrow/external; and narrow/internal (Figure 10.3). Certain situations require a broad attentional focus so that one can be sensitive to a wide variety of cues. Other situations require a narrow focus. Hitting a baseball, for instance, requires a narrow/internal focus. In American football, playing the quarterback position requires one to develop a broad/external focus of attention, unlike playing offensive guard, which requires a narrower type of focus.

Generally, when the environment is dynamic and complex, a narrow attentional style is important. When decision-making requires reflection, analysis, and synthesis, internal attentional style is important. When one is involved in a competitive performance environment, the general mode of behavior results from a narrow and internal attentional style. The skill to change attentional styles at appropriate moments in open environments becomes critical for successful performance.

The ability to flow from one attentional style to another also depends upon the individual's level of arousal (Nideffer, 1979). When anxiety and arousal levels elevate, one's ability to flow from one attentional style to another efficiently and effectively is limited (Landers, 1980). This phenomenon might be explained by **cue utilization theory** (Easterbrook, 1959): The breadth of stimuli an individual can attend to is narrowed when the individual is in a high state of arousal, and the ability to determine the relevancy of the stimuli is diminished. For example, those who are inexperienced in

Cue utilization theory
a paradigm in which the breadth of stimuli to which an individual can attend is narrowed when arousal is high and ability to determine relevance of the stimuli is lower

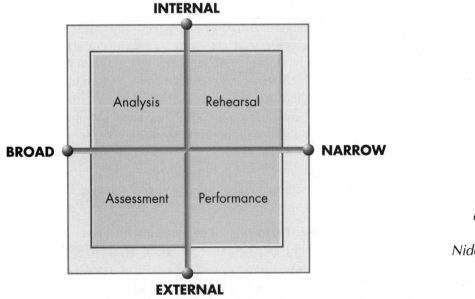

Attentional dimensions (based on Nideffer, 1976)

10.3
FIGURE

skilled movement (e.g., swimming, pistol shooting, and golf) may be inundated with external stimuli to select from, and they may have difficulty focusing attention because they do not know what information is relevant (Nideffer, 1976; Richards & Landers, 1981; Kirschenbaum & Bale, 1980; Feltz, 1982).

In open environments (e.g., field hockey, volleyball, team handball), the use of specific attentional styles proves beneficial (Fisher, 1984). One might use a broad/external focus to be aware of teammates, opponents, and where the object of interest is. Open environments may also require one to assume a broad/internal focus, whereby performances are stored as they relate to the dynamics of the playing environment. A narrow/internal focus may also be required in order to actually perform the movement. Finally, a narrow/external focus may also be used when performing the movement while relating it to other individuals or objects.

Optimizing arousal levels for successful learning and performance is a cornerstone of multidimensional learning. A highly organized and consistent pattern for preparing to perform in self-paced activities is one of the meaningful building blocks (Boutcher & Crews, 1987).

SELF-PACED ACTIVITIES

Self-paced activities activities in which individuals can participate at their own rate that involves a relatively stable environment, predictable situations, and little need for rapid changes

Many motor behaviors involve self-paced activities and externally paced activities. **Self-paced activities** usually occur in situations involving relatively stable environments, predictable situations, and situations in which there is little need for rapid changes. The individual has sufficient time to perceive the relevant stimuli in the situation, develop an action plan, and execute the movement with control. Putting a golf ball, bowling for the strike, serving a racquetball, shooting an arrow, and hitting in tee-ball are examples of self-paced activities.

A five-step strategy has been developed (Singer, 1993) to facilitate learning through performance in self-paced activities:

1. **Readying.** Performance expectations must be positive. Prepare for the performance by associating it with things that have been positive in previous performances. Develop consistency in the technical performance of the skill.

2. **Imaging.** Visualize going through a perfect performance. See it, feel it, and smell it.

3. **Focusing.** Center thoughts on a specific aspect of the activity, such as the shape of the ball as it approaches.

4. **Executing.** Initiate the movement when ready. Stay in the present moment by focusing.

5. **Evaluating.** For the next performance, compare this performance outcome to the goal and the previous four steps. Adjust the strategy appropriately.

Externally paced activities are those that involve another person (partner/opponent) or an object. These external elements create dynamic environmental conditions. Responses, therefore, must be made quickly, accurately, and efficiently. Returning service in volleyball, tennis, badminton, or racquetball, playing goalie in ice or field hockey, soccer, or team handball, and playing defense in basketball, football, or water polo provide examples of externally paced activities.

Externally paced activities
activities that are influenced by another person (partner/opponent), or an object

As people try to concentrate throughout their motor performances, difficulties in the duration and intensity of concentration often arise. These states generally revolve around fluctuating levels of attentional focus. The individual may continue to rehearse what has just happened or may be preparing for a future play or situation rather than concentrating on the situation at hand. "Should have" statements are indicators of focusing on the past. These can include:

"I should have contacted the ball lower. . . ."

"I should have passed the ball to my teammate sooner. . . ."

"I should have waited to go in for the 'kill'. . . ."

"What if" statements are indicative of focusing on the future. These include:

"What if I blow the putt?"

"What if she sets me?"

"What if we cannot get the ball back?"

We may also try to attend to too many cues. Because there are many distractions in any environment, it can be simple to lose focus on that which is relevant. The individual can "lock" into a broad/external focus, allowing a number of stimuli to present themselves. Basketball spectators, for example, have been known to affect free throw shooting success. In gymnasiums where spectators sit close to the endline of the court, they wave pom poms or towels as the shooter prepares to release the shot in order to create visual "noise." At professional football games, crowds have significantly increased the auditory "noise" in an attempt to derail the quarterback's snap count with the offensive line. The results might include poor choices on the part of those who try to attend to too many conflicting cues.

MENTAL PRACTICE

Objective: To develop vivid and controlled images while increasing self-perceptions of personal performance.

Equipment and Preparation: A chair; quiet area

Experience: **One** — Select a close friend. Ask the person to sit in a chair in front of you. Look at the person intensely, focusing on getting a sharp image of the individual. Picture the details of the person: facial contours, mannerisms, expressions, the type of cologne used, a particular style of wearing apparel, etc. Picture the individual speaking. Notice the person's face and facial expressions used; hear the person's voice. Think about how you feel about this person. Recreate the emotions that you feel when you are in the presence of this person.

Two — Place yourself in a familiar area where you usually perform your sport or physical activity. It is empty except for you. Stand in the middle of the area and look around everywhere. Notice how quiet it is. Select as many details about the area as possible, looking from floor to ceiling (or sky to ground), wall to wall (or boundary to boundary). Picture the same setting with 1,000 spectators present. Focus on the sights, sounds, smells, and feelings you experience when getting ready to perform in front of the spectators.

Three — Select a piece of equipment used in your sport or physical activity. Focus on the object. Picture every detail of the object. Use your hands to feel the object, and look carefully at every part of it. Feel its texture and outline. Picture using the object in your sport or physical activity. Focus on seeing yourself performing the activity well. Repeat the skill again and again. Listen to the sounds that are involved with the movement. Combine the feel of the movement and the equipment used in movement with the sound of the movement. Clarify the picture of you performing the movement by combining sight, smell, and sound involved in the completion of the performance.

Assignment: After completing each of the above experiences, write down, in detail, the process you used to provide vividly controlled images. Did it become easier to mentally rehearse or image each experience? Why or why not?

The free throw shooter places too much force behind the ball; the tailback rushes forward, causing the center to prematurely snap the ball, and the exchange is fumbled.

The internal "feel" of the movement is another focus that an individual can "lock" into. When learning a new motor skill, determining the "feel" of the movement through proprioceptors in the initial learning stage is an important part of the multidimensional learning process. Once the individual has learned the motor skill and performance has become automatic, a narrow/internal focus should only be used infrequently. "Locking" into this focus provides a detailed analysis of technique and movement patterns that generally inhibits performance success (i.e., "paralysis by analysis").

A behavioral outgrowth of attentional difficulties is the notion of **choking**. Choking is a difficult construct to define but involves a decrease in performance at critical times. Perhaps the best way to define choking is through the identification of behavioral characteristics. Table 10.1 provides this construct in detail.

Choking is generally thought of as a poor performance in crucial situations. For example, at important times of a game or match, the

Choking
when motor performance repeatedly deteriorates in crucial situations, characteristics of which include increased heart rate, sweating, breathing rate, and muscular tension; inappropriate situational flexibility, narrow focus, internal focus; disruption of coordinated movement, increased muscle tension and fatigue, timing detriment, and relevant cues unattended to

---

TABLE 10.1

The Construct of Choking

Situations Preceding Choking

1. Meaningfulness of competitive importance
2. Turning points in the event
3. Awareness of importance of performance

Physical Dynamics

1. Increased heart rate
2. Increased sweating
3. Increased breathing rate
4. Increased muscular tension

Attentional Dynamics

1. Inappropriate situational flexibility
2. Narrow focus
3. Internal focus

Detriment in Performance

1. Disruption of coordinated movement
2. Increased muscle tension and fatigue
3. Timing(too fast/too slow; too early/too late)
4. Relevant cues unattended to

individual pitches a ball instead of a strike; rolls a spare instead of a strike; misses a relatively easy putt; rims the free throw; or kicks the ball wide of the goal. In short, a pattern of behavior is established that exhibits itself when importance is related to the motor behavior. Heart rate, blood pressure, and sweating are manifestations of a biological alteration that is associated with the attentional level.

Several psychologists (Luria, 1961; Galperin, 1969; Wohl, 1977) have developed models that identify three phases in voluntary motor behavior. These phases include: (1) actions that are controlled and augmented by encouragement from significant others (such as parents or coaches); (2) expressive, audible self-talk generated by the individual; and (3) self-talk, internalized, that develops into self-regulating behavior. Based on this work, one strategy to change a person's focus is through self-talk.

Self-talk refers to one's ability to shape emotional responses that factor into multidimensional learning through motor behavior. The individual can provide one of two types of self-talk to enhance learning: positive self-talk or negative self-talk. **Positive self-talk** is that which helps one to focus thoughts on the present through motivational or instructional elements. Negative self-talk is the type that elicits dramatic anxiety responses and provides negatively self-fulfilling prophecies. Table 10.2 provides examples of positive and negative self-talk.

Self-talk can be performed by developing meaningful *cue words* that describe the desired behavioral outcome. When one is learning

Self-talk
silent monologue that enables a person to shape emotional responses that factor into multidimensional learning through motor behavior

Positive self-talk
silent speaking to oneself that assists in focusing thoughts on the present through motivational or instructional elements

TABLE

10.2 *Self-Talk Scenarios*

Situation	Positive Self-Talk/Result	Negative Self-Talk/Result
Hitting the object just outside the sideline (tennis/volleyball/ badminton/baseball/softball)	"Next time, swing faster and stronger. Be patient for the next chance." / Increase in focus, control, and energy	"How stupid is that?? I will never be able to do that again." / Increase in tension, heightened anxiety
Throwing the object just out of bounds (darts/softball pitch/ hammer, javelin/layup shot)	"Focus, breathe, and relax." /Improved effort, focus	"I just can't get the ball in the hoop." / Anger, withdrawal of effort

a hook ball in bowling, cue words might include *focus*, *energize*, and *complete*. These words provide instructional self-talk that focuses attention in the moment and through the completion of the skill.

Cue words that facilitate speed of action can also be used effectively. A batsman in cricket can increase bat speed by using *fast bat* or *quick bat*; a long jumper can increase velocity by using *explode* or *bullet* when driving with the takeoff leg on the takeoff board.

MOTIVATION AND ITS INFLUENCE ON MOTOR BEHAVIOR

Another topic related to the individual's sphere of focus is motivation and its role in multidimensional learning and motor behavior. Simply put, **motivation** is the effort used to direct and energize behavior (Roberts, 1992). Direction implies what a person is attracted to or attends to. Intensity describes how much effort a person exhibits toward the attraction. For example, one person might attend karate classes for a semester. Someone else might attend karate, kung fu, and tai chi classes during the same semester. Direction of motivation suggests an attraction to participation in martial arts. Taking three classes suggests an individual's intensity of motivation. Theories of motivation ask the question why an individual elicits a particular behavior.

Motivation
the effort applied to direct and energize behavior

Motivation and arousal are not synonymous. Motor behavior professionals sometimes mistakenly believe they can motivate players by telling them to beat on lockers during halftime or by providing inspirational speeches between games of a match. These strategies, when used for arousal purposes, may actually contribute to detrimental performances (Roberts, 1992), because arousal levels may be too high or too low.

It has also been determined that motivation and motor behavior are learned (Ames, 1992; Roberts, 1982; 1984). The integration of cognition and motivation in human movement provides the setting for a discussion of **achievement motivation**. This construct (Murray, 1938) addresses one's efforts to behave competently, to take pride and display excellence in that competence, and to overcome adversity to do so. Put another way, achievement motivation refers to the efforts involved in choosing an activity, striving (intensity or trying hard), persisting (continuing intensity or trying hard), and excelling

Achievement motivation
an individual's efforts to behave competently, taking pride and displaying excellence in that competence, and overcoming adversity to do so

(outcome of performance) in the accomplishment of a task. Many people strive to achieve personal bests when running a mile or a marathon, swimming a mile, or completing more push-ups in one minute than ever before. The characteristics or behaviors associated with achievement motivation include trying harder, concentrating more intensely, performing better, persisting in the face of failure, paying more attention, and choosing to practice or participate longer in activities (Maehr & Braskamp, 1986).

Competitiveness
achievement motivation in the context of motor behavior with social evaluation

Also, additionally important to the discussion of achievement motivation is the notion of **competitiveness** (Martens, 1976), which is achievement motivation in the context of motor behavior with social evaluation (Martens, 1976). It plays a major factor in multi-dimensional learning. Because achievement motivation influences one's learning and competitiveness influences learning in environments where others are involved, both constructs are important to the discussion in this chapter. In Section IV, a better understanding of the application of this construct will be presented.

Although they are performance-based, achievement motivation and competitiveness are processes that are learned. Four basic areas of achievement motivation have been identified: (1) choosing an activity, (2) striving (intensity), (3) persisting (continuing intensity when failure is a possibility), and (4) excelling (outcome of performance). Choosing an activity might refer to a decision to select rugby instead of American football or to play with those who are of similar ability, lesser ability, or better ability. Striving refers to how hard one pursues goals; persisting describes efforts to continue through difficulties; and excelling relates to the attainment of those goals.

Categories of achievement motivation devised by theorists include need achievement (Murray, 1938), test anxiety (Mandler & Sarason, 1952), expectancy of reinforcement (Crandall, 1963), and social cognitive (Bandura, 1977). Theories that are of significance to multidimensional learning and motor behavior have been selected for inclusion in this chapter: need achievement theory, attribution theory, perceived confidence theory (social cognitive), and achievement goal theory (social cognitive).

Need achievement theory
an interactive paradigm in which personal and situational characteristics serve to predict behavior

Need achievement theory (Atkinson, 1957; McClelland, 1961) is an interactive one in which personal and situational characteristics serve to predict behavior. The theory centers around the idea that people are motivated to either achieve success or avoid failure (personality factors) based on the likelihood of success in a given situation or the value of the success (situational factors). Those who are motivated to achieve success also approach success with a sense of pride of accomplishment. Those who are motivated to avoid failure approach success by attempting to avoid the shame of failure. Corresponding behaviors mirror the intent: Those who are motivated to achieve success look for situations in which they can succeed with at least some risk; those who are motivated to avoid failure avoid risks and challenges or perform poorly in difficult situations so that the shame of failure is minimized by those who evaluate the perceived shame (Roberts, 1972). This theoretical model has provided the basic roots from which the study of achievement motivation has blossomed and grown.

Extending from the need achievement theory is **attribution theory**. The premise of this theory is that people ascribe causes for their successes and failures (Heider, 1958; Weiner, 1985, 1986). The theory describes the processes people use to explain their behaviors. An underlying assumption of this theory is that the individual processes information and controls performance. Most of the attributions people make about their successes or failures in sport revolve around winning and losing. The general premise is that attributions one makes about an outcome affect future failures or successes, and the cycle continues (Biddle, 1993). People predict sport outcomes using the environmental information available to them, and they try to determine cause and effect (Roberts, 1982). These attribution processes can be placed into two basic groups: stability and control (Weiner, 1985). Stability ranges from stable to unstable, while control ranges from internal to external control. For example, a rider in an equestrian event involving jumps might attribute performance success or failure to ability or talent (stable) or to luck (unstable). The rider may also attribute the success or failure to fantastic focus during the last two jumps (internal) or lack of other skilled riders, creating an easy competition (external). Finally, the rider might also attribute performance success or failure to a strategically planned jump schedule or other horses' abilities to clear the jump.

Attribution theory
what individuals attribute their successes or failures to

The meaningfulness of this theoretical approach to explain behavior is helpful to the motor behavior professional in at least two ways: (1) If one determines his performance to be related to a stable cause, such as well-developed skill, then he will expect to do well in the future in similar situations. This type of future success expectancy can assist in self-efficacy and perceived competence, thereby creating an internal environment more conducive to learning. (2) If one determines the cause of her performance to be related to internal or under-control categories, emotional reactions of shame or pride will be generated. The interrelationship of attributions and achievement motivation are summarized in Table 10.3.

Attribution theory has provided the basis for social cognitive approaches to motivation (Duda, 1981) that have proven beneficial to the study of motor behavior (Roberts, 1992; McAuley, 1991). These approaches have presented the individual as dynamic and using processes that connect cognition and motor performance to achieve motor performance–related goals. Two of these paradigms will be discussed: perceived confidence or ability and achievement goals.

In broad terms, goal achievement through motor performance is an integral part of multidimensional learning (Duda, 1993; Nicholls, 1984). At least two areas converge to provide an individual with conditions that explain motor behavior from a social cognitive perspective: achievement goals and perceived confidence (Duda, 1993). **Perceived confidence**, a multidimensional construct that includes cognitive, social, and motor areas, provides an individual with direction. This perception of confidence or ability is determined by particular orientations that represent success: outcome orientation or task orientation. **Outcome orientation** is the perspective that determines the worth of one's performance by comparing it with the performance of others. For example, someone who competes in Greco-Roman wrestling sets an achievement goal to be the best in his age group at the local YMCA. This, to him, means beating all those who are not only on the team during practice, but at the next meet. With this orientation, he is focused on the outcome, so that when he wins his perceived confidence is high; when he loses, his perceived confidence is low.

Perceived confidence
perception of ability determined through orientations which mean success

Outcome orientation
the perspective that determines the worth of one's performance by comparing it to the performance of others

TABLE

10.3

Attribution/ Achievement Motivation Relationship

Degree of Stability	
Excellent	Anticipated future success
Poor	Anticipated future failure
Polarity of Cause	
Internal	More shame or pride
External	Less shame or pride
Degree of Control	
Under control	More motivation
Little or no control	Less motivation

In contrast, perceived confidence can also be directed by **task orientation**. In this case, one uses prior personal performances as the yardstick by which success is measured. The individual who competes in Greco-Roman wrestling sets an achievement goal to improve performance by successfully executing a pin at the next practice session. This accomplishment is not directly related to others' performances.

From a motor behavior professional's perspective, it is important to note that those individuals who are more task oriented tend to exhibit persistence, intensity, and a strong desire to pursue excellence that is based upon the realistic perception of their abilities (Duda, 1993). Those who are more outcome oriented have difficulty in sustaining reasonable perceptions of perceived confidence, quit trying in the face of adversity, or find unrealistic reasons to explain their lack of success.

The final dimension to be discussed as it relates to achievement motivation involves achievement goals. This construct is based on a continuum in sport involving mastery of a goal and competitiveness. On one side, an individual is focused on performing a particular task or skill with competence (Ames, 1987; Nicholls, 1984). This is similar to task orientation, discussed earlier. On the other side, competitiveness is derived from comparing self with others. This perspective is directed in a social context.

Researchers have provided the motor behavior professional with enlightening information about the role of the learning environment in this regard (Ames, 1992; Ames & Archer, 1987; Roberts, 1992). If an individual has been placed in an environment where task orientation has been encouraged, the individual may develop a mastery orientation based upon competence through self-comparison. If an individual is in an environment where competitiveness with others is encouraged, the individual may develop a competitive orientation based upon comparison with and against others. The social dynamics will be discussed more thoroughly in Section IV.

It has been determined that achievement motivation and competitiveness are learned and occur in sequential phases (Scanlan, 1988; Weinberg & Gould, 1995): (1) autonomous competence phase; (2) social comparison phase; and (3) integrated phase. The autonomous phase occurs between birth and four years of age. In this phase the individual constantly interacts with, challenges, and competes with the environment. There is little concern for competition with others, only the desire to master the environment. For

Task orientation
the use of prior personal performances as the yardstick by which success is measured

example, a two-year-old twin is generally concerned about getting higher to reach the top of the counter to grab the cookie there rather than being the first twin to reach the top of the counter.

The second phase, social comparison, generally occurs once the person has begun kindergarten. The sphere of concern becomes a comparison of self with others. It now becomes important for the twins to see who is more flexible, more agile, jumps higher, or runs faster. The final phase, that of integration, involves a dynamic combination of the first two phases. This phase includes the determination of when which phase is the more appropriate to exhibit. The twins view it as important to compare themselves to others while also determining what is appropriate to achieve individually.

FEEDBACK

Augmented feedback
feedback that is
provided externally
to the individual

Providing individuals with appropriate feedback and reinforcement is yet another perspective of motor behavior. The sensory feedback mechanisms have been discussed previously in this and other sections (vision, audition, and somatosensation). Another form of feedback, **augmented feedback,** will be included to enhance the understanding of feedback. Figure 10.4 provides a graphic of the

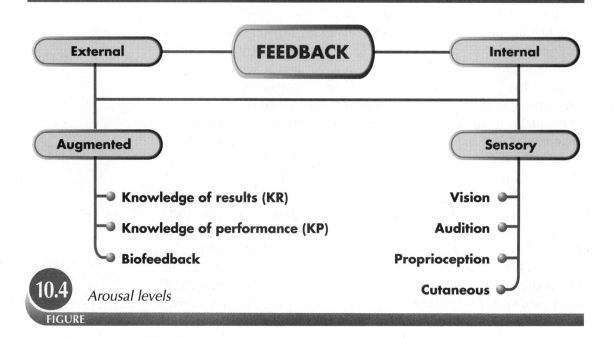

10.4
FIGURE

Arousal levels

unique contributions that each construct of feedback in the overall concept of learner feedback.

Augmented feedback refers to information that is provided outside the individual from a variety of sources during and after performance. Several types of feedback are available. Among these are *knowledge of performance* (KP), or information that is provided about movement quality, *knowledge of results* (KR), or information that is provided about the movement outcome, and *augmented sensory feedback* (biofeedback), a part of KP, or sensory information that is provided to the individual immediately and continuously through the use of instruments.

It is important to understand that (1) augmented feedback is needed when learning some types of motor skills, shortening learning time, and/or facilitating heightened performance; (2) it is not needed when learning other skills; and (3) there are situations where the provision of augmented feedback inhibits motor performance. A closer examination of each of these points will help you to understand the role of feedback in multidimensional learning and motor behavior.

The point has been made by several theorists (Schmidt, 1975; Adams, 1971; Rink, 1985) that augmented feedback is necessary for motor skill learning to occur. Additional information (Lee & Magill, 1983; Salmoni, Schmidt, & Walter, 1984) has led to a paradigm shift in thinking about how augmented feedback influences the learning of motor skills.

It has been determined that some skills require augmented feedback in order for learning to occur. Specifically, through the withdrawal of KR under laboratory conditions, investigators determined that moving a lever to a specific position without the aid of vision was severely inhibited or nearly impossible if KR was taken away too early or if KR was not provided at all (Bilodeau, Bilodeau, & Schumsky, 1959). The learners did not know the goal. Investigators also determined that learning to move a lever to a specific position in a specific amount of time, with the aid of vision, was severely inhibited when KR was provided on only two trials. They found that improvement in accuracy was related to the number of trials in which KR was provided (Newell, 1974). KR was used to develop memory of limb position and movement speed that was used to produce the desired performance (Adams, 1971). This closed-loop model is now regarded as outdated.

A critical piece of information gleaned from this research involves the absence of sensory information. When sensory information is unavailable or severely inhibited while the skill is being performed, the role of augmented feedback is quite important in learning. When speed is involved, the learner is hard-pressed to integrate time, space, force, and flow without the assistance of KR. When learning a new skill, the learner is also in need of KR to facilitate the understanding of the goal of the skill along with its motor performance.

There are also skills for which augmented feedback is not necessarily required in order to learn the skill. Investigators (Magill, Chamberlin, & Hall, 1991; Newell, 1974) discovered that in laboratory-based studies involving the phi phenomenon (the illusion that a series of lights flashing sequentially represents motion) and coincidence anticipation, subjects did not need augmented KR to learn when to anticipate the exact moment a sequential series of lights arrived at a target light. These findings help us to understand the relationship between the timing of apparent motion and its target. Information was gleaned from internal feedback mechanisms rather than from augmented ones.

In addition, when augmented feedback is provided through model performances, individuals may need little or no additional augmented feedback once the model is seen demonstrating the skill appropriately (Kernodle & Carlton, 1992; Swinnen, Walter, Lee, &

LAB EXERCISE

FEEDBACK AND LONG JUMP PERFORMANCE

Objective: To determine the role of feedback in performance through standing long jump performance.

Equipment and Preparation: Roll/fold mat that is at least seven feet long; partner; tape measure; marking pen; masking tape. Mark off a total distance of seven feet, using inches, from the mat's end.

Experience: To prevent the mat from slipping, someone holds the mat in place. Partner (performer) stands with his or her back to the end of the length of the mat. When ready, estimates the distance the first jump will be. The performer then turns and jumps. The distance is measured to the nearest inch and compared to the estimated jump. Repeat the estimation and jump four additional times.

Assignment: Note any changes in the performer's movement by trial as well as by estimation. How did feedback and memory play roles in performance?

Serrien, 1993). When those who receive KP as a form of augmented feedback are compared to those who observe a model, the results are similar (Magill, 1994). In either case, the individual forms a model to which internal feedback can be compared in future trials.

There are other skills that can be learned more efficiently or performed at an elevated level when augmented feedback is available. Investigators (Stelmach, 1970; Wallace & Hagler, 1979) have determined that certain factors associated with augmented feedback, when present, enhance learning. It was found that many skills have internal feedback mechanisms at basic levels of performance. For example, once a two-point shot is learned in basketball, the performance of a three-point shot holds within it internal feedback based upon the two-point shot. There is, however, an upper level of performance that may not be surpassed without the assistance of augmented feedback. The relevance of the augmented feedback, however, needs to be determined so that the individual can understand the meaning of the change in behavior that is being sought to enhance performance.

Finally augmented feedback can be detrimental to multidimensional learning and motor behavior. Several researchers (Buekers, Magill, & Hall, 1992; Magill, Chamberlin, & Hall, 1991; Winstein & Schmidt, 1990) have indicated that when erroneous KR was given, a negative effect resulted. The detriment came from the fact that the KR was full of error. For example, when an individual was consistently misinformed that responses were early when they were late or late when they were early, performance deteriorated. Because of the misinformation, individuals developed a different set of goals from which to compare previous performances and develop strategies for future ones.

Those who have investigated augmented feedback have also determined that the *frequency* of presentation of augmented feedback can create detrimental results (Lee, White, & Canahan, 1990). The performance of those subjects who received augmented feedback on every trial deteriorated compared to that of subjects who were given augmented feedback with a systematic reduction of frequency (faded schedule of presentation). Providing augmented feedback, then, after every trial is actually detrimental to performance enhancement. It is possible that the individual develops an expectation that augmented feedback will be provided; therefore, the individual attends less frequently and persistently to internal feedback and standards of performance from within.

Summary feedback, another way to reduce the frequency of KR, can be provided after trials during practice. During the time when no KR is given, the individual can cognitively process information and compare it in working memory. KR is used to compare sensory feedback-based performance.

Based upon this information about the relevance of augmented feedback, the motor behavior professional must learn to evaluate motor skills on the basis of specific factors we have discussed. To summarize these points, if an individual needs sensory feedback information to perform the skill appropriately, then augmented feedback should be provided. The level of feedback depends on the skill of the learner. As the learner's performance improves, so does the level of KR specificity. For example, if someone learning to bowl could not see the pins, some type of augmented feedback would be needed to facilitate learning. Once the individual has learned the process of performing a strike, KR specificity as it relates to throwing the strike becomes more meaningful. If an individual is presented with a novel task (something that represents a new construct involving time, space, force, or flow), such as juggling four kitchen knives for the first time, augmented feedback would facilitate learning. If the individual has the opportunity to view the skill by observing an appropriate model, augmented feedback might not be needed. For example, initially balancing a hackey sack on the top of the left foot while hopping on the other foot might only require observing the motor behavior to accomplish it. If, however, the dynamic balancing of the hackey sack on the top of the left foot was changed to alternately kicking the hackey sack from left foot to right foot, left knee to right knee, left elbow to right elbow, and head back to left foot, the individual might require augmented feedback. The provision of feedback in this setting would facilitate time, space, force, and flow requirements of coordination.

BIOFEEDBACK

Technology continues to facilitate our understanding of motor behavior through the use of instruments designed to assess the performance of the autonomic and central nervous systems. The awareness of heart rate, blood pressure, respiratory rate, muscular tension, and central nervous system messages (through EEG or pupillary responses) from the somatosensory systems has enabled people to learn to monitor, control, and alter their states. *Biofeedback* refers to the immediate display of an individual's biological signals (Trachtman & Kluka, 1993), while **biofeedback training** refers to programs that have been designed to alter or maintain those bio-signals. The use of electromyography (EMG) for altering or main-taining muscular tension has produced mixed results (Budzynski & Stoyva, 1975; Zaichkowski, Dorsey, & Mulholland, 1979). The use of electroencephalography (EEG) and visual accommodation have produced encouraging results (Trachtman & Kluka, 1993), but more research needs to be conducted to substantiate the role of biofeedback as an augmented feedback mechanism.

Biofeedback training
programs that have been designed to alter or maintain biosignals

Biofeedback becomes particularly helpful once an individual be-comes familiar with sensory feedback cues (Zaichkowsky & Fuchs, 1989). It can facilitate sensory feedback to alter and enhance the in-ternal standards that future performances will be compared to by changing or strengthening physiological and cognitive networks during and after performances.

One final issue of importance will be discussed as it relates to multidimensional learning and motor behavior. Observation and learning seem to be innately interwoven into an individual's sphere of focus.

OBSERVATIONAL LEARNING

Observational learning is another perspective that influences overall motor skill acquisition. Its role is important in the learning process for both the individual and the motor behavior professional.

When creating a learning environment, the motor behavior pro-fessional must select meaningful ways to present material effectively. This can be achieved through **observation**, or viewing a movement performed by another person before learning that movement. People's dependence on vision in motor skill acquisition has been mentioned throughout this text. We can learn to perform motor skills effectively as a result of watching others perform the move-ment prior to our attempting it.

Observation
viewing a movement another person performs before learning that movement

Several variables must be considered before using modeling to facilitate learning. Figure 10.5 provides an inclusive paradigm (McCullagh, Weiss, & Ross, 1989) of all that is involved in the demonstration/observation process. The demonstration/observation paradigm has been divided into six general areas: those factors affecting the observer; perceptions of the observer and the demon-strator; parts of the demonstration; rehearsal strategies used by the observer; behavioral action; and feedback involving the observer, the demonstrator, and behavioral action.

Of these six, it is important to elaborate on three of them to provide a better understanding of the paradigm. The word *performance* literally refers to an act at a moment in time. Although a

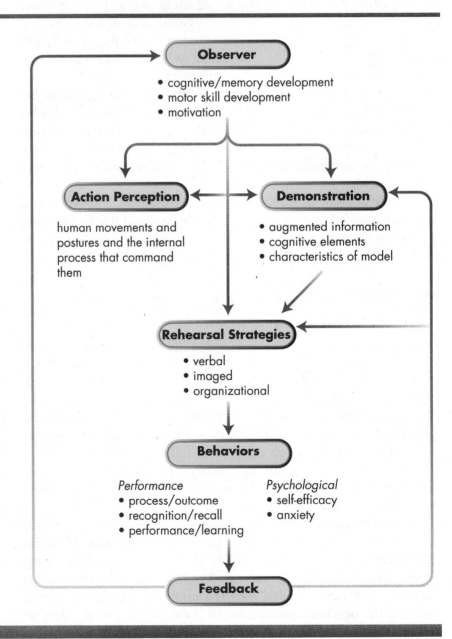

Paradigm for demonstration/ observation

10.5
FIGURE

performance is completed uniquely, people viewing that performance each perceive it quite differently and assimilate that which is important differently. Some of the variables that cause individuals to differ in their perceptions include what stage of cognitive and memory development they are in, where in the motor skill acquisition process they are, and how motivated they are to learn the skill.

Children, age four to seven years reported difficulty organizing the information received through demonstration/observation (Weiss & Klint, 1987). Therefore, it is important to provide verbal cues along with modeling in order to help create a cognitive rehearsal strategy (Weiss & Klint, 1987).

As youngsters mature physically, height, weight, timing, coordination, strength, and flexibility also change. The individual who grows five inches in four months and weighs twenty-five additional pounds must continuously make adjustments in that which has been learned since the skill was introduced.

There seem to be a number of sex differences that manifest themselves throughout the life span that may affect modeling. Male and female prepubescents seem to progress on a steady continuum in motor skill acquisition. Several researchers (Clark & Ewing, 1985; Seefeldt & Haubenstricker, 1982; Sigelman & Shaffer, 1995) have noted that as children age, larger variations in motor skill acquisition between the sexes occur. This may, however, be a product of the quality and quantity of movement experiences as well as socialization rather than an indictment of sex at birth. Most of the research on sex differences in motor skill acquisition throughout the life span was completed during the 1980s. With the institutionalization of federal laws providing equal opportunity to organized sport for both sexes in the United States (Title IX of the Education Act, 1972), more detailed investigations must be conducted to provide updated information about the role cultural socialization has upon motor skill acquisition.

The importance of the motivational set of the observer cannot be understated. Individuals must understand why learning a particular skill is important, they must participate in an environment that is positively charged with reasons to learn, and they must be provided with encouraging feedback. The use of drills, experiences, or games that provide elements of success and fun can increase one's motivational set. It is also important to use demonstrators who are similar to those involved in the learning process. An individual who is similar in appearance (skill ability, age, sex, height, weight, race, etc.) can instill confidence in the observer (McAuley, 1985), thereby providing additional motivation for success.

Three other key elements are included in the demonstration/ observation process model. Characteristics of the individual used as the model, supplementing the model's image with verbal cues, and cognition complexity affect overall learning. There seems to be some support for the notion that the demonstrator should have a level of performance ability closely resembling efficiency and effectiveness as they relate to the goal of the skill (Magill, 1993; Schmidt, 1991). The observer creates a "perceptual blueprint" (as was discussed in Section I; Sheffield, 1961). The danger, however, lies in the observer's perception of the demonstrator's credibility. It could be perceived that the demonstrator is perceived as such an expert that the observer could never possibly perform the movement that well. Additionally, the observer, while initially learning, may be unaware of which cues are important for performance.

There is also some support for the use of models who are relatively unskilled (Lee & White, 1990). These models have been referred to as *learning models* (Rose, 1997). The key to the successful use of someone relatively unskilled in the performance is the analysis made after observation. Research supports the notion that the observer plays a more active role in the learning process when observing a learning model. The motor behavior professional must, however, follow up the demonstration with questions that lead the observer to determine what produced efficient and effective or inefficient and ineffective movement. Without that important feedback, the observer is no better off in the learning process.

What seems to be agreed upon is whether or not the demonstrator is a learning model or a skilled model is that observers benefit from the use of demonstration.

SYSTEMATIC OBSERVATION SKILLS AND THE MOTOR BEHAVIOR PROFESSIONAL — FACILITATING THE LEARNING PROCESS

Motor behavior professionals who can select critical environmental and technical cues in a short period of time are those who can most effectively analyze movement and provide appropriate feedback to learners. How can the motor behavior professional swiftly and accurately assess the movement, providing constructive, efficient, and effective feedback? In other words, (1) what should the individual continue to do? (2) what should the individual stop doing? (3) what should the individual start doing?

Professionals can develop and refine the skills of cue acquisition, cue interpretation, and analysis. The following checklist has been devised to assist the professional in learning more efficient and effective observational skills:

- Classify each of the sport-specific skills.
- Understand the physics associated with skills and how they are used within the context of the game.
- Chunk each skill into phases.
- Focus on key body areas.
- Interpret meaningful information.
- Provide effective and efficient feedback.

In order to acquire and interpret cues, the professional must initially learn to classify movement. Poulton (1957) devised a method of classifying skills on a continuum from closed to open. To review, closed skills occur in a stationary or controlled environment. Open skills are those that occur in a dynamic environment. Closed skills include the dimension of internal timing. Internal timing involves the appropriate sequencing of movements throughout the body, facilitating a coordinated performance. In open skills, the dimension of spatial relationship is added through external timing. External timing has the component of body/object relationships. Understanding the timing proves beneficial to skill analysis.

A thorough understanding of the biomechanics involved in each skill and how the skill is framed within the context of the game is also meaningful. Learning biomechanical principles, studying films, texts, and research articles, watching efficient performances, using mental imagery to visualize efficient performances, and using coding skills provides the basis for cue acquisition (James & Dufek, 1993; Kluka, 1997). Each skill and the human body are coded, having individual components, in combination with timing from within and from without (between individuals/ objects).

By developing a visual/mental model of the skill, based upon biomechanical principles, the motor behavior professional can use the technique of external mental imagery to facilitate cue acquisition and interpretation. Each skill can be coded into:

- the ready position just before skill initiation,

- the preparation or backswing phase,
- the action,
- the follow-through, and
- the preparation for the next move.

For example, the high outside attack in volleyball requires the professional to focus upon:

- the initial starting position and dynamic body balance,
- the foot positioning as it relates to body angle, looking up the body to the coiling of the hitting arm,
- the uncoiling of the hitting arm as it contacts the ball,
- the visual release of the ball at contact to the core of the body, viewing its dynamic balance upon landing, and
- looking again at torso/head/limb movement in preparation for further play.

When observing the performer, the professional must stay far enough away to be able to see the entire movement in relationship to other events in the environment. Reiterating what was presented in Section III of this text, only three degrees of visual angle are in focus (a thumb's width); other movements are observed by peripheral vision. (The small angle of clarity is the result of photoreceptors being packed more densely in the fovea centralis than in any other portion of the retina.) The performer's movement should be observed at least three times, once from the front, once from the back, and once from the side (at a ninety-degree angle), before any attempt is made to provide analysis.

Focus on the core of the body, specifically on the area from the navel to the nose. Peripheral vision can assist in cue acquisition/interpretation. Shifting focus from the torso/head to the limbs adds meaningful data elements for interpretation. To interpret cues, ask yourself the following questions (Barrett, 1979):

- How is the alignment of the head/torso?
- What is the head position and what impact does it have on the movement?
- Is there dynamic stability in relationship to side/side, front/front/back, up/down?
- What role did the arms/legs play?

- What contributed to the production of force?
- Where is the center of the body during the skill?
- Does the center of gravity change during the skill?
- Where is the body weight during the ready position, the preparation, the action, the follow-through, and preparation for the next movement phase?
- Where is the head throughout? Where are the eyes fixed? (e.g., on the ball, on the target, or in between?)
- How wide is the base of support?
- If hip movement is important, what are the amounts and directions?
- Where are the shoulders in relation to the hips?
- Where is the hand in relation to the desired outcome just before and during contact with the ball?
- What is the extent of the follow-through?
- What is the range of movement within each joint that contributes to the production of force?
- What is the outcome of the movement?

The interpretation of meaningful information facilitates analysis. One means by which this skill can be developed is through the use of videotape analysis. By videotaping the movement from the front, side, and back, more complete information can be obtained.

By viewing the actions in slow motion, the professional can then answer the previous questions. Also, by stopping the video during

QUALITATIVE ANALYSIS OF MOVEMENT EXPERIENCE

LAB EXERCISE

Objective: To qualitatively analyze a movement based upon visual observation.

Equipment and Preparation: Partner; clipboard, paper, and pencil

Experience: Select a closed skill for the partner to perform that requires only the use of the body and the environment.

Assignment: Following the format in the text, analyze the movement and provide visual, auditory, and tactile feedback to the partner.

the preparation phase and during the action, the professional can try to predict what the results will be. By continuing the videotape, the professional can view the outcome and can rerun the action to determine what contributed to the result. Finally, the professional can be provided with footage to observe the effects of spectators and officials on the game. Viewing the tape repeatedly will help the professional to determine what behaviors contributed to the results.

Providing efficient and effective feedback based upon skill classification, biomechanical concepts, skill codification, observation of key body areas, and the interpretation of meaningful information completes the observational skills checklist. The professional and the performer also need to determine effective verbal and visual cues that provide meaning to the performer. Short, feeling-filled or area-related words (e.g., *crush, reach, shape, explode*) can be used to enhance effectiveness. Auditory and visual cues are the easiest to communicate. By using short, meaningful verbal cues at least three seconds prior to movement initiation, the performer can process the cues and trigger an appropriate motor program response. For example, if a drop shot becomes appropriate in badminton, using the verbal cue "drop" as the performer initiates the backswing should give the player enough time to focus on hitting the drop shot and running the appropriate motor program to do so.

Cues based in somatosensory experience can also be used as verbal cues. If the performer needs to swing the racket faster (as in the case of badminton), the cue "explode" or "crush" may be used to focus the performer internally to feel the arm moving faster. Using the visual cue of a one-inch dot on a section of net tape could facilitate the learning of zone net attacks.

The development of observational skills enables the motor behavior professional to select information for detailed processing to appropriately analyze performance. The approach provides the professional with important tools to facilitate the learning and performance of individuals and teams.

KEY POINTS

- Characteristics of the learner that have multidimensional implications include sex, age, experience level, capability, and learning style.

- Chronological age plays an important role in learning motor skills.

- In the initial stage of learning, learners try to get the general notion of the movement. At the next level, they try to determine and perform what it takes to integrate cognitive and motoric efforts into coordinated, purposeful movement. At the highest level, they try to refine that purposeful movement into action that is repeatable, flexible, and automatic.

- Physical and physiological characteristics such as skeletal size, weight, muscular power, strength and endurance, agility, flexibility, and cardiovascular and muscular endurance contribute to the learner's characteristics and readiness to learn motorically.

- Learning styles have also been found to influence motor behavior.

- Concentration is central to the discussion of learning from a multidimensional perspective.

- Attention can be viewed as alertness, as a limited capacity or resource, and as selectivity.

- Attentional focus refers to a state of focus in which irrelevant stimuli are removed and relevant ones are enhanced.

- Attentional focus can be viewed two-dimensionally: direction and breadth of focus.

- Self-paced activities involve a relatively stable environment, predictable situations, and little need for rapid changes. Externally paced activities are those that involve another person or object.

- Choking refers to one's inability to repeatedly perform in stressful situations.

- Self-talk can be positive or negative and can shape motor behavior.

- Motivation is the effort used to direct or energize behavior.

- Achievement motivation refers to the efforts involved in choosing an activity, striving, persisting, and excelling in the accomplishment of a task.

- There are several theories of achievement motivation.

- Achievement motivation and competitiveness are learned and occur in sequential phases.

- Augmented feedback involves information that is provided from outside the individual through a variety of sources during and after performance.

- Knowledge of performance (KP) is information that is provided about the movement's quality.
- Knowledge of results (KR) refers to information that is provided about the movement's outcome.
- Biofeedback refers to the immediate display of one's biological signals; biofeedback training involves programs that enable one to alter or maintain those biosignals.
- Observational learning influences overall motor skill acquisition.

DISCUSSION QUESTIONS

1. Discuss one of the following sports and provide an example of a situation in which shifts in attentional focus can be explained, according to Nideffer's model: basketball, tennis, archery, golf, team handball, soccer.

2. Discuss what contributes to choking; describe the process of choking and a strategy that enables one to avoid it.

3. Describe the differences between achievement motivation and competitiveness.

4. Determine the difference between outcome and task goal orientation. Which should be emphasized in physical education settings? In sport settings? Why?

5. Describe the importance of modeling for motor skill learning. What characteristics does the motor behavior professional need in order to be a competent observer?

ADDITIONAL READINGS

Glencross, D. J., Whiting, H. T. A., & Abernethy, B. (1994). Motor control, motor learning, and the acquisition of skill: Historical trends and future directions. *International Journal of Sport Psychology, 25*, 32–52.

Magill, R. A. (1994). The influence of augmented feedback on skill learning depends on characteristics of the skill and the learner. *Quest, 46,* 314–327.

REFERENCES

Adams, J. A. (1971). A closed-loop theory of motor learning. *Journal of Motor Behavior, 3,* 111–149.

Ames, C. (1987). The enhancement of student motivation. In D. A. Klieber & M. Maehr (Eds.), *Advances in motivation and achievement* (pp. 123–148). Greenwich, CT: JAI Press.

Ames, C. (1992). Achievement goals, motivational climate, and motivational process. In G. C. Roberts (Ed.), *Motivation in sport and exercise* (pp.161–176). Champaign, IL: Human Kinetics.

Ames, C., & Archer, J. (1987). Mothers' beliefs about the role of ability and effort in school learning. *Journal of Educational Psychology, 79,* 409–414.

Atkinson, J. W. (1957). Motivational determinants of risk-taking behavior. *Psychological Review, 64,* 359–372.

Bandura, A. (1977). Self-efficacy: Toward a unifying theory of behavioral change. *Psychological Review, 84,* 191–215.

Barrett, K. (1979). Observations for learning and coaching. *JOPERD, 50*(1), 23–25.

Bertelson, P. (1967). The time course of preparation. *Quarterly Journal of Experimental Psychology, 19,* 272–279.

Bertelson, P., & Tisseyre, F. (1968). The time course of preparation with regular and irregular foreperiods. *Quarterly Journal of Experimental Psychology, 20,* 297–300.

Biddle, S. (1993). Attribution research and sport psychology. In R. N. Singer, M. Murphey, & L. K. Tennant (Eds.), *Handbook of research on sport psychology* (pp. 437–464). New York: Macmillan.

Bilodeau, E. A., Bilodeau, I. M., & Schumsky, D. A. (1959). Some effects of introducing and withdrawing knowledge of results early and late in practice. *Journal of Experimental Psychology, 58,* 142–144.

Borwinick, J., & Thompson, L. W. (1966). Premotor and motor components of reaction time. *Journal of Experimental Psychology, 71,* 9–15.

Boutcher, S. H., & Crews, D. J. (1987). The effect of a preshot attentional routine on a well-learned skill. *International Journal of Sport Psychology, 18,* 30–39.

Briner, W. W., & Ely, J. B. (1999). Volleyball injuries at the 1995 U. S. Olympic Festival. *International Journal of Volleyball Research, 1*(1), 1–5.

Budzynski, T. H., & Stoyva, J. M. (1975). *EMG-Biofeedback bei unspezifichen und spezifischen Angstzustanden.* In H. Legewie & Nusselt (Eds.), Biofeedback Therapie (pp. 163–185). Munich: Urban & Schwarzenberg.

Buekers, M. J., Magill, R. A., & Hall, K. G. (1992). The effect of erroneous knowledge of results on skill acquisition when augmented information is redundant. *Quarterly Journal of Experimental Psychology, 44A,* 105–117.

Carter, R. C. (1982). Visual search with color. *Journal of Experimental Psychology: Human Perception and Human Performance, 8,* 127–136.

Clark, J. E., & Ewing, M. (1985). A meta-analysis of gender differences and similarities in the gross motor skill performances of prepubescent children. Paper presented at the annual meeting of the North American Society for the Psychology of Sport and Physical Activity. Gulfport, MS.

Clark, N. (1997). *Sports nutrition guidebook,* (2nd ed.). Champaign, IL: Human Kinetics.

Crandall, V. C. (1963). Achievement. In H. W. Stevenson (Ed.), *Child psychology* (pp. 415–459). Chicago, IL: University of Chicago Press.

Del Rey, P. (1989). Training and contextual interference effects on memory and transfer. *Research Quarterly for Exercise and Sport, 60,* 342–347.

Del Rey, P., Whitehurst, M., & Wood, J. (1983). Effects of experience and contextual interference on learning and transfer. *Perceptual and Motor Skills, 56,* 581–582.

Del Rey, P. Wughalter, E., & Whitehurst, M. (1982). The effects of contextual interference on females with varied experience in open skills. *Research Quarterly for Exercise and Sport, 53,* 108–115.

Duda, J. L. (1981). A cross-cultural analysis of achievment motivation in sport and the classroom. Unpublished doctoral dissertation. Univesity of Illinois.

Duda, J. L. (1993). Goals: A social-cognitive approach to the study of achievement motivation in sport. In R. N. Singer, M. Murphey, & L. K. Tennant (Eds.), *Handbook of research on sport psychology* (pp. 421–436). New York: Macmillan.

Duffy, E. (1962). Activation and behavior. New York: Wiley.

Easterbrook, J. A. (1959). The effect of emotion on cue utilization and the organization of behavior. *Psychological Review, 66,* 183–201.

Farmer, E. W., & Taylor, R. M. (1980). Visual search through color displays: Effects of target-background similarity and background uniformity. *Perception and Psychophysics, 27,* 167–272.

Feltz, D. (1982). Path analysis of the causal elements in Bandura's theory of self-efficacy and an anxiety based model of avoidance behavior. *Journal of Personality and Social Psychology, 42,* 764–781.

Fisher, A. C. (1984). Sport intelligence. In W. F. Straub & J. M. Williams (Eds.), *Cognitive sport psychology* (pp. 42–50). Lansing, NY: Sport Science Associates.

Galperin, P. J. (1969). Stages in the development of mental arts. In M. Cole & I. Maltzmann (Eds.), *A handbook of contemporary Soviet psychology* (pp. 249–273). New York: Basic Books.

Gentile, A. M. (1972). A working model of skill acquisition with application to teaching. *Quest,* Monograph XVII, 3–23.

Goode, S. L., & Wei, P. (1988). Differential effects of variations of random and blocked practice on novice learning an open motor skill in D. L. Gill and J. E. Clarke (Eds.), *Abstracts of research papers,* 1988 (p. 80). American Alliance for Health, Physical Education, Recreation and Dance Annual Convention, Kansas City, MO. Reston, VA: AAHPERD.

Heider, F. (1958). *The psychology of interpersonal relations.* New York: Wiley.

James, R., & Dufek, J. (Oct., 1993). Movement observation: What to watch for and why. *Strategies,* 17–19.

Jelsma, O., & Pieters, J. M. (1989). Practice schedule and cognitive style interaction in learning a maze task. *Applied Cognitive Psychology, 3,* 73–83.

Jelsma, O., & Van Merrienboer, J. J. G. (1989). Contextual interference interactions with reflection-impulsivity. *Perceptual and Motor Skills, 68,* 1055–1064.

Jonides, J., & Gleitman, H. (1972). A conceptual category effect in visual search. *Perception and Psychophysics, 12,* 457–460.

Kernodle, M. W., & Carlton, L. G. (1992). Information feedback and the learning of multiple-degree-of-freedom activities. *Journal of Motor Behavior, 24* (2), 187–196.

Kirschenbaum, D. S., & Bale, R. M. (1980). Cognitive-behavioral skills in golf: Brain power golf. In R. M. Suinn (Ed.), *Psychology in sports: Methods and applications* (pp. 334–343). Minneapolis: Burgess.

Kluka, D. (1997). Observation skills: Qualitative analysis for competitive excellence. *FIVB The Coach, 3,* 24–27.

Landers, D. M. (1980). The arousal-performance relationship revised. *Research Quarterly for Exercise and Sport, 51,* 77–90.

Lansing, R. W., Schwartz, E., & Lindsley, D. B. (1956). Reaction time and EEG activation. *American Psychologist, 11,* 433.

Lee, T. D., & Magill, R. A. (1983). Activity during the post-KR interval: Effects upon performance or learning? *Research Quarterly for Exercise and Sport, 54,* 340–345.

Lee, T.D., White, M. A., & Canahan, H. (1990). On the role of knowledge of results in motor learning: Exploring the guidance hypothesis. *Journal of Motor Behavior, 22,* 119–208.

Luria, A. (1961). *The role of speech in the regulation of normal and abnormal behaviors.* New York: Liveright.

Maehr, M., & Braskamp, L. A. (1986). *The motivational factor: A theory of personal investment.* Lexington, MA: Lexington Books.

Magill, R. A. (1993). *Motor learning: Concepts and applications* (4th ed). Madison, WI: Brown & Benchmark Publishers.

Magill, R. A. (1994). The influence of augmented feedback on skill learning depends on characteristics of the skill and the learner. In R. A. Magill (Ed.), *Quest: Communicating information to enhance skill learning* (pp. 314–328). Champaign, IL: Human Kinetics.

Magill, R. A., Chamberlin, C. J., & Hall, K. G. (1991). Verbal knowledge of results as redundant information for learning an anticipation timing skill. *Human Movement Sciences, 10,* 485–507.

Mandler, G., & Sarason, S. B. (1952). A study of anxiety and learning. *Journal of Abnormal and Social Psychology, 47,* 166–173.

Martens, R. (1976). *Competitiveness in sport.* Paper presented at the International Congress of Physical Activity Sciences. Quebec City.

McAuley, E. (1985). Modeling and self-efficacy: A test of Bandura's model. *Journal of Sport Psychology, 6,* 283–295.

McAuley E. (1991). Efficacy, attributional, and affective responses to exercise participation. *Journal of Sport and Exercise Psychology, 13,* 382–393.

McClelland, D. C. (1961). *The achieving society.* New York: Free Press.

McCullagh, P., Weiss, M. R., & Ross, D. (1989). Modeling considerations in motor skill acquisition and performance: An integrated approach. In K. B. Pandolf (Ed.), *Exercise and sport science reviews* (vol. 17, pp. 475–513). Baltimore: Williams & Wilkins.

Murray, H. A. (1938). *Explorations in personality.* New York: Oxford University Press.

Newell, K. M. (1974). Knowledge of results and motor learning. *Journal of Motor Behavior, 6,* 235–244.

Nicholls, J. G. (1984). Achievement motivation: Conceptions of ability, subjective experience, task choice, and performance. *Psychological Review, 91,* 328–346.

Nideffer, R. (1976). Test of attentional and interpersonal style. *Journal of Personality and Social Psychology, 34,* 394–404.

Nideffer, R. (1979). The role of attention in optimal athletic performance. In P. Klavora & J. V. Daniel (Eds.), *Coach, athlete and the sport psychologist* (pp. 99–112). Toronto, Ontario: University of Toronto.

Pearl, A. J. (Ed.). (1993). *The athletic female.* Champaign, IL: Human Kinetics.

Posner, M. I., & Boies, S. J. (1971). Components of attention. *Psychological Review, 78,* 391–408.

Poulton, E. C. (1957). On prediction in skilled movements. *Psychological Bulletin, 54,* 467.

Richards, D. E., & Landers, D. M. (1981). *Test of attentional and interpersonal style scores of shooters.* Unpublished manuscript, Pennsylvania State University, University Park, PA.

Rink, J. (1985). *Teaching physical education for learning.* St. Louis: Times Mirror/Mosby.

Ripoll, H. (1988). Analysis of visual scanning patterns of volleyball players in a problem solving task. *International Journal of Sport Psychology, 19,* 9–25.

Roberts, G. C. (1972). Effect of achievement motivation and social environment on performance of a motor task. *Journal of Motor Behavior, 4,* 37–46.

Roberts, G. C. (1982). Achievement motivation in sport. In R. Terjung (Ed.), *Exercise and sport science reviews* (Vol. 10) (pp. 237–269). Philadelphia, PA: Franklin Institute Press.

Roberts, G. C. (1984). Achievement motivation in children's sport. In J. Nicholls (Ed.), *The development of achievement motivation* (pp. 251–281). Greenwich, CT: JAI Press.

Roberts, G. C. (1992). Motivation in sport and exercise: Conceptual constraints and convergence. In G. C. Roberts (Ed.), *Motivation in sport and exercise.* Champaign, IL: Human Kinetics.

Rose, D. J. (1997). *Multilevel approach to the study of motor learning and control.* Boston, MA: Allyn and Bacon.

Salmoni, A. W., Schmidt, R. A., & Walter, C. B. (1984). Knowledge of results and motor learning: A review and critical reappraisal. *Psychological Bulletin, 95,* 355–386.

Scanlan, T. K. (1988). Social evaluation and the competition process: A developmental perspective. In F. L. Smoll, R. A. Magill, & M. J. Ash (Eds.), *Children in sport* (3rd ed.) (pp. 135–148). Champaign, IL: Human Kinetics.

Schmidt, R. A. (1975). A schema theory of discrete motor skill learning. *Psychological Review, 82,* 225–260.

Schmidt, R. A. (1991). *Motor learning and performance: From principles to practice.* Champaign, IL: Human Kinetics.

Seefeldt, V., & Haubenstricker, J. (1982). Patterns, phrases, or stages: An analytical model for the study of developmental movement. In J. A. S. Kelso & J. E. Clark (Eds.), *The development of movement control and coordination* (pp. 309–318). New York: Wiley.

Shapiro, D. C., & Schmidt, R. A. (1982). A schema theory of discrete motor skill learning. *Psychological Review, 82,* 225–260.

Sheffield, F. N. (1961). Theoretical considerations in the learning of complex sequential tasks from demonstrations and practice. In A.A. Lumsdaine (Ed.), *Student response in programmed instruction* (pp. 13–32). Washington, DC: National Academy of Sciences, National Research Council.

Sigelman, C. K., & Shaffer, D. R. (1995). *Life-span human development.* Belmont, CA: Wadsworth.

Singer, R. (May 11, 1993). UF research shows success in sport involves much more than movement skills. *University of Florida Digest,* 7.

Stelmach, G. E. (1970). Learning and response consistency with augmented feedback. *Ergonomics, 13,* 421–425.

Stelmach, G. E., & Hughes, B. (1983). Does motor skill automation require a theory of attention? In R. A. Magill (Ed.), *Memory and control of action* (pp. 67–92). Amsterdam: North-Holland.

Stroop, J. R. (1935). Studies of interference in serial verbal reactions. *Journal of Experimental Psychology, 18,* 643–662.

Swinnen, S. P., Walter, C. B., Lee, T. D., & Serrien, D. J. (1993). Acquiring bimanual skills: Contrasting forms of information feedback for interlimb decoupling. *Journal of Experimental Psychology: Learning, Memory, and Cognition, 19*(6), 1328–1344.

Trachtman, J. N., & Kluka, D. A. (1993). Future trends of vision and peak sport performance. *International Journal of Sports Vision, 1*(1), 1–7.

van Rossum, J. H. A. (1987). *Motor development and practice: The variability of practice hypothesis in perspective.* Amsterdam: Free University Press.

Wallace, S. A., & Hagler, R. W. (1979). Knowledge of performance and the learning of a closed motor skill. *Research Quarterly, 50,* 265–271.

Weinberg, R. S., & Gould, D. (1995). *Foundations of sport and exercise psychology.* Champaign, IL: Human Kinetics.

Weinberg, R. S., & Ragan, J. (1978). Motor performance under three levels of trait anxiety and stress. *Journal of Motor Behavior, 10,* 169–176.

Weiner, B. (1985). An attributional theory of achievement motivation and emotion. *Psychological Review, 92,* 548–575.

Weiner, B. (1986). *An attributional theory of motivation and emotion.* New York: Springer-Verlag.

Weiss, M. R., & Klint, K. A. (1987). "Show and tell" in the gymnasium: An investigation of developmental differences in modeling and verbal rehearsal of motor skills. *Research Quarterly for Exercise and Sport, 58,* 234–241.

Winstein, C. J., & Schmidt, R. A. (1990). Reduced frequency of knowledge of results enhances motor skill learning. *Journal of Experimental Psychology: Learning, Memory, and Cognition, 16,* 677–691.

Wohl, A. (1977). *Bewegung und Sprache.* Schorndorf: Hofmann.

Yerkes, R. M., & Dodson, J. D. (1908). The relationship of strength of stimulus to rapidity of habit formation. *Journal of Comparative Neurology and Psychology, 18,* 459–482.

Zaichkowsky, L. D., Dorsey, J. A., & Mulholland, T. B. (1979). The effects of biofeedback assisted systematic desensitization in the control of anxiety and performance. In M. Vanek (Ed.), *IV sretovy kongress, ISSP* (pp. 809–812). Prague: Olympia.

Zaichkowsky, L. D., & Fuchs, C. Z. (1989). Biofeedback-assisted self-regulation for stress management in sports. In D. Hackfort & C. D. Spielberger (Eds.), *Anxiety in sports* (pp. 235–245). Washington, DC: Hemisphere.

Social Perspectives

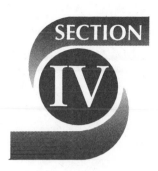

Jody Conradt is the winningest women's college basketball coach in the United States. She is the first women's basketball coach to win 600 games and the first to win 700 games, the first to coach a women's team to an undefeated season and a national championship, and held a 12-year undefeated dynasty in Southwest Conference play (183 consecutive victories against Southwest Conference teams). The practice environment established at The University of Texas at Austin provided much of the "right stuff" for those Conradt coached to performance excellence. At The University of Texas at Austin, Conradt's teams qualified for the NCAA National Tournaments 14 times since 1983 and won the national championship in 1986 by going a perfect 34–0. In 1991 she was honored with the National Association for Girls and Women in Sport's (NAGWS) Guiding Woman in Sport Award for her national leadership. In 1998, she was inducted into the Naismith Memorial Basketball Hall of Fame in Springfield, Massachusetts. What could be some of the components that contributed to Conradt's performance success from a social perspective?

Dynamics of the Practice Environment

*T*he precise manner in which to arrange practice environments is still under discussion. **Practice environment** refers to the surroundings and conditions used to rehearse motor behavior performances. As was discussed in the previous chapter, motor behavior from learning to performance is multidimensional. Because people and practice conditions change, it is impossible to generate

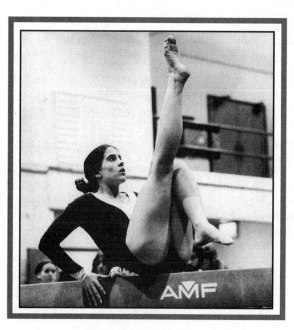

Practice environment
the surroundings and conditions used for rehearsal of motor behavior performances

Classical conditioning
shaping the relationship between stimulus and response, how a stimulus or a response is associated with another stimulus, and the conditions under which stimulus and response are independently assessed

Extinction
the process of phasing out a behavior; the length of time between presentation of the original stimulus to evoke a response and the new stimulus to evoke the same response

Schedule of reinforcement
a program to selectively reinforce behavior through positive and negative rewards

Positive reinforcement
rewards that the recipient perceives as pleasurable

Negative reinforcement
rewards that the recipient perceives as unpleasant

Fixed rate reinforcement
a type of schedule of reinforcement that is given after predesignated trials

statements about motor behavior that are absolute. We know more about how to sustain life on a space station than we do about how individuals learn and perform motorically. It is possible, however, to provide perspectives that are based on research. It is also evident that additional research is needed in several areas of interest to provide greater understanding of the impact that the practice environment has on human motor behavior.

Much of the information that was first used to determine the difference between learning and performance came from animal experimentation. In the early 1900s, the notion of **classical conditioning** was devised (Pavlov, 1927). Pavlov used dogs to test conditioned reflexes. The dogs' salivation, brought on initially by the introduction of food, activated a lever connected to a pen. The pen, attached to a rod that was suspended onto a revolving drum, provided a graphic representation of each drop of saliva. In one experiment, the dog was conditioned to salivate when it saw a circle, thereby replacing the food with the circle. The dog was then shown an ellipse, but given no food. The dog soon learned to discriminate between an ellipse and a circle. Then it was shown a series of ellipses, progressively circular in appearance. When the ellipses became almost circular, the dog changed its behavior markedly; it barked and growled and refused to eat any of the food it was given. This type of research design identified a relationship between stimulus and response, how a stimulus or a response could be associated with another stimulus, and the conditions under which stimulus and response had to be independently assessed. The learning effect, which was achieved by removing the unconditioned stimulus (food), was determined by how often the conditioned stimulus (circle) evoked the response (salivation). The length of time it took to eliminate a conditioned response by lack of reinforcement was known as the period of **extinction**.

The work conducted by Pavlov led to a number of research studies of learning through reinforcement. Behavior was reinforced selectively (using **schedules of reinforcement**), with **positive** (something pleasurable) and **negative** (something unpleasant) **reinforcement**. Typically, positive reinforcement for animals was food; negative reinforcement was a mild electric shock. Schedules of reinforcement were used each time an appropriate behavior was exhibited, or after clusters of appropriate responses. For example, reinforcement was given after every third response (**fixed rate reinforcement**) or after the average of three responses (**variable rate** reinforcement). By assessing varying types of practice conditions, researchers determined the strength and length of retention of the learned behavior. Animal investigations involving reflexive behavior and the impact of practice conditions on learning and performance, while quite different from the acquisition of voluntarily controlled skilled action, laid the groundwork for understanding the differences between the measurement of learning and performance.

In animal experimentations, rewards for specific behaviors were often used to mold an animal's response. For example, food was used as a positive reinforcer to a rat to run a maze, taking a particular path. Food was provided every time the rat would perform the route (or a part of the route) appropriately. Schedules of reinforcement were varied (food might be used on every third response or every fifth response) to determine which practice conditions would create the longest learned response. These programs of conditioning by varying schedules of reinforcement helped us to understand the differences between learning and performance. It was determined (McGeoch, 1927, 1929, 1931) that although one type of reinforcement schedule may produce superior performance while the skill is being acquired, that same schedule may not be the best to produce outstanding performance when individuals are evaluated later.

RETENTION, TRANSFER, AND PRACTICE

The relationship of retention and transfer were detailed in Section I of this text. The degree to which skilled motor behavior is generalizable has met with limited support. There seems to be, however, an unsubstantiated viewpoint among many non-motor behavior professionals (Singley & Anderson, 1989) that some have a predisposition for superior "general motor abilities," thereby influencing their ability to perform well motorically.

On the other hand, the identical elements theory described in Section I referred to specific transfer (Thorndike, 1903), the idea that the more similar the elements that comprise individual tasks are, the greater the transfer of learning between them. Researchers (Schmidt, 1988; Adams, 1987) have suggested that the ability to learn and perform motor skills is highly specific. Transfer of skills would be expected to be highly specific as well.

A third position, which accepts something of both of the above-mentioned positions, refers to the notion of processing information that is *appropriately transferrable* (Bransford, Franks, Morris, &

Variable rate reinforcement
a schedule of reinforcement after an average of trials, thereby making the rate varying

LAB EXERCISE

PRACTICE, RETENTION, TRANSFER

Objective: To explore differences in practice, retention, and transfer as they relate to performance.

Equipment and Preparation: Two partners; 5 racquetballs; 2 pieces of rope, each four feet long; blindfold; tape measure; masking tape. Place a line, measuring two feet in length, on the floor, using the masking tape. Measure the distances of 10 and 12 feet from the tape mark. Place small pieces of tape to mark the spots. With the rope, make circles on the floor around the spots so that the spots become the circles' centers.

Experience: While blindfolded, Partner One tosses a total of 10 (practice) racquetballs in an underhand motion so that they bounce inside the circle. Record all trials as successful or unsuccessful. Partner Two retrieves the balls. Partner Three hands balls to Partner One. Partner Two then tosses 10 balls in the same manner, without being blindfolded. Everyone then rests for an additional 5 minutes after Partner Three is finished. Using the same performance schedule, each performer is blindfolded and and tosses 5 balls from 10 feet (retention) and 5 from 12 feet away (transfer). No feedback should be given throughout the trials.

Assignment: Determine the number of successful attempts for each performer under the following three conditions: (1) practice conditions;
(2) retention conditions;
(3) transfer conditions.

Calculate the mean for each. Using a bar graph, plot the means for each performer. Discuss the findings as they relate to practice, retention, and transfer.

Stein, 1979). This perspective provides the added dimension of information processing as a preselection for that which is to follow. For example, the more appropriate the learning and the better the fit for motor skill transfer are, the greater the transfer later. In other words, the closer the practice environment is to the actual transfer test, the higher the likelihood of transfer.

Bilateral transfer
a concept that holds that performing a motor skill using one side of the body will also increase performance when using the other side of the body to perform the same movement

BILATERAL TRANSFER AND PRACTICE

Within the construct of retention of learning and transfer lies an interesting phenomenon: **bilateral transfer**. Simply put, performing a motor skill using one side of the body will also improve performance for the same movement when it is done with the other side of the body. For example, when a layup shot in basketball is initially practiced and performed using the right side of the body from the right side of the basket, the shot, taken with the left hand and from the left side of the basket, is also enhanced (Hicks, Gualtieri, & Schroeder, 1983).

It has been determined that bilateral transfer is neuromuscularly and cognitively rooted. Neuromuscularly, *schema theory* (Schmidt, 1975) supports findings of corresponding EMG readings found when an individual performs a task with one side of the body in appendages on the other side of the body (Hicks, Frank, & Kinsbourne, 1982).

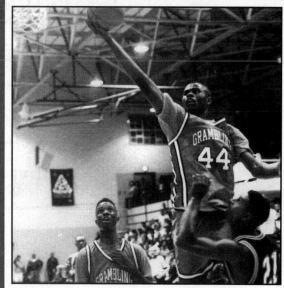

A layup shot, practiced with the right hand, can enhance the shot when the left hand is used.

It has also been suggested that if a person practices with one appendage and then performs a mirror image of the task with the other appendage, greater positive transfer is likely to occur. On simple tasks, such as using a pursuit rotor with the preferred hand, it was found that there was greatest bilateral transfer when subjects used the mirror-image technique rather than same-direction or opposite-direction responses (Hicks, Gualtieri, & Schroeder, 1983).

Cognitively, bilateral transfer can occur from processing within the central nervous system that may bypass the neuromuscular system (Kohl & Roenker, 1983). This perspective received credence based upon information gleaned from experiments involving mental rehearsal, in which EMG readings were produced in the limb that was involved in the mental rehearsal (Feltz & Landers, 1983; Feltz & Riessinger, 1990) and not in the one on the opposite side. This cognitively based perspective does not negate the inclusion of the neuromuscular system; it suggests that there is an interconnection between the cognitive and neuromuscular perspectives that facilitates bilateral transfer. Additionally, when mental practice is used in conjunction with physical practice, it has been suggested that the use of both techniques may facilitate the greatest amount of bilateral transfer (Kohl & Roenker, 1980; 1983).

FACTORS INFLUENCING LEARNING AND PERFORMANCE IN A PRACTICE ENVIRONMENT

Several factors influence learning and performance in a practice environment. One has to do with the *structure* of the practice session; another refers to the way in which the practice is *organized*; and the third concerns the effect the first two have on the individual, or the *amount/distribution* of practice.

PRACTICE STRUCTURE

The quality and quantity of motor skill practice has been considered, discussed, analyzed, debated, and argued over for over three centuries by motor behavior professionals. Jody Conradt undoubtedly has considered, discussed, analyzed, debated and argued over practice structure during her professional career. What is important is to consider the context in which particular motor skills are to be performed. The motor behavior professional who can best determine what the environment most appropriately resembles will be able to structure a practice that leads to successful performance. For example, the gymnast who performs a side horse routine is in an environment that is extremely stable: the horse, the pommels, and the judges all remain in the same proximity to one another and are relatively immovable. The table tennis player is provided with a rather dynamic environment, where the speed of the ball and spins placed on it vary greatly; the table and net, however, are quite stable. The team handball goalie is provided with quite a dynamic environment, where ball speed and trajectory, offense and defense strategies, and number of players involved fluctuates from moment-to-moment. This type of environment produces a high level of uncertainty, especially when compared to the side horse event in gymnastics.

Practice variability changes in the practice environment to provide variety

In any of these environments, the notion of **practice variability** is an important one (Schmidt, 1975) as a basis for structuring the practice of discrete skills. From an applied perspective, *schema theory* suggests that if an individual experiences motor skills multidimensionally and in a variety of situations, a set of principles are developed from which movement can be selected based upon the dynamics of the environment. For example, the following practice experiences can be devised for individuals to experience a variety of ways in which to dribble in field hockey:

- Dribble clockwise in a circle that is 3 m (10 feet); dribble counterclockwise in a circle that is 3 m;

- Dribble clockwise in a circle that is 1 m (3 feet); dribble counterclockwise in a circle that is 1 m;

- Dribble forward 5 m (15 feet); dribble diagonally forward to the right 5 m; dribble diagonally forward to the left 5 m;

- Dribble from the left of the top of the striking circle and shoot for the right back corner of the goal; dribble from the right of the top of the striking circle and shoot for the left back corner of the goal.

Dribble for 3 m, pass left to a teammate, run ahead, receive a pass from that person, dribble 3 m, pass right to another teammate, run ahead, receive a pass from that person, dribble and drive for the back right corner of the goal.

It has been found (Gould & Weiss, 1987; Smoll, Magill, & Ash, 1988; Weiss & Ebbeck, 1995) that children benefit greatly from the use of variety in the practice structure to accommodate for shorter attention spans and less performance skill under a variety of conditions. Children should learn basic motor patterns such as skipping, hopping, jumping, and leaping. Experiences that are designed by the motor behavior professional to practice those skills in a variety of movement zones (high, medium, and low), in a variety of timing sequences (sustained, midspeed, and percussive), and in various directions (forward, backward, upward, downward, right, left) are important for developing patterns that can be transferred to meet environmental demands.

Part of the motor behavior professional's responsibility is to provide learning and performance experiences that promote the linkage of one motor skill practiced in one setting to another motor skill in another setting. For example, the Louisiana School for the Blind provides myriad opportunities for adults to have movement experiences that closely link movement patterns together with real-world environments without the use of vision. Many participate in sport and physical activity experiences, using alternative sensory information (olfaction, audition, kinesthesis, tactile, and gustatory) to guide motor behavior success.

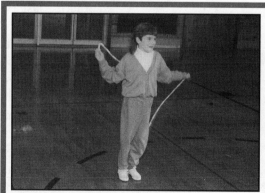

Learning the basic motor pattern of jumping is beneficial to children.

When to introduce variations in the practice structure is one of the motor behavior professional's considerations. One of the models presented previously included two basic stages of learning: *stage one,* to develop an overall idea of the skills, and *stage two,* depending upon the environment, to diversify or fixate movement. Considering these two constructs carefully, the motor behavior professional can surmise that, until the individual has gotten the idea of the skill, varying practice would have limited meaning in the motor learning process. By creating a practice environment that initially contains repeatedly similar experiences (on the continuum of closed to open skilled behavior), the individual can better find the meaning and relevance of movement.

In stage two of the model, the determination of environmental demands can easily provide the format from which meaningful and appropriately varied experiences can be created. When the environment requires diverse skills, providing experiences that vary from similarly repeated trials becomes a necessity. When the environment requires fixation of skills, experiences that vary from exact routine are also important, as attention can easily wax and wane, thereby reducing the quality of the learning experiences.

Following are two examples of ways in which the motor behavior professional can structure the practice environment to include practice variability based upon the two-stage motor learning model (Gentile, 1972):

● **Gymnastics** — *Floor exercise (relatively closed, internally paced, stable environment)*

Practice tumbling passes in isolation of dance movements; practice last two tumbling tricks from initial pass into dance movements and into second tumbling pass; practice opening pose through first tumbling pass and dance movements; practice final tumbling pass through final pose; practice final pass, ending in a less difficult skill/more difficult skill (less difficult skill = tuck back somersault; more difficult skill = double tuck back somersault); practice the last one-third of the routine first; practice the first one-third of the routine last; practice the middle one-third of the routine first; practice the entire routine with no music playing; practice the entire routine with no one else moving or speaking in the gymnasium; practice tumbling passes and/or dance movements in tandem with another gymnast.

Through varieties of experiences in varying sequences, the gymnast is provided with opportunities to focus attention and quality of practice on portions of the routine. She is also able to practice alternatives in case hand or foot placement is inappropriate to succeed in difficult tumbling passes, rather than bailing out of a move with no alternative previously rehearsed.

• **Beach volleyball attack in four-person** *(relatively open, externally paced, dynamic environment)*

Practice a short middle attack off a pass from the back row; practice a left side high-outside attack from a pass coming from left back, coming from right back; practice a right side high-outside attack from a pass coming from left back, coming from right back; practice a shoot set from a pass coming from right back; practice a right side attack, but dumping the ball into the left back area; use two blockers on the opposite side of the net for these sequences; mix these up so that they are randomly performed within the practice environment.

By creating variations in ball velocity, angle, direction, height, and distance, the beach player is provided with challenging experiences that more closely resemble the dynamic environment of beach volleyball. Players are afforded opportunities to experience variations of the basic attack movement.

Despite the detailed discussion of practice variability, a second pressing issue must also be considered: Is there a best way to organize practice that is most conducive for learning and enhancing performance?

PRACTICE ORGANIZATION

Because of its level of interest for motor behavior professionals and researchers, the issue of how to organize practice continues to be discussed. Through the work of several researchers (Battig, 1966, 1972, 1977; Shea & Morgan, 1979; Lee & Magill, 1983; Goode & Magill, 1986), this topic has become one of the most investigated in motor behavior.

Logic used by the motor behavior professional would dictate that practices could easily be organized by similar skills rehearsal; that is, **blocked practice**, whereby players practice many repetitions

Blocked practice training in which individuals practice many repetitions of the same skill before going on to another skill

of the same skill before going on to another skill. For example, players have shot and made 100 free throws after practice; players have performed 50 tennis serves in a row; or players have completed 30 down-the-line serves in volleyball. Using the blocked practice approach, a typical blocked practice schedule might look like this in indoor volleyball (two-hour practice session):

- 15 minutes — warmup
- 15 minutes — serving
- 15 minutes — passing
- 15 minutes — setting/hitting
- 15 minutes — hitting/blocking/transition
- 30 minutes — simulated game
- 15 minutes — conditioning/cool down

This blocked practice schedule approach, however, has been seriously challenged by a theoretical framework (Battig, 1966) considered a classic in the facilitation of learning and interference within a context (**contextual interference**). The theory was developed to explain the effects of randomized task presentation on verbal skills acquisition. Basically, learning through performance is better retained when the practice environment contains elements of high contextual interference. Although low–contextual interference practice sessions produce great initial performances, practice sessions fraught with high contextual interference produce longer-lasting performance retention. To apply this notion to motor learning, a paradigm-shifting investigation was conducted (Shea & Morgan, 1979) involving two groups who used quick hand and arm movements. One group practiced three different movements in blocked order, completing a total of 54 trials: 18 trials of the first movement, followed by 18 trials for the second, and finishing with 18 trials of the third. The other group also completed a total of 54 trials, but each pattern was randomly interspersed in the total number of trials. Initially, subjects using the blocked practice schedule showed substantially more improvement than the random practice schedule group. However, when a randomly

Contextual interference
the use of different contexts to practice several skills

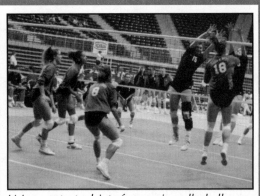

Using contextual interference in volleyball practice is advantageous at the elite level.

designed test for learning followed ten days later, the group that used the random practice schedule had superior retention.

Although blocked practice schedules help players in their initial decision-making and performance enhancement, when interference is introduced to simulate real-world conditions, learning becomes less efficient. Under conditions where the environment is dynamic and the player must adapt to variations, random practice schedules are superior to blocked practice sessions for retaining motor skills. The learner, however, is quite likely to perform worse during practice, but better days afterward in the real-world environment of the game or match. The motor behavior professional must use patience, understanding, and creativity to enhance learning. An additional and important perspective is that random practice benefits most those who use different motor programs to accomplish the goals of tasks (Schmidt, 1988; Magill & Hall, 1990). Those who perform skills requiring the same basic motor program may benefit more from blocked practice schedules. Additional research needs to be conducted in ecologically based investigations to definitively prove this perspective.

A possible revision to the blocked practice schedule for volleyball shown earlier would incorporate conditioning into all drills so that a separate time would not need to be parceled out. Additionally, only drills that incorporate a minimum of three volleyball-related skills should be used in practice, because the game flows with a minimum of three skills per action. Practice sessions could be arranged using the most difficult cognitively based skills interspersed with those requiring limited decision-making time. Drills that require players to practice leadership, decision-making, and match management under stress should also be interspersed throughout the practice time.

Other factors should be considered when determining the level of contextual interference to be used in the practice environment. They include individual variations in intellectual capability, age, experience, and learning style (Magill & Hall, 1990).

Variations in Intellectual Capability

In discussions of learning, retention, and performance, individual variations in intellectual capability must be considered. Information is sparse about the effects of blocked and random practice schedules with individuals with reduced intellectual capabilities. Additional investigations using players with Down syndrome, those involved in Special Olympics, and those who have sustained head trauma would substantially add to our knowledge base. What *is* known has been determined from two published investigations (Edwards, Elliott, & Lee, 1986; Heitman & Gilley, 1989). These studies focused on learning to anticipate under three conditions, using groups of adolescents with and without Down syndrome. Both groups experienced blocked and random practice schedules. The group without Down syndrome benefited more from random practice; the group with Down syndrome benefited about equally from blocked and random practice schedules. With the limited information available, we cannot reach firm conclusions about the usefulness of random or blocked practice schedules for people with reduced intellectual capabilities. It would seem, however, that blocked and random practice schedules can be successfully used with those who possess Down syndrome.

Variations in Age

Generally, when working with children, investigators have found quite mixed results. In some investigations (Del Rey, Whitehurst, & Wood, 1983; Pigott & Shapiro, 1984), blocked practice sessions have proven superior for skill practice sessions. In other investigations (Pollock & Lee, 1990; Edwards, Elliott, & Lee, 1986), random proved more effective than blocked. From a practical perspective, the motor behavior professional may have to experiment with both types of practice schedules to determine what tasks, task difficulty, and age groups are more conducive to one type of session or the other until additional research is conducted.

With university-aged (18 to 25 years) or older adults (65 to 92 years), it has been determined that random practice scheduling is superior to blocked practice for retention of motor skills (Del Rey, 1989; Proteau, Marteniuk, Girouard, & Dugas, 1987). A substantial positive effect was found (Del Rey, 1982) in active rather than sedentary older adults; the benefit of random practice, however, was significant with all older adults.

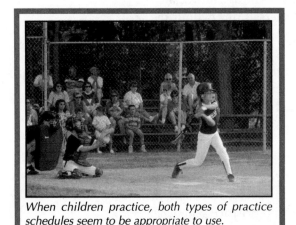

When children practice, both types of practice schedules seem to be appropriate to use.

Variations in Experience

Several investigations have been conducted involving individuals' levels of experience and the amount of contextual interference incorporated into the practice environment (Del Rey, 1982; Del Rey, 1989; Del Rey, Wughalter, & Whitehurst, 1982; Del Rey, Whitehurst, & Wood, 1983; Goode, 1986). The categorization of individuals was similar to that which has been used in the development of the expert-novice paradigm referred to in Section III of this text. Within the expert-novice paradigm, one of the characteristics of the expert is that of

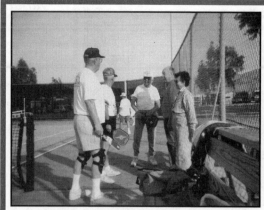

Random practice seems to be superior to blocked practice for older adults.

detailed perceptual knowledge of the skill and what it takes to perform it in a variety of contexts. The novice, on the other hand, is still trying to become familiar with the general concept of the skill as it relates to the goal. In these investigations, those who had limited or no perceptual knowledge of how to perform the skill and had never before performed the skill were considered to be novices. Based upon the two-stage model of learning (Gentile, 1972), it would seem logical that if the individual has not gotten the idea, that person would not benefit from contextual interference imbedded in a random practice schedule. The investigations support this notion.

One additional investigation might provide one important piece of information for the motor behavior professional to consider. Investigators (Goode & Wei, 1988) used a mixed approach that was devised (Lee & Magill, 1983) to combine blocked and random practice schedules into the learning and retention process. It was determined that if novice adults initially used a blocked practice schedule when learning to anticipate and followed it with a random practice schedule, long-term transfer and performance were enhanced. This is helpful in retention.

Considering these factors, the motor behavior professional must again factor in individuals' experience with specific skills or related skills in order to more appropriately determine when higher contextual interference can be added to the practice environment. It is also worthwhile to consider combining the two forms of practice organization when working with novice adults.

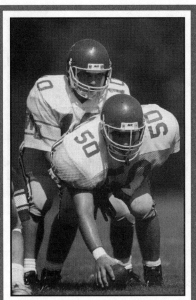

Variations in experience affect the amount of contextual interference used in the practice environment.

Variations in Learning Style

Cognitive learning style, as discussed earlier (Section III), may also affect an individual's response to the type and form of contextual interference used in the learning process. A somewhat limited number of investigators (Jelsma & Pieters, 1989; Jelsma & Van Merrienboer, 1989) have discerned that when tasks require accuracy as well as speed, the style of learning one is most comfortable with may affect the level of contextual interference needed for greatest retention.

The investigators found that those who were comfortable with impulsive or reactive learning styles gave up accuracy for speed. On the other hand, those with reflective or proactive learning styles gave up speed for accuracy. High levels of contextual interference, generally prevalent in random practice schedules, seemed to be best for those who were comfortable with reflective learning styles, as random practice requires greater decision-making and reflection strategies. Those with impulsive learning styles benefited more from blocked practice schedules. It should be obvious, however, that much more research needs to be conducted before we can conclude what influence learning style has on the learning and performance of motor skills that require speed and accuracy.

To summarize, focusing on relevant environmental cues has been shown to be of great importance to learning success.

LAB EXERCISE

VERBAL INSTRUCTION

Objective: To determine the importance of verbal instruction in skill performance.

Equipment and Preparation: Paper and pencil.

Experience: Develop a set of instructions for presenting the forward roll to a group of freshmen in high school; develop a set of instructions for presenting the forward roll to a group of first graders.

Assignment: Determine their similarity and their differences. What is their prospective effectiveness with students?

Routine Effectiveness

It has been shown that practice with distractions (contextual interference) present is important. A systematic presentation of distractors is helpful in creating a gamelike practice environment. The establishment of routines before, during, and after performances can also affect learning and the retention of motor skills. The effectiveness of routines is well documented (Cohn, Rotella, & Lloyd, 1990; Lobmeyer, & Wasserman, 1986; Orlick, 1986; Schmidt, 1975). Motor behavior professionals can help individuals to develop pre-performance routines during practice that can be easily transferred to performance environments. Two examples are listed in Table 11.1.

SPEED/ACCURACY TRADEOFF AND PRACTICE ORGANIZATION

A debate that arises when determining how best to control the dynamics of the practice environment is what the goal should be for motor skills that require both speed and accuracy. One of the most useful paradigms devised on the topic is known as **Fitts' law** (Fitts, 1954). Fitts' law suggests that there is a tradeoff between speed and accuracy. When speed is emphasized, accuracy is reduced; when

Fitts' Law
a principle involving the tradeoff between speed and accuracy: When speed is emphasized, accuracy is reduced; when accuracy is emphasized, speed is reduced

TABLE
11.1

Pre-Performance Routines

Volleyball Serve

1. Determine the desired placement of the serve.
2. Place body and feet in an optimum position behind the endline.
3. Visually image and kinesthetically feel a successful serve.
4. Take a deep breath and exhale.
5. Wait for the referee's whistle for service.
6. Toss the ball, focusing on the point of contact, and serve it.

Bowling Delivery

1. Take a deep breath and exhale.
2. Look at the pins and determine what is required for success.
3. Position the body and feet appropriately behind the foul line.
4. Visually image and kinesthetically feel the approach, swing, and release of the successful ball.
5. Focus on the target, begin the approach, swing, and release the ball.
6. Hold the follow-through and observe the ball's arrival.

SPEED AND ACCURACY

Objective: To determine what is most effective for performance accuracy.

Equipment and Preparation: Archery target; cement block wall; ten tennis balls; masking tape; tape measure; clipboard; pencil; three archery target models (one representing speed, one accuracy, and one speed and accuracy). Measure off twelve feet from the wall and mark it with masking tape on the floor. Tape the archery target to the wall so that the bull's-eye is at eye level.

Experience: Throw the tennis balls at an archery target, ten for speed, ten for accuracy, and ten for both speed and accuracy.

Assignment: Using an *X*, record the contact location of each tennis ball on the archery target models. Graph accuracy of each relative to the center. What is the best approach for accuracy?

accuracy is emphasized, speed is reduced. To determine the relationship between speed and accuracy, a tapping test was used. Using a stylus in their preferred hand, subjects were asked to alternately tap metal plates (targets) as rapidly as possible. The distance between the plates was varied; the sizes of the plates also varied. Movement time was recorded between each tapping of targets. It was found that as the need for accuracy decreased, speed of movement could be increased. To summarize, as the distance of targets increases, movement time increases; as target size decreases, movement time increases; if the distance between targets remains the same and target size remains the same, movement time remains essentially the same; and if target distance and target size change, movement time changes proportionately.

Fitt's law has several important implications for motor behavior professionals designing a practice environment. Table 11. 2 provides important information to consider.

If the goal of the movement involves primarily spatial accuracy (the "where to . . . ," such as throwing darts at a target), movements should be made more slowly to reduce spatial errors. To avoid spatial error, experiences that are initially closer to the target are helpful (e.g., if the goal is a down-the-line serve in volleyball, initially moving the server closer to the net; dart throwing; target archery).

Goal	Movement	Examples	TABLE 11.2
Spatial accuracy	Decrease speed or distance	Down-the-line serve in volleyball; dart throwing; target archery	*Speed/Accuracy Paradigm*
Temporal accuracy	Increase speed; decrease movement time	Cricket batting; tennis drive; badminton smash	

If the movement goal primarily involves temporal accuracy (the "timing" of the skill, such as when to swing the bat at the ball in cricket), increasing the speed of the movement will reduce errors in timing accuracy. Additionally, the longer the movement time is, the more likely it will be that temporal errors will occur (Newell, Carlton, Carlton, & Halbert, 1980). When movement distance is increased, so is speed (Schmidt, Zelaznik, Hawkins, Frank, & Quinn, 1979). This has little, if any, effect on temporal accuracy.

If the movement goal is to generate huge amounts of force (e.g., kicking a football from the 40-yard line; executing a smash in badminton or a forehand drive in tennis), speed can be increased by decreasing movement time. Adding slightly more weight to the movement can also decrease error, as in using a racket that weighs more.

In situations where implement-to-object contact is important (such as baseball, softball, badminton, tennis, jai alai, cricket), the swing to contact should be initiated and completed with high levels of muscular involvement; therefore, the swing should be performed at a high rate of speed. Practice can also be enhanced by slightly increasing the weight of the implement. For example, by increasing the weight of a bat by a few ounces, cumulative speed will be increased. Muscle fiber recruitment increases and this helps muscles and joints to vary speed. If, however, the intent is to quicken the speed of the swing, decreasing the length of the implement and/or shortening movement time would facilitate this as well.

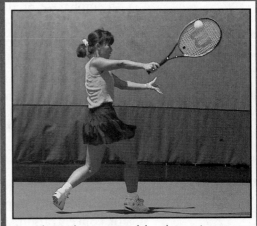

Speed can be increased by decreasing movement time.

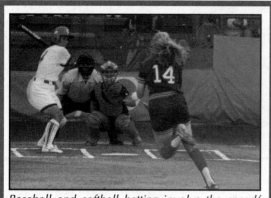
Baseball and softball batting involve the speed/accuracy paradigm.

To illustrate this point succinctly: Baseball batting has been rather thoroughly investigated (Hubbard & Seng, 1954; Slater-Hammel & Stumpner, 1950; Bahill & LaRitz, 1984). Schmidt (1991) relates the following scenario: A baseball, pitched at approximately 90 mph, travels from release to the plate in approximately 450 ms. The movement time of a bat averages 160 ms. The eyes and brain signal the swing approximately 160 ms prior to the initiation of the movement. Regarding the decision whether to swing at the ball or not, decision time and movement time must be factored into the equation (in this case, 160 ms [for the decision] + 160 ms [for the movement time] = 320 ms). Because the ball takes 450 ms to be delivered and because 320 ms of that are used to signal and execute the swing, there remains only 130 ms to decide whether or not to swing. From a practical perspective, the decision to swing or not would have to be made in approximately the first one-fourth (0.29) of the trajectory after the pitcher's release. The batter waiting to decide until the pitch has traveled halfway to the plate has waited too long to limit temporal error.

Because much of the necessary information about the environment must be gleaned from conditions that precede the initiation of movement, it is also important for the motor behavior professional to emphasize predictive cues (detailed in Section III) that will facilitate advance information. It is also important for the individual to begin each movement from a basic "ready" position so that the motor behavior elicited becomes somewhat consistent. With repeated performances as an inherent part of the practice environment, it is important to consider yet another element when designing instruction: physiological fatigue.

FATIGUE AND MOTOR BEHAVIOR

Physiological fatigue affects an individual's motor learning and performance multidimensionally. One of the affected dimensions is that of concentration. (Concentration was discussed in Section III.) An average marathoner, for example, completes the 26.2-mile journey in three to three-and-a-half hours. Researchers investigating the cognitive strategies of elite marathon runners (Silva & Applebaum, 1989; Schomer, 1986) discovered that those who were faster used a combination of associative and disassociative attentional strategies, while those who finished later used disassociative attentional strategies almost exclusively. **Associative attentional strategy** refers to focus upon heart and breathing rates as well as muscular tension; **disassociative attentional strategy** refers to denying physiological feedback from the body in order to cope with fatigue, abdominal cramping, or "hitting the wall." The motor behavior professional who can help individuals to learn when to associate and when to disassociate effectively will facilitate experiences that are generally without injury and will maximize efficiency and effectiveness.

Most of the research conducted on fatigue and its relationship to learning and the performance of motor skills has focused on decreases in performance rather than impact on learning (Caplan, 1969; Stelmach, 1969; Poulton, 1988). Based upon theories of motor control proposed in the 1960s (see Section I for details), fatigue is a by-product of retroactive inhibition, or a lack of sufficient stimulus to perform the task at hand. This type of fatigue may have an impact on the learning of a motor skill. Other investigators (Carron, 1972; Nunney, 1963; Godwin & Schmidt, 1971; Dwyer, 1984) have tried to determine states of fatigue through the use of step tests, bicycle ergometers, and treadmills. This type of fatigue may have an impact on performance.

Associative attentional strategy
focusing on items that associate with a motor behavior, such as heart and breathing rates as well as muscular tension, while running a marathon

Disassociative attentional strategy
focusing on items separate from motor behavior, such as denying physiological feedback from the body to cope with fatigue, abdominal cramping, or "hitting the wall" when running a marathon

Fatigue and the Performance of a Motor Skill

In general, the higher the level of fatigue, the more detrimental the performance outcome. Theorists view this as being similar to the inverted-U hypothesis (Yerkes & Dodson, 1908), whereby motor skill performance is actually enhanced by low to moderate levels of fatigue. Investigators have tried to induce low to moderate levels of fatigue to illustrate this point (Williams & Singer, 1975; Carron, 1972; Richards, 1968). Once fatigue has reached a particular level, performance begins to plummet, declining to the point of total failure. Other investigators have tried to quantify the upper limits of fatigue to illustrate the near-failure of performance (Carron, 1972; Richards, 1968; Cobb, 1994).

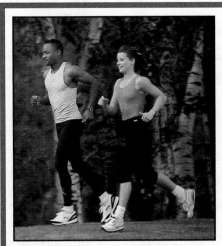

Variations in practice facilitates learning and performance.

Low to moderate levels of fatigue seem to have no effect on learning but may lead to decreases in performance. High levels of fatigue may affect both. It has been determined that performance deteriorates for several reasons: (1) lactate levels in the blood rise enough to produce an environment in which there is insufficient muscular innervation to produce optimal muscular contraction (Cobb, 1994; Richards, 1968); (2) there is insufficient neural circuitry functioning to promote neuromuscular coordination (Richards, 1968); and (3) there is insufficient attentional focus for the continuation of the activity (Allard, 1982). From a motor behavior professional's perspective, it would seem logical that levels of factors that contribute to fitness (i.e., cardiorespiratory strength and endurance, muscular strength and endurance, flexibility, dynamic and static balance, and agility), would play a substantial role in performance. These factors, however, have not been quantitatively applied to research designs in this area of interest.

What *has* been determined is that performance is more seriously affected if fatigue is introduced early into the practice setting rather than later in practice; muscular fatigue can be isolated to parts of the body (e.g., legs or arms) (Caplan, 1969; Cobb, 1994); and muscular fatigue can also be a by-product of psychological distress (Weinberg, 1989). There has remained some controversy, however, over the probability of fatigue in isolated body parts alone. Depending upon the level of fatigue and the fitness of the individual, it has also been determined (Nunney, 1963) that fatigue, induced by bicycle ergometers, treadmills, or step tests, produced similar effects on manipulative tasks (e.g., mirror tracing, pursuit rotor): fatigue created a detriment in performance. Because some investigators have reported conditions of fatigue to be detrimental to performance and others have not, this area requires further study. It would be particularly useful for investigators to also consider the role of baseline fitness and the novelty of skills used when they try to determine the impact of fatigue on motor skill performance.

A practical example of the challenge fatigue presents to motor skill performance involves the sport of biathlon. The goal of biathlon is to cover a distance through the snow, using cross country skis, and shoot for accuracy with a rifle at targets placed along particular junctures of the path, as quickly as possible. The combining of gross and fine motor movements, speed and accuracy, and physiological and psychological fatigue make the sport one of the most challenging both for participants and for motor behavior professionals trying to facilitate performance.

Fatigue and the Learning of a Motor Skill

In Section I, we described the learning of a motor skill. It is difficult to determine the effects of fatigue on the learning of a motor skill. The information available is mixed: some researchers have concluded that fatigue is not a factor in learning, while others have determined that it is a factor. Perhaps the mixed results are due as much to the ways in which the investigations were conducted as to anything else. For example, several of the investigations may have produced fatigue levels that were insufficient to warrant substantive fatigue (Alderman, 1965; Schmidt, 1969; Carron, 1969). These investigators did not mention the assessment of any conditions that would provide meaningful data about fatigue levels, such as blood glucose levels, blood lactate levels, cardiorespiratory states, or blood pressure. They did not sequence the workloads to induce fatigue based upon exercise physiological principles of fatigue, nor was recovery time built into the work protocol.

Investigators who have documented high levels of fatigue (Caplan, 1969; Carron, 1972; Thomas, Cotten, Spieth, & Abraham, 1975) indicate decrements in performance resulting from fatiguing conditions. They designed protocols that factored in exercise bouts and evaluated skill throughout the exercise that produced fatigue (repeated measures format). For example, a subject might be asked to ride a bicycle ergometer for one hour, with a workload devised to produce a high amount of fatigue. During that hour, a pretest using the specific task to be investigated (like juggling), and tests at 15, 30, 45, and 60 minutes (posttest) might be conducted.

Additionally, a few investigators have determined that some amount of low-level fatigue may actually enhance the learning of motor skills (Pack, Cotten, & Biasiotto, 1974; Williams & Singer, 1975). Individuals with low-level fatigue performed better at initial learning and on retention tests a few days later. It is plausible to assume that the inverted-U hypothesis of fatigue and performance might be involved with these types of findings. It may also be plausible to assume that the psychological phenomenon of association/disassociation plays a role in these findings.

When to induce fatigue has also been of interest. It would make sense, based upon the findings just discussed, that inducing low levels of fatigue early in the practice session might enhance perform-ance. Inducing high levels of fatigue early in the session has yielded findings that reflect a decrement in initial learning. It would there-fore make sense to determine what effect inducing fatigue late in the learning process might have. Those investigators who did so (Alder-man, 1965; Carron, 1969; Schmidt, 1969) reported no detrimental effects on learning, probably because most of the learning had al-ready taken place.

It should also be noted that the complexity (multisequenced, timing, accuracy, decision-making) of the skills used in investiga-tions involving the effects of fatigue on learning must also be con-sidered. If, for example, skills are somewhat novel and simple, it would be logical to expect most learning to occur initially. Con-versely, if the skills are novel and complex, learning may take longer. Classifications of skills by their complexity may also affect learning. When speed and accuracy were investigated as variables, speed was detrimentally affected by fatigue; accuracy, however, was enhanced with the onset of fatigue. These two findings provide credence to the idea presented earlier that physiological fatigue hampers speed, and cognitive/central processing fatigue hampers accuracy.

Unfortunately, there is still insufficient information to state con-clusively what the effects of fatigue are on the learning of motor skills based upon complexity of the skills. More research is needed to delineate practice organization based upon skill complexity.

A final statement on the effects of fatigue on learning seems appropriate. If a person is trying to learn new skills while in a fatigued state, it is possible for inefficient and ineffective motor pat-terns to be practiced that will certainly be detrimental to learning and performance later. On the other hand, it may be advantageous for the person to learn the skill in a fatigued state so as to more closely approximate performances within a game environment. A drill used in volleyball requires the attacker to contact as many vol-leyballs as possible within a three-minute time period. As soon as the attacker has hit a ball, another one is delivered, so that the indi-vidual must laterally adjust, approach, attack, land, back up, and repeat the procedure between thirty and fifty times. The motor be-havior professional must weigh the advantages and disadvantages of the drill and determine whether and how to use it to enhance the learning/performance process. Obviously, more research also needs to be conducted in this area to determine the viability of learning and retention in various states of fatigue that simulate gamelike conditions.

AMOUNT AND DISTRIBUTION OF PRACTICE

The number of practice sessions, the length of each practice session, how each practice session is divided, and how much practice is beneficial for optimum learning are issues of great interest to the motor behavior professional. Several decisions must be made about practice: How much time is available to present the activity (three months, three weeks, three days)? How often is the activity to be presented (daily, once per week, twice per week, three times per week)? How long will it be presented daily (half hour, one hour, two hours, three hours)? What is the fatigue/rest factor involved with this activity?

Several important perspectives must be presented so that we may better understand the complexity of each of these questions. The first of these is the massed or distributed practice perspective. Functionally, **massed practice** is that practice which involves little or no rest between attempts and functions rather continuously (Magill, 1993). A **distributed practice** is one that contains rest components between attempts so that there are noticeable breaks in the practice of specific skills (Magill, 1993).

There would seem to be some logic in the notion that distributed practice would be superior to massed practice because of the issue of physiological and cognitive fatigue. A brief examination of investigations should confirm or deny this perspective.

Several researchers have found that distributing practice sessions and distributing intensified motor skill work within a practice session are better for learning and retention than massed practices (Ellis, 1978; Schmidt, 1988; Lee & Genovese, 1988). Other researchers have determined that massed practice has only proven detrimental to performance, not to learning (Adams, 1987; Magill, 1993; Singer, 1980). It has also been pointed out (Baddeley, 1990) that researchers have begun to learn that distributed practice sessions may facilitate neuromuscular innervation and hardwiring of the brain for long-term memory storage by providing more time for the person to physiologically and neurochemically adjust to the changing nature of the cellular environment. This area requires much more intensified investigation.

Massed practice
practice that involves little or no rest between attempts and functions rather continuously

Distributed practice
practice that contains rest components between attempts so the practice of specific skills has no noticeable breaks

MANIPULATING THE PRACTICE ENVIRONMENT EXPERIENCE

Objective: To determine which model of massed and distributed practice is most appropriate based upon skill and ability.

Equipment and Preparation: Paper and pencil. Use 20 massed/distributed practice trials to construct a practice strategy for the scenarios below. (Example: Trials 1–10 massed; trials 11–15 distributed; trials 16–20 massed).

Experience: Determine the best practice presentation for each of these scenarios:
– Beginning performers who are learning to play the piano;
– Beginning performers who are learning to serve volleyballs;
– Beginning performers who are learning to perform handstands;
– Experienced performers who are practicing putts in golf;
– Experienced performers who are practicing a floor exercise routine;
– Experienced performers who are practicing basketball free throws.

Assignment: Devise as many combinations of massed and distributed practice as possible. Determine the best practice presentation for each of the above scenarios.

Intertrial rest interval
the duration of rest between attempts

There is rather substantial disagreement over whether massed or distributed practice is more appropriate. This more than likely stems from the manner in which experimentation has been conducted over the years. One of the variables most easily manipulated is that of how much rest is given between attempts — the **intertrial rest interval**. Because no golden standard of rest interval length has ever been determined based on the task and the learner, it is almost impossible to compare results from investigation to investigation. In its purest sense, massed practice historically referred to that which had no rest periods at all. Therefore, any experiment conducted with a rest bout of any length (even as little as fifteen seconds) was considered a distributed practice session.

Of important note was a meta-analysis conducted on the literature published on the topic (Lee & Genovese, 1988). Two important pieces of information were found as a result of the investigation: by the end of practice, those subjects who were involved in distributed practice performed better than those who were involved in massed practice; and after an intertrial rest interval, performance improvement was minimal when compared to massed practice. This information, coupled with other findings (Bourne & Archer, 1956;

Kimble & Bilodeau, 1949; Plutchik & Petti, 1964) produced the perspective that there may be an optimal intertrial rest interval. There seemed to be the most benefit when rest intervals were approximately sixty seconds long. The literature, fraught with inconsistencies in protocol, thus far only provides a thumbnail sketch of the topic. Much more research must be conducted to determine the optimal length of rest intervals.

Much of the existing literature can be categorized by task. The most frequently investigated motor skills using massed and distributed practice conditions were continuous skills. The **pursuit rotor** was the most popular instrument used to assess learning and performance. Essentially, the pursuit rotor was a record player–type turntable that revolved clockwise or counterclockwise. The individual was to keep a stylus, held by the hand, in contact with a disk, positioned on top of the turntable. The goal was to keep the stylus in contact for as long as possible while the turntable speed varied. Because this task was quite uncomplicated, it proved to be simple to assess massed and distributed practice conditions. It was determined by several researchers using this approach in the early 1950s (Adams & Reynolds, 1954; Denny, Frisbey, & Weaver, 1955) that distributed practice was better than massed practice sessions for continuous skills, particularly because massed practice has a deleterious effect on performance and on learning.

Pursuit rotor
an instrument designed to assess learning and performance using a record -player type of turntable that revolves clockwise or counterclockwise

Investigations using discrete skills have not produced any substantive findings about massed or distributed practice conditions, particularly since none of the experiments were ecologically based. Massed practice has been shown to benefit discrete skill learning (Carron, 1969; Lee & Genovese, 1988) by massing the distribution of those attempts. It is important to note that all experiments were conducted in laboratory settings, generally using a pursuit rotor. The complexity of the skill was negligible when compared to something like a tennis serve.

This lack of decisive information is important for the motor behavior professional. It is incumbent upon the professional to take into account the following when trying to determine what is the most appropriate condition to use: learning characteristics of the individual, the type of skill, the goal of the skill, and the goal of the practice. In softball, for example, a member of the 1996 United States gold medal–winning softball team is ready to practice batting. The goal of the practice session is to contact as many fastballs that are within the strike zone as possible. Choices must be made. For

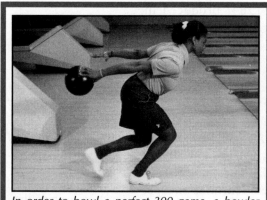

In order to bowl a perfect 300 game, a bowler executes a hook ball for greatest success.

instance, the player can practice batting in a massed context (sixty balls consecutively as quickly as possible) or in a distributed context (sixty balls total, in groups of five, with a sixty-second rest in between). Because the goal is to contact as many fastballs as possible, the massed context might be preferred. If, however, hitting through the "sweet spot" of the ball is the practice goal, distributed practice might be selected.

In general, the more complex the discrete skill, the more likely it will benefit from distributed practice. When cognitive decision-making plays an important role in the successful performance of a motor skill, sufficient time must be given to analyze, synthesize, and adjust both cognitively and physiologically to the dynamics of practice.

Additionally, when one is learning to make modifications in previously learned skills, it may also be prudent to use a distributed practice approach. For example, you have learned to throw a bowling ball successfully down the lane and produce a strike using a straight ball delivery. In order to bowl a perfect 300 game, you must eventually learn to throw the ball using a hook delivery. Distributed practice, which would allow for cognitive reflection, analysis, and synthesis, would be the preferred choice.

Finally, for working with people whose attention spans are less than optimal, distributed practice sessions could be beneficial. The intensity of focus can be optimized in short periods of time to create a cumulative effect of successful performance rather than a decrement in performance based upon massed practices.

Another issue with the amount and distribution of practice involves the way in which skills are presented. Most motor skills involve complex, interdependent, and interrelated movements of the entire body for optimal performance. Whether complex motor skills should be presented and practiced as an entire unit (**whole-task practice**) or be broken down and presented and practiced in parts (**part-task practice**) has been richly discussed and is of tremendous interest to motor behavior professionals. Each perspective has its benefits as well as its liabilities. Before decisions can be made about the most appropriate presentation for practice, information about each is helpful.

Whole-task practice
motor skills presented and practiced as an entire unit

Part-task practice
motor skills presented and practiced in parts

Which type of practice is more feasible depends partly on the resultant behavior as it relates to the entire skill. For example, a tennis serve is a rather complex motor skill, requiring a ball toss, coordinated weight shift through legs, torso, arm, hand, wrist, and fingers, plus an arm swing attached to a hand that grips a racket, contact of that tossed ball, and a follow-through to enhance power and avoid injury. Much debate has centered around the presentation and practice of the skill as one unit versus breaking it down to a sequential combination of ball toss and weight shift, arm and racket reach, contact, and follow-through.

Investigations conducted on this topic have provided mixed results (Naylor & Briggs, 1963; Stammers, 1980; Wightman & Lintern, 1985; Newell, Carlton, Fisher, & Rutter, 1989). Results were presented either in terms of task specificity, the capabilities of the individual, or how the part practice was organized (Chamberlain & Lee, 1993).

The specificity of the task has provided interesting information for motor behavior professionals. Tasks have included skills that possess elements of prediction (Naylor & Briggs, 1963), skills that involve tracking and simulation (Wightman & Lintern, 1985), and skills that are used during video games (Newell, Carlton, Fisher, & Rutter, 1989). It has been determined that the more interdependent skills are, the more important their presentation and practice as a unit (whole-task practice) is. It is interesting to note that the tasks have fair numbers of spatial and temporal components; hence, it would also seem logical that the less interdependent the skills are, the more their presentation and practice could be developed into parts (part-task practice).

Some motor skills are so interrelated that it is only logical to present and practice them as a unit. In parachuting, for example, the rehearsal of landing and rolling, though two distinct skills, are better practiced as a unit for timing and safety purposes. In parasailing, the importance of keeping the craft relatively horizontal to maintain flight is critical to success. The components of pitching and rolling must continuously be monitored and adjusted for. It would only be logical to maintain these as a unit, rather than isolate either as a part of the parasailing experience. In short, when the task requires high interdependence of skills that, if separated, would result in failure to achieve the goal of the skill, the task could be presented and practiced as a whole. The less interdependent the skills of the task are for ultimate success, the more the task could be presented and practiced in parts.

The capability of the individual to perceptually process the information needed to complete the task is another consideration for the motor behavior professional. It is important to determine the existing skill ability as the individual begins practicing. A youngster or an adult inexperienced with the motor skill may be better served by part-task practice to the extent that it is possible to develop and present parts of the task. The *River Dance* is a detailed contemporary folk dance with a series of intricate parts. Major passages are connected through a series of break steps. Because of its somewhat novel rhythm, speed, and precision, parts of the dance can easily be presented and practiced, then strung together to a whole-task practice component. Additionally, when first learning how to make the ribbon move in rhythmic gymnastics, one might benefit from a part-task practice perspective. Any motor skill movements choreographed into routines would be inappropriate without the ribbon continually moving.

Generally, the better able one is to perform basic locomotor patterns, the more quickly parts can be taken into wholes. Most human movement has components of one of more of the following basic locomotor patterns: running, hopping, skipping, jumping, leaping, galloping, and walking. Most human movement has components of one or more of the following basic arm patterns as well (if upper body parts are involved in the movement): underarm, sidearm, and overarm. Team handball is a game in which many basic locomotor skills are combined with basic arm patterns for performance success. One of the ways to advance the ball down the court is by dribbling. The skill of dribbling, similar to that used in basketball, combines the basic patterns of walking or running and the use of upper body parts to maneuver the ball from one place to another. The motor behavior patterns that comprise team handball appear to be examples of part-task practice appropriateness.

PART-TASK PRACTICE ORGANIZATION

Using the information-processing model to explain motor behavior, there is some validity to the proposition that part-task practice is effective because it provides limited amounts of information to be processed. It also seems plausible that, using a limited attention capacity model of learning, a person can base motor performance decisions on smaller amounts of stimuli. It also appears that the individual can concentrate in greater detail on complex motor behavior patterns that are often associated with part-task practice. With these concepts in mind, there seem to be at least three ways in which part-task practice can be organized (Wightman & Lintern, 1985). They include simplification, fractionation, and segmentation.

Simplification involves the modification of movements to the basics of the skill within a particular environment; that is, what is absolutely necessary for the skill to resemble the pattern of movement. When a ten-year-old practices a free throw shot, the height of the goal and the size of the ball might be reduced in order to provide more appropriate relationships between the height of the person and the basket and the size of the ball and the hand. The act may also be simplified by the youngster using a two-handed shot if strength seems to be a factor. Altering the speed of the skill but not altering the relative timing is another way in which to apply the construct of simplification to the enhancement of motor behavior. In tee-ball, batting the ball from a tee eliminates the concern about timing an approaching ball-to-bat contact; the swing is coordinated with appropriate force through the center of the ball for distance and accuracy. Lead-up games for exposure and experience of skills also used in baseball or softball combine the skills of running and fielding, fielding and throwing, and throwing and catching.

Fractionation involves the dismantling of the coordination of a skill into several parts. One such skill that might benefit from fractionation is a modification of a jumping jack (coordinated jumping jack). In this type of jumping jack, the legs move in three-fourths time (out-in-in, out-in-in) while the arms move in two-fourths time (up-down, up-down). Practicing the legs first until the rhythm is established, then the arms until the rhythm is established, then starting the legs in rhythm, then adding the arms can prove successful. With both parts being rather unrelated, fractionation can be an effective strategy for practice. The more interrelated the movement pattern, however, the less fractionation is effective.

A third form of part-task practice applies the notion of **segmentation**. In this approach, a skill is divided into parts based upon temporal and spatial characteristics and levels of performance. Each of the designated parts is then combined with other parts, leading to the performance of the entire skill. For example, the Czech national (folk) dance, the *Beseda*, is comprised of a series of eight coordinated movement parts set to music that, when combined with a break step, is performed for approximately one-half hour. One way to present the lengthy performance would be to practice the break

Simplification
modifying movements to the simplest basics of the skill within a particular environment

Fractionation
dismantling the coordination of a skill into several parts

Segmentation
dividing skills into parts based upon temporal and spatial characteristics and levels of performance; then combining each of the parts with other parts, leading to performance of the entire skill

step, then practice Part I and the break step, then practice Part II, then practice the break step and Part II, then practice Part I, the break step, and Part II, followed by Part II and the break step, etc. This type of sequencing of part-task practice can be used effectively in closed skills that require a set progression.

There is yet another way in which practice can be organized to provide the appearance of part-task practice while providing whole-part practice. It is the construct of **attentional cueing**. This strategy provides opportunities for practicing the entire skill while concentrating on only one or two parts of it. It is, by the way, important to give the person the opportunity to understand the whole movement as it relates to a larger context before attentional cueing can be beneficial.

Attentional cueing
a strategy that provides opportunities for practicing an entire skill while concentrating on only one or two parts of it

Finally, the issue of how much practice is needed to create optimum learning must also be addressed. The amount of practice time spent beyond the amount of time needed to attain a particular level of performance based upon preestablished criteria (Magill, 1993) is called **overlearning**. This term, however defined, seems to be a misnomer. Skills cannot really be overlearned; they can, however, be *overpracticed* (Magill, 1993). Melnick (1971) performed an investigation to answer the questions of whether additional practice after meeting a performance-based criteria level was beneficial or not and whether there was a preferred amount of additional practice that could enhance performance. Two groups practiced stabilometer balancing until they achieved specific predetermined levels of performance. Once they attained that criterion score, they either discontinued practice or were asked to practice half again as many trials (50 %) the same number (100 %), or twice as many trials (200 %) as before. A test for retention was administered one week later. The results were fascinating: groups who were asked to do additional practice performed better on the retention tests than did those who stopped after reaching the criterion score. More interestingly, those who were in the group practicing half again as many repetitions did as well as those who completed the same number or twice again the number originally done. In other words, there was a rate of diminishing returns (Magill, 1993). This perspective suggests that once a particular skill is learned, practicing half again as much can provide practice time well invested for retention. Other investigators have found similar effects (Goldberger & Gerney, 1990; Shea & Kohl, 1990). A highly complex sequence of discrete skills requires an increased amount of practice as well.

Overlearning (overpractice)
practice time spent above the amount of time needed to attain a level of performance based upon preestablished criteria

The motor behavior professional can incorporate these concepts into the decision-making process about organizing the practice environment. Criterion-based performance levels should be used in motor skill learning. Once the level of performance has been reached, 100 percent more attempts may be sufficient to overpractice the skill (Melnick, 1971). Because there seems to be a point of diminishing returns, setting criterion-based levels that are attainable is important so that individuals can experience success and reach an overpractice setting. A common-sense approach used by motor behavior professionals for many years has been to construct performance curves of motor skills. In this way, the professional *and* the individual discover when performance (inferring learning) has plateaued at particular levels of efficiency. As we will discuss in Section V, performance curves resemble snapshots of performances on the road to efficient learning. Once a plateau has been reached, either performance has stabilized or the learner does not have the correct strategy to progress.

Practicing a skill repeatedly can provide great meaning for the individual. Psychologically, it can produce a sense of confidence and competence in one's ability to perform the skill. As a parallel consideration, however, the *amount* of practice of a motor skill is not the only important variable in motor behavior. Also important to consider are other constructs that have been detailed in this section, like the variability of practice to focus attention and the types of meaningful feedback provided.

KEY POINTS

- Motor behavior from learning to performance is multidimensional.
- The notion of classical conditioning (Pavlov, 1927) identified the relationship between stimulus and response.
- The period of extinction was the length of time it took to eliminate a conditioned response by lack of reinforcement.
- Using schedules of reinforcement (selectively reinforced behavior) with something pleasurable (positive reinforcement) and with something unpleasant (negative reinforcement), learning can occur.
- The variable of reinforcement (reward) for specific behaviors was used to mold an animal's response.

- Types of conditioning programs helped us to understand differences between learning and performance.

- The closer the practice environment is to the actual transfer test, the higher the likelihood of transfer.

- Performing a motor skill using one side of the body will also increase performance when the other side of the body is used to perform the same movement. This is called bilateral transfer.

- Schmidt (1975) determined that bilateral transfer is neuromuscularly and cognitively rooted.

- It has been suggested that combining mental practice with physical practice will facilitate the greatest amount of bilateral transfer.

- Structure, organization, and the amount and distribution of practice influence learning and performance in a practice environment.

- Practice variability is an important principle for structuring the practice of discrete skills.

- Children benefit greatly from the use of variety in the practice structure to accommodate their shorter attention spans and to elicit skilled performance under a variety of conditions.

- Two basic stages of learning are to develop an overall idea of the skills and to diversify or fixate movement (depending upon the environment) (Gentile, 1972).

- Under conditions where the environment is dynamic and the individual is required to adapt to variations in the surroundings, random practice schedules are superior to blocked practice sessions for the retention of motor skills.

- Variations in intellectual capability, age, experience, and learning style should be considered when determining the level of contextual interference to be used in the practice environment.

- Focusing on relevant environment cues has been shown to be of great importance to performance success.

- A systematic presentation of distractors is of benefit in a gamelike practice environment.

- Physiological fatigue affects an individual's motor learning and performance multidimensionally.

- Massed practice involves little or no rest between attempts and functions rather continuously.

- Distributed practice contains rest components between attempts so that there are noticeable breaks in the practice of specific skills.

- Overlearning of motor skills connotes the overpracticing of motor skills.

- Three ways in which part-task practice can be organized are simplification, fractionation, and segmentation.

DISCUSSION QUESTIONS

1. How does the construct of contextual interference relate to variability of practice?

2. Cite two examples of contextual interference used to vary practice.

3. Discuss the notion of attentional cueing and its role in understanding a movement in its entirety.

4. Present a functional definition of overpractice. Determine how its meaning would be used to design a practice setting for learning the skill of serving in tennis.

5. Describe how the speed/accuracy tradeoff would affect an individual playing ice hockey as a forward and shooting for goal.

6. Design a practice setting for a team sport, incorporating the concept of prepractice routine. Design one for an individual sport.

ADDITIONAL READINGS

Chamberlin, C., & Lee, T. (1993). Arranging practice conditions and designing instruction. In R. N. Singer, M. Murphey, & L. K. Tennant (Eds.), *Handbook of research on sport psychology*, (pp. 213–241). New York: Macmillan.

Magill, R. A. (Ed.). (1994). *Quest: Communicating information to enhance skill learning,* 46(3), Champaign, IL: Human Kinetics.

Magill, R. A., & Hall, K. G. (1990). A review of the contextual interference effect in motor skill acquisition. *Human Movement Science, 9,* 241–289.

REFERENCES

Adams, J. A. (1987). Historical review and appraisal of research on learning, retention and transfer of human motor skills. *Psychological Review, 101,* 41–74.

Adams, J. A., & Reynolds, B. (1954). Effects of shift of distribution of practice conditions following interpolated rest. *Journal of Experimental Psychology, 47,* 32–36.

Alderman, R. (1965). Influence of local fatigue on speed and accuracy in motor learning. *Research Quarterly, 36,* 131–140.

Allard, F. (1982). Cognition, expert performance, and sport. In M. Whiting (Ed.), *New paths to sport learning* (pp. 22–26). Ontario: Coaching Association of Canada.

Baddeley, A. D. (1990). *Human memory. Theory and practice.* Boston: Allyn & Bacon.

Bahill, A. T., & LaRitz, T. (1984). Why can't batters keep their eyes on the ball? *American Scientist, 72,* 249–253.

Battig, W. F. (1966). Facilitation and interference. In E. A. Bilodeau (Ed.), *Acquisition of skill* (pp. 215–244). New York: Academic Press.

Battig, W. F. (1972). Intratask interference as a source of facilitation in transfer and retention. In R. F. Thompson & J. F. Voss (Eds.), *Topics in learning and performance* (pp. 131–159). New York: Academic Press.

Battig, W. F. (1977). Reaction to Schutz. In D. Mood (Ed.), *The measurement of change in physical education* (pp. 101–104). Boulder, CO: University of Colorado Press.

Bourne, L. E., Jr., & Archer, E. J. (1956). Time continuously on target as a function of distribution of practice. *Journal of Experimental Psychology, 51,* 25–32.

Bransford, J. D., Franks, J. J., Morris, C. D., & Stein, B. S. (1979). Some general constraints on learning and memory research. In L. S. Cermak & F. I. M. Craik (eds.), *Levels of processing in human memory* (pp. 331–355). Hillsdale, NJ: Erlbaum.

Caplan, C. S. (1969). *The influence of physical fatigue on massed versus distributed motor learning.* Unpublished doctoral dissertation, University of California, Berkeley.

Carron, A. V. (1969). Performance and learning in a discrete motor task under massed vs. distributed practice. *Research Quarterly, 4,* 481–489.

Carron, A. V. (1972). Motor performance and learning under physical fatigue. *Medicine and Science in Sport, 4,* 101–106.

Chamberlain, C., & Lee, T. D. (1993). Arranging practice conditions and designing instruction. In R. N. Singer, M. Murphey, & L. K. Tennant, (Eds.), *Handbook on research in sport psychology,* (pp. 213–241). New York: Macmillan.

Cobb, T. (1994). *The effect of blood lactate and relationship of blood glucose levels on contrast sensitivity function in female athletes.* Unpublished master's thesis, The University of Alabama at Birmingham.

Cohn, P. J., Rotella, R. J., & Lloyd, J. W. (1990). Effects of cognitive-behavioral intervention on the preshot routine and performance in golf. *The Sport Psychologist, 4,* 33–47.

Del Rey, P. (1982). Effects of contextual interference on memory of older females differing in levels of physical activity. *Perceptual and Motor Skills, 55,* 171–180.

Del Rey, P. (1989). Training and contextual interference effects on memory and transfer. *Research Quarterly for Exercise and Sport, 60,* 342–347.

Del Rey, P., Whitehurst, M., & Wood, J. (1983). Effects of experience and contextual interference on learning and transfer. *Perceptual and Motor Skills, 56,* 581–582.

Del Rey, P., Wughalter, E., & Whitehurst, M. (1982). The effects of contextual interference on females with varied experience in open skills. *Research Quarterly for Exercise and Sport, 53,* 108–115.

Denny, M. R., Frisbey, N., & Weaver, J., Jr. (1955). Rotary pursuit performance under alternate conditions of distributed and massed practice. *Journal of Experimental Psychology, 49,* 48–54.

Dwyer, J. (1984). Influences of physical fatigue on motor performance and learning. *Physical Educator, 41,* 130–136.

Edwards, J. M., Elliott, D., & Lee, T. D. (1986). Contextual interference effects during skill acquisition and transfer in Down's Syndrome adolescents. *Adapted Physical Activity Quarterly, 3,* 250–258.

Ellis, H. C. (1978). *Fundamentals of human learning, memory, and cognition* (2nd ed.). Dubuque, IA: Wm. C. Brown.

Feltz, D. L., & Landers, D. M. (1983). The effects of mental practice on motor skill learning and performance: A meta-analysis. *Journal of Sport Psychology, 5,* 25–57.

Feltz, D. L., & Riessinger, C. A. (1990). Effects of in vivo emotive imagery and performance feedback on self-efficacy and muscular endurance. *Journal of Sport & Exercise Psychology, 12,* 132–143.

Fitts, P. M. (1954). The information capacity of the human motor system in controlling the amplitude of movement. *Journal of Experimental Psychology, 47,* 381–391.

Gentile, A. M. (1972). A working model of skill acquisition with application to teaching. *Quest,* Monograph XVII, 3–23.

Godwin, M. A. & Schmidt, R. A. (1971). Muscular fatigue and learning a discrete motor skill. *Research Quarterly, 42,* 374–382.

Goldberger, M., & Gerney, P. (1990). Effects of learner use of practice time on skill acquisition of fifth grade children. *Journal of Teaching Physical Education, 10,* 84–95.

Goode, S. L. (1986). *The contextual interference effect in learning an open motor skill.* Unpublished doctoral dissertation, Louisiana State University, Baton Rouge.

Goode, S. L., & Magill, R. A. (1986). Contextual interference effects in learning three badminton serves. *Research Quarterly for Exercise and Sport, 57,* 308–314.

Goode, S. L., & Wei, P. (1988). "Differential effects of variations of random and blocked practice on novice learning an open motor skill" (Abstract). In D. L. Gill and J. E. Clarke (Eds.). *Abstracts of research papers, 1988* (p. 80). AAHPERD Convention, Kansas City, MO.

Gould, D., & Weiss, M. R. (1987). *Advances in pediatric sport sciences, Vol. 2: Behavioral issues.* Champaign, IL: Human Kinetics.

Heitman, R. J., & Gilley, W. F. (1989). Effects of blocked versus random practice by mentally retarded subjects on learning a novel skill. *Perceptual and Motor Skills, 69,* 443–447.

Hicks, R. E., Frank, J. M., & Kinsbourne, M. (1982). The locus of bimanual skill transfer. *Journal of General Psychology, 107,* 277–281.

Hicks, R. E., Gualtieri, C. T., & Schroeder, S. R. (1983). Cognitive and motor components of bilateral transfer. *American Journal of Psychology, 96,* 223–228.

Hubbard, A. W., & Seng, C. N. (1954). Visual movements of batters. *Research Quarterly, 25,* 12–22.

Jelsma, O., & Pieters, J. M. (1989). Practice schedule and cognitive style interaction in learning a maze task. *Applied Cognitive Psychology, 3,* 73–83.

Jelsma, O., & Van Merrienboer, J. J. G. (1989). Conceptual interference interactions with reflection-impulsivity. *Perceptual and Motor Skills, 68,* 1055–1064.

Kimble, G. A., & Bilodeau, E. A. (1949). Work and rest as variables in cyclical motor learning. *Journal of Experimental Psychology, 39,* 150–157.

Kohl, R. M., & Roenker, D. L. (1980). Bilateral transfer as a function of mental imagery. *Journal of Motor Behavior, 12,* 179–190.

Kohl, R. M., & Roenker, D. L. (1983). Mechanism involvement during skill imagery. *Journal of Motor Behavior, 15,* 197–206.

Lee, T. D., & Genovese, E. D. (1988). Distribution of practice in motor skill acquisition: Learning and performance effects reconsidered. *Research Quarterly for Exercise and Sport, 59,* 59–67.

Lee, T. D., & Magill, R. A. (1983). The locus of contextual interference in motor-skill acquisition. *Journal of Experimental Psychology: Learning, Memory, and Cognition, 9,* 730–746.

Lobmeyer, D. L., & Wasserman, E. A. (1986). Preliminaries to free throw shooting: Superstitious behavior? *Journal of Sport Behavior, 9,* 70–78.

McGeoch, J. A. (1927). The acquisition of skill. *Psychological Bulletin, 24,* 437–466.

McGeoch, J. A. (1929). The acquisition of skill. *Psychological Bulletin, 26,* 457–498.

McGeoch, J. A. (1931). The acquisition of skill. *Psychological Bulletin, 28,* 413–466.

Magill, R. A. (1993). *Motor learning: Concepts and applications* (4th ed.). Madison, WI: Brown & Benchmark.

Magill, R. A., & Hall, K. G. (1990). A review of the contextual interference effect in motor skill acquisition. *Human Movement Science, 9,* 241–289.

Melnick, M. J. (1971). Effects of overlearning on the retention of a gross motor skill. *Research Quarterly, 42,* 60–69.

Naylor, J., & Briggs, G. (1963). Effects of task complexity and task organization on the relative efficiency of part and whole training methods. *Journal of Experimental Psychology, 65,* 217–244.

Newell, K. M., Carlton, L. G., Carlton, M. J., & Halbert, J. A. (1980). Velocity as a factor in movement timing accuracy. *Journal of Motor Behavior, 12,* 47–56.

Newell, K. M., Carlton, M. J., Fisher, A. T., & Rutter, B. G. (1989). Whole-part training strategies for learning the response dynamics of microprocessor driven simulators. *Acta Psychologica, 71,* 197–216.

Nunney, D. N. (1963). Fatigue, impairment, and psycho-motor learning. *Perceptual and Motor Skills, 16,* 369–375.

Orlick, T. (1986). *Psyching for sport: Mental training for athletes.* Champaign, IL: Leisure Press.

Pack, M., Cotten, D., J., & Biasiotto, J. (1974). Effect of four fatigue levels on performance and learning of a novel dynamic balance skill. *Journal of Motor Behavior, 6,* 191–198.

Pavlov, I. P. (1927). *Conditioned reflexes.* (Transl. and ed. by G. V. Anrep.). London: Oxford University Press.

Pigott, R. E., & Shapiro, D. C. (1984). Motor schema: The structure of the variability session. *Research Quarterly for Exercise and Sport, 55,* 41–45.

Plutchik, R., & Petti, R. D. (1964). Rate of learning on a pursuit rotor task at a constant work rest ratio with varying work and rest periods. *Perceptual and Motor Skills, 19,* 227–231.

Pollock, B. J., & Lee, T. D. (1990). Contextual interference in motor learning: Dissociated effects due to age. *Research Quarterly for Exercise and Sport,* 256–260.

Poulton, E. C. (1988). The *Journal of Motor Behavior* in the 1960s and the 1980s. *Journal of Motor Behavior, 20,* 75–78.

Proteau, L., Marteniuk, R. G., Girouard, Y., & Dugas, C. (1987). On the type of information used to control and learn an aiming movement after moderate and extensive training. *Human Movement Science, 6,* 181–199.

Richards, D. K. (1968). A two factor theory of the warmup effect in jumping performance. *Research Quarterly, 39,* 668–673.

Schmidt, R. A. (1969). Performance and learning a gross muscular skill under conditions of artificially induced fatigue. *Research Quarterly, 40,* 185–191.

Schmidt, R. A. (1975). A schema theory of discrete motor skill learning. *Psychological Review, 82,* 225–260.

Schmidt, R. A. (1988). *Motor learning and control: A behavioral emphasis* (2nd ed.) Champaign, IL: Human Kinetics.

Schmidt, R. A. (1991). *Motor learning and performance: From principles to practice.* Champaign, IL: Human Kinetics.

Schmidt, R. A., Zelaznik, H. N., Hawkins, B., Frank, J. S., & Quinn, J. T. (1979). Motor-output variability: A theory for the accuracy of rapid motor acts. *Psychological Review, 86,* 415–451.

Schomer, H. (1986). Mental strategies and the perception of effort of marathon runners. *International Journal of Sport Psychology, 17,* 41–59.

Shea, J. B., & Kohl, R. M. (1990). Specificity and variability of practice. *Research Quarterly for Exercise and Sport, 61,* 169–177.

Shea, J. B., & Morgan, R. L. (1979). Contextual interference effects on the acquisition, retention, and transfer of a motor skill. *Journal of Experimental Psychology: Human Learning and Memory, 5,* 179–187.

Silva, J. M., & Applebaum, M. I. (1989). Association and dissociation patterns of United States Olympic Marathon Trial Contestants. *Cognitive Therapy and Research, 13,* 185–192.

Singer, R. N. (1980). *Motor learning and human performance* (3rd ed.). New York: Macmillan.

Singley, M. K., & Anderson, J. F. (1989). *The transfer of cognitive skill.* Cambridge, MA: Harvard University Press.

Slater-Hammel, A. T., & Stumpner, R. L. (1950). Batting reaction time. *Research Quarterly American Association Health Physical Education, 21*(4), 353–356.

Smoll, F. L., Magill, R. A., & Ash, M. J. (1988). *Children in sport* (3rd ed.). Champaign, IL: Human Kinetics.

Stammers, R. B. (1980). Part and whole practice for a tracking task: Effects of task variables and amount of practice. *Perceptual and Motor Skills, 50,* 203–210.

Stelmach, G. E. (1969). Efficiency of motor learning as a function of inter-trial rest. *Research Quarterly, 40,* 198–202.

Thomas, J. R., Cotten, D. J., Spieth, W. R., & Abraham, N. L. (1975). Effects of fatigue on stabilometer performance and learning of males and females. *Medicine and Science in Sports, 7,* 203–206.

Thorndike, E. L. (1903). *Educational psychology.* New York: Lemke & Buechner.

Yerkes, R. M., & Dodson, J. D. (1908). The relationship of strength of stimulus to rapidity of habit formation. *Journal of Comparative Neurology and Psychology, 18,* 459–482.

Weinberg, R. S. (1989). Anxiety, arousal, and motor performance: Theory, research, and applications. In D. Hackfort & C. D. Spielberger (Eds.), *Anxiety in sports: An international perspective* (pp. 95–115). New York: Hemisphere.

Weiss, M. R., & Ebbeck, V. (1995). Self-esteem and perceptions of competence in youth sport: Theory, research, and enhancement strategies. In O. Bar-Or (Ed.), *The encyclopedia of sports medicine, Vol VI: The child and adolescent athlete.* Oxford: Blackwell Scientific.

Wightman, D. C., & Lintern, G. (1985). Part-task training for tracking and manual control. *Human Factors, 27,* 267–283.

Williams, J., & Singer, R. N. (1975). Muscular fatigue and the learning and performance of a motor control task. *Journal of Motor Behavior, 7,* 265–270.

Group Dynamics and Motor Behavior

CHAPTER FOCUS

- The nature of groups
- Group interaction, structure, size, goals, cohesiveness, temporal change
- The makings of a team
- Forming, storming, norming, performing
- A model for determining group performance
- Individual performance and group effort
- Attributing successes and failures — Achievement attributions
- Social facilitation and the practice environment
- Goal setting
- Group cohesion and group performance
- Strategies for building team cohesion

*H*uman movement relates not only to the individual, but also to the inter-action and interdependence of individuals as they move through multidimensional time and space. There is a need, particularly at the undergraduate level, to discuss the impact other humans have upon the processes involved in

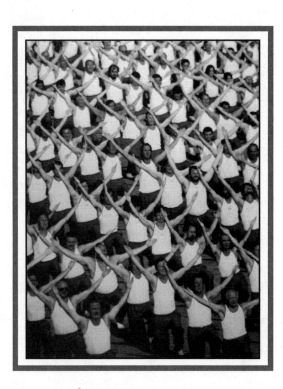

motor learning so that motor behavior professionals can more fully understand the importance of learning and performance environments on those in the environments.

To provide a snapshot of the world as it approaches the third millennium, an interesting ratio was developed by an anonymous source (1997):

If the world's population was shrunk to a village of 100 females and males, but maintained the existing human ratios, the village would have the appearance of:

- 57 Asians
- 21 Europeans
- 14 Western Hemispheric people (North and South Americans)
- 8 Africans
- 70 nonwhite
- 30 white
- 70 non-Christians
- 30 Christian
- 70 unable to read
- 50 malnourished
- 80 living in substandard housing
- 1 university graduate
- 50 percent of the world's wealth would be in the hands of six people . . . all citizens of the United States of America

With this as a backdrop, one of the amazing threads that is common to this village of human beings is the medium of human movement. Despite its diversity, the villagers, reflected through motor behavior, function dependently, independently, and interdependently for life and growth. Human movement is often conducted in the presence of others and is often influenced by the behavior of others. This chapter involves understanding the nature of groups, how individuals relate to groups, and how groups influence motor behavior.

THE NATURE OF GROUPS

Interdependence
mutual influence of two or more individuals in a relationship

From a motor behavior perspective, it is important to determine that which characterizes a group. A group is not just a collection of individuals. One of its distinctive markers is the characteristic of **interdependence**. Interdependence refers to a mutual influence of two or more people that creates an effect on the relationship. Other characteristics might include interaction, structure, size, goals, unity, and temporal change.

Interaction encompasses the ways in which group members influence each others' behaviors. For example, the captain of the team (who was determined to be responsible for warmups) enters the gymnasium, fashionably late, while another member led warmups. Until that time, the other members appeared to be sluggish to begin warmup. Immediately upon arrival there is a noticeable change in the behavior of all of the others in the gym. As the captain assumes position of leading warmups, the others begin to put forth effort.

The structure of the group can be identified in terms of *role*, *status*, and *attraction*. Members of a group will assume roles of support, leadership, or opposition. Roles can be formal or informal. A *formal role* could be that of teacher, coach, captain, setter, quarterback, striker, or center. An *informal role* can be that of peacemaker, confidante, or critic. Finally, some are better liked, more respected, or more popular.

The size of the group can vary considerably. Group size has been divided into dyads (2), triads (3), small group (4 to 20), society (20 to 30), and large group (more than 40) (Simmel, 1902). The size of the group is worth noting, because influence and communication play roles in the success or failure of groups. Frequently, the social units in organized sport are small groups or are dissected into small groups, as defined here.

Goals facilitate the need for and the formation of groups. Typically, group members will unite to pursue common goals. For example, individuals will create a group based on the desire to win a state championship in ice hockey. Goals can be used to assist in role clarification. When roles are clarified, players seem to accept them.

The extent to which the group links its members to each other and to the group is called **cohesiveness**. Individuals can be "bound" to one another as well as to the group. A gymnast may be attracted to those who, like him, participate on parallel bars; he may also be attracted to the gymnastics team as a whole.

Interaction
the ways in which group members influence each others' behaviors

Cohesiveness
close linking of group members

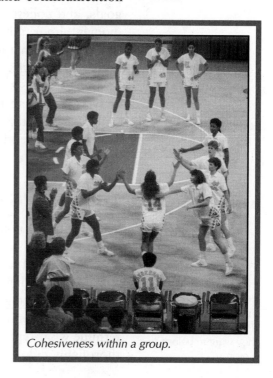
Cohesiveness within a group.

Temporal change involves a little of all of the characteristics we have discussed, placing the characteristics in a dynamic environment. A true story probably best illustrates the characteristic of temporal change. Members of a rugby team (Read, 1974) traveling in a chartered airplane to an international competition in South America crashed in the Andes Mountains. They were able to survive subzero temperatures only by working and staying together as a group. Each person had individual responsibilities, like cleaning, finding water, or taking care of those who were injured. One person was designated as the coordinator of these activities: the rugby team's captain. Unfortunately, he was killed in an avalanche, thereby making the leadership role available. Three individuals assumed the role. With little chance of survival, group decisions were made: those who hoped to survive needed food. There was none except from those members who had already died. After more than one and one-half months, near death, the group decided that two individuals should try to seek help by traversing down the mountain. After walking for nearly fourteen more days, they found their way to a small farm. After seventy days, help was on its way to the remaining fourteen rugby team members who managed to survive. The temporal change involving interdependence, interaction, structure, size, goals, and cohesiveness vacillated most assuredly from moment to moment, hour to hour, day to day, and week to week.

The word that may best represent the process that takes place in a group is *dynamic*. Selected by a noted theorist (Lewin, 1948), its meaning implies that groups have power rather than weakness, are active rather than passive, are fluid rather than static, and provide synergy rather than lethargy. The term **group dynamics**, then, connotes the influential processes and their study that occur within groups.

Group dynamics
the influential processes within groups

THE MAKINGS OF A TEAM

With regard to motor behavior, a collection of individuals does not make a team. There seem to be four stages in the process of team development (Tuckman, 1965). They are referred to as forming, storming, norming, and performing.

In the first stage, **forming**, individuals must make decisions as to whether or not they want to belong to a group. They must also determine what types of roles they are willing to fill. A youngster who thoroughly enjoys doing cartwheels, backward rolls, and tinsicas in

Forming
the first stage in team development, in which individuals must make decisions as to whether they want to belong to a group

the back yard is encouraged to become a member of the gymnastics team at the local YMCA. The first decision to be made is to attend one of the practices. Once there, the youngster determines that it is fun and might be worth continuing. The child begins to interact with others while participating in tumbling drills. By the end of the first session, the child has two new friends and is eager to be a member of the team.

The second stage, **storming**, is the "testing of power" phase. Discussions about decisions surface, conflicts occur, and disharmony prevails as roles, responsibility, and status are established within the group. This phase can produce overt motor behaviors that are aggressive and exhibit rage, anger, and frustration in a sporting environment. Because this stage is one in which multidimensional dynamics occur, the motor behavior professional must provide consistency in decision-making and behaviors and discussion about individual abilities and team roles in order to reduce the arousal that has manifested itself as anxiety.

Storming
the second, "testing-of-power" stage in the process of team development involving discussions about decisions, conflicts, and disharmony as roles, responsibilities, and status are established within the group

Norming, the third stage, is the "calm after the storm," when group members begin to get a sense of ease so that they can perform at a particular level and work together. The group becomes increasingly cohesive and task focused, using individual strengths to benefit the common good of the team. Still somewhat dynamic in its demeanor, the group divides responsibilities more effectively and exhibits solidarity. It is particularly important for the motor behavior professional to include each member in the decision-making process to determine the levels of expectation at this stage.

Norming
the third stage in team development, when group members begin to get a sense of ease so they can perform at a given level and work together

The pinnacle stage is that of **performing**. In this stage, focus and actions envelop the notion of team success. This is the most stable of the stages. Members function well in roles, each striving to make their unique contributions to the greater good of the group, thereby providing synergy to one another to accomplish the mission. In general, the greater the interaction and cooperation needed, the more important the group process becomes; the less important the level of interaction and cooperation, the less important the group process.

Performing
the last stage in the process of team development when focus and actions envelop the notion of team success and team members function well in roles

The motor behavior professional can facilitate the team-building process by considering the following research-based perspectives:

- Design situations for interaction that requires group members to be physically close to one another (Weinberg & Gould, 1995). When individuals are close to one another, they are more apt to interact and to find commonalities that can build team unification rather than divisiveness.

- Design situations in which other members of the group can provide opportunities to listen, spiritual and emotional support, constructive assessments, and empathy (Albrecht & Adelman, 1984). An environment where nurturance, tolerance, understanding, and acceptance prevails can be extremely advantageous, especially during times of crisis.

- Define team identity through uniqueness or something that sets the group apart from all others. For example, encouraging the team to decorate ball carts, nets, and balls or printing slogans on practice shirts builds team identity and uniqueness (Kluka, 1991).

- Design a strategy that will encourage openness, honesty, trust, and ethical behavior in your relationships with all those you are responsible to. Judgments will be made involving the coach's communication skills, the perception of the contributions of the coach and players to the team, and the perception that the coach is trying to help each player to improve (Anshel, 1990). The greater the perception of fairness between players and coach, the greater the level of commitment and enjoyment.

- Despite the diversity that can be experienced on a team (refer to the village scenario early in this chapter), determine the common tenets that members can relate to and believe in. For example, several fundamental human tenets seem to transcend age, ability, sex, race, sexual orientation, culture, ideology, economics, politics, and religion: personal strength; balance of the qualities of body, mind, and spirit; fairness; justice; integrity; and trust (Kluka, 1996).

A MODEL FOR DETERMINING GROUP PERFORMANCE

In an attempt to directly associate individual abilities with group performance, a model (Steiner's model) was developed to illustrate how members interact (Steiner, 1972). The model is based on a prediction formula that depends on the resources of group members and task demands:

Actual productivity =
Potential productivity − Losses through faulty group process

This formula is based upon the notion that a group's best performance (potential productivity) should be that which is based upon each individual's best performance with no duplication of effort between members of the group. The losses refer to motivation and coordination. Motivation losses happen when group members display less effort when performing within the group. Coordination losses occur when timing or strategies are not in sync within the group. For example, during the third game of the 1998 National Basketball Association Championship series between the Utah Jazz and the Chicago Bulls, all five of the starting players for the Bulls performed brilliantly, and they trounced the Jazz by forty points. Motivation and timing losses for the Jazz were extremely high, while timing losses were kept to a minimum by the Bulls. According to this model, when the group efficiently and effectively uses its available resources, combined with task demands, actual productivity will be maximized.

INDIVIDUAL PERFORMANCE AND GROUP EFFORT

One of the more interesting phenomena for the motor behavior professional to understand involves the notion of what happens to individual abilities when group effort is required for a task. The answer to the notion is known as the **Ringelmann effect** (Ingham, Levinger, Graves, & Peckman, 1974). Ringelmann conducted an investigation in the late 1800s that involved the task of pulling a rope by individuals and by groups (two to eight people). It was hypothesized that if each individual pulled 100 pounds, groups of two could pull 200, groups of three could pull 300, and groups of eight could pull 800 pounds. Unfortunately, when the test was conducted, as the number in the group increased, individual performance decreased. The two-person groups pulled only 93 percent of the total hypothesized weight, while the eight-person group only pulled 49 percent. The investigation was replicated to determine the viability of results (Ingham, et al., 1974). The results were quite similar in groups of two and three: performance of each group member decreased as group size increased. The effect was further validated; the more contemporary investigators determined that the reason for the decrease was decreased individual motivation.

The Ringelmann effect has become the basis for the term **social loafing**. Theorists (Harkins, Latane, & Williams, 1980) intimated

Ringelmann effect
member's performance in each group decreases as group size increases; the basis for the term "social loafing"

Social loafing
performance of each group member decreases as the number of individuals within the group increases

Allocational strategy
a technique whereby individuals make a total effort when working alone and mask individual performance when working in a group

Minimizing strategy
a technique whereby individuals within the group save energy because they believe their lack of effort will go undetected

that social loafing may be the result of where individuals place their efforts — that is, their **allocational strategies**. When working alone, individuals realize that they are responsible for the total effort; when working in a group, individual performance is masked. Also, individuals within the group may believe that their lack of effort will go undetected, so they are saving energy — they are practicing a **minimizing strategy**. Additionally investigations (Latane, Williams, & Harkins, 1979) have determined that when individuals believe their performance is identifiable, no social loafing occurs. Further, another group of investigators (Huddleston, Doody, & Ruder, 1985) determined that even when individuals knew ahead of time about the social loafing phenomenon, individual results on relay teams were slower than individual runs of the same distance.

After surveying fifty-two studies of sex differences in group performance, it was determined (Wood, 1985) that two factors seem to be relevant in the determination of which sex, male or female, excels. The two factors are task content and style of interaction. Groups of men seemed better at tasks that involved mathematical competence or physical strength. Women seemed better at tasks that involved verbal competence. Also, because men seem to behave using a task-oriented interaction style, and women behave using an interpersonally oriented interaction style, men perform better than women when success is determined by task activity; women perform better than men when success is determined on a high level of social activity. The effect of social loafing in sport-related endeavors seems, however, to be equal in males and females, across age groups, and in different cultures (Jackson & Williams, 1990). This may be due to the nature of task involvement leading toward quantitative success (wins/losses). Researchers have suggested that motor behavior professionals can find ways to reduce the consequences of the effect:

● Identify individual contributions to the group effort through appropriate evaluation (Kerr & Bruun, 1981).

● When those working through group effort find what they are doing interesting, challenging, and meaningful, they are less likely to loaf; therefore, make practices interesting and challenging through goal-setting and other motivational techniques (Brickner, Harkins, & Ostrom, 1986).

● When contributing to a group effort, some individuals work only as hard as they perceive others in the group are. This is known as the **free-rider effect**. The establishment of criteria-based levels of performance for all might be helpful with perceptions involving work intensity (Kerr, 1983).

- Once individuals become members of groups, their perceptions of personal responsibility may decrease. This known as **diffusion of responsibility** (Latane & Darley, 1970). It is important that each person's contribution be valued so that they see that their contributions have some impact on the results.

Free-rider effect
the concept that some individuals in a group work only as hard as they perceive that others in the group work

Diffusion of responsibility
decreased perceptions of personal responsibility once individuals become members of groups

ATTRIBUTING SUCCESSES AND FAILURES — ACHIEVEMENT ATTRIBUTIONS

Attributions refer to how individuals explain the causes of behaviors and events to themselves and to others. It is also important, for an understanding of groups, to describe **attribution theory** and its role in group outcome and performance. Much of what is known about attribution theory in sport stems from research on achievement motivation (Weiner, 1979). Weiner developed a predictive model for the results of attributions. Based on that model, research was conducted on attributions in sport. Table 12.1 provides a representation of individual responses to specific events. *Internal factors* are those that affect the outcome because of the individual's personal ability and/or effort. *External factors* are those over which the individual has limited or no control.

In several sport-related investigations (Bukowski & Moore, 1980; Bird, Foster, & Maruyama, 1980; Johnson & Biddle, 1988),

Attribution theory
what individuals attribute their successes or failures to

	Causes	
	Within self (internal)	Outside of self (external)
In control	Ability	Coaching, others close to the events
	Control	
Limited/ no control	Effort practice	Luck ease of task officials

TABLE
12.1

Sport Attribution Model

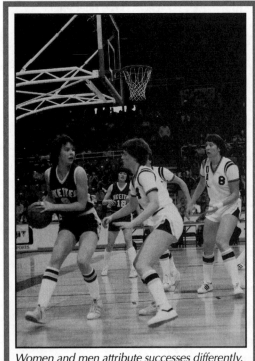
Women and men attribute successes differently.

team success was perceived to be internally attributed to individual and team skill, team effort, and dedication to quality practice. Team failure was perceived to be externally attributed to poor officiating or the difficulty of communication between coach and team. Additionally, attributions about team performance were related to team cohesiveness. More research needs to be conducted in the area of group attributions and group success.

Some of the literature has provided information between men and women in how they make attributions about sport successes and failures. It was mentioned earlier that Deaux (1984) found that women tended to attribute success in sport to luck, good coaching, or external causes, and failures to internal lack of ability. Men, on the other hand, tended to attribute success to internal factors such as skill and determination; they attributed failure to external factors such as poor officiating or poor coaching. More recently, sport attribution research has revealed little difference between women and men in their internal and external attributions for success and failure (Biddle & Hill, 1988; Weiss, McAuley, Ebbeck, & Wiese, 1990; Rudisill, 1988). This may be the result of a quarter of a century of women's participation in sport; women's achievement goals have begun to more closely resemble men's.

Very little research has been conducted on the effects of culture, race, and ethnicity on attribution theory. One researcher (Duda, 1986), using a cross-cultural perspective, found that members with different cultural backgrounds residing in the United States viewed the term *success* quite differently than the Eurocentric model that has been used for investigation. Four major categories were found to be important for success in research involving white, black, and Hispanic teens: self-improvement (task competence); winning/losing (competition with others); social approval (recognition of performance by others); and friendships (relationships within the group). It was determined that white males valued competitive goals, Hispanics preferred self-improvement goals, black females preferred friendship goals, and black males preferred self-improvement goals.

An additional investigation (Whitehead, 1986) focused on the achievement goals and attributions of adolescents from the United Kingdom and the United States. The subjects were all white youngsters. Results were quite similar for both groups in two categories: winning/losing and self-improvement. There was disparity, however, on the social approval category, with American youngsters perceiving it to have far greater importance.

These types of investigations are critically important when determining the success of groups in sportive environments. It may be that culture has an impact on the attributions people make about their successes and failures in sport. More research is needed in this area to provide greater insight into the causes of these differences so that strategies can be designed to enhance motor skill acquisition and group performance success.

From a social context, significant others can play important roles in influencing achievement motivation (discussed in Section III) and achievement attributions. Motor behavior professionals can directly and indirectly influence learning and practice environments. In the choices about tasks and games, competition and cooperation, the determinations about individuals and groups, and the perceived importance of goals, much is defined (Roberts, 1993). Five questions have been devised to help the motor behavior professional to design practice environments conducive to optimum performance (Weinberg & Gould, 1995):

- What is the interaction of personal and situational factors in influencing achievement behavior?

- Will task/mastery goals be emphasized rather than outcome goals?

- Will attributional feedback be given and then adjusted?

- Will individuals' attributions be assessed and inappropriate ones corrected?

- Will individuals be provided with the opportunity to determine when to be competitive and when to focus on individual improvement?

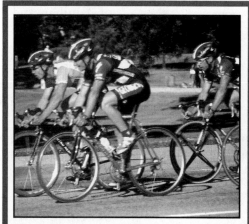

The interaction of personal and situational factors influence achievement in cycling.

When a person fails to meet goals, the motor behavior professional can provide appropriate attributional feedback by putting the encouragement to try harder in the context of the individual's personal goals and abilities. The person must believe that the goal can be accomplished (Horn, 1985). When a person succeeds in meeting the expressed goals, that success can be equated to the individual's ability and effort. The use of attributions that connote luck, lack of ability, or the simplicity of the task are counterproductive to a learning environment based upon sound research.

The performance of individuals alone and in groups has been documented for a century. Of particular interest is yet another theory, that of social facilitation.

SOCIAL FACILITATION

One of the earliest investigations of the topic of social facilitation involved bicyclists (Triplett, 1898). During cycling races, it was noted that the cyclists achieved different speeds when they raced against the clock than when they were paced by motorcycles. When the cyclists were paced by someone, their times seemed to be better. On the notion that performances might improve when someone else was present, other experiments were conducted (Triplett, 1898; Allport, 1920; Travis, 1925). The original notion developed into the concept of **social facilitation**.

Social facilitation
competition with someone else rather than with time to improve performance

Social facilitation theory was further investigated (Zajonc, 1965) to determine social facilitation results when tasks were simple or familiar and required *dominant responses* versus when tasks were unfamiliar or complex and therefore required *nondominant responses*. A comprehensive review of the available research (Bond & Titus, 1983) indicated that although the quality of performance might not improve with an audience, the rate of production did. It was also determined that an audience can produce a level of arousal that inhibits the performance of complex tasks that may not yet be sufficiently learned. This is called **social inhibition**. An audience helps the individual when tasks have been well-learned or are fairly simple.

Social inhibition
an audience's producing a level of arousal in the individual that detracts from performance

SOCIAL FACILITATION AND THE PRACTICE ENVIRONMENT

During practice, it is important to introduce audiences gradually to novices. To create a relatively stable environment initially, the motor behavior professional might want to severely limit or eliminate audiences during practice when complex skills or new skills are introduced.

Another way to achieve group success is to use the concept of goal setting.

GOAL SETTING

Goal setting involves translating vision into achievable action. It has been shown that setting specific goals has a substantial impact on motor behavior (Mento, Steel, & Karren, 1987). Goal setting must be systematic, directed, and measurable. Three basic questions can be asked when setting a goal: What is the goal? This focuses on growth and contribution. Why set the goal? This focuses on the motivation to do it. How is the goal to be set? This focuses the decision to control or release it.

The goals set should have several components: (1) They should be specific. Setting a goal of making six out of ten free throws is better than a goal of trying harder. (2) They should be challenging. If no effort is needed to achieve a goal, the goal becomes meaningless. It must have worth to the individual or the group. (3) They should be attainable. If the goal is so difficult that producing a flawless performance is the only way to achieve it, the goal may not be attainable. (4) They should be measurable. Performance-related goals are those that are quantifiable. Ten serves to the opponent's backhand within the match is a measurable goal. (5) They should be multiple. By using multiple goals, the probability of achievement is increased. If only one goal is set, and the goal is not reached, then positive motivation wanes. (6) They should be personal. Individuals in the group must have their own goals to achieve each day, each week, each year.

Goals can be set in a variety of areas (Weinberg & Gould, 1995). They can include individual motor skills, team skills, fitness, enjoyment, and psychological skills. Examples of each of these are shown in Table 12.2.

Interestingly, the effectiveness of setting individual and group goals may have some basis in culture differences. Several investigations (Mackie & Goethals, 1987; Zander, 1982; Wheeler, Reis, & Bond, 1985) have been conducted to determine the role of collective

Goal setting
translating vision into achievable action

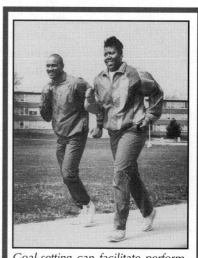

Goal-setting can facilitate performance.

TABLE 12.2 Goal Setting Areas		
Individual motor skills	I will increase my serving ability by six serves per match.
Team skills	The swim team will improve times on each event by 1 percent.
Fitness	I will improve my cardiovascular endurance by lowering my preexercise heart rate from 68 bpm to
	65 bpm by jogging for three miles each day, five days a week, at a pace 70 percent of my maximum for six months.
Enjoyment	When I return a serve it is fun. I will acknowledge that joy ten times by raising my hand and patting myself on the back.
Psychological skills	I will visualize myself being successful in putting out on the fifth hole.

Individualism
concern for personal needs, interests, goals, and achievements

Collectivism
concern for group needs, interests, goals, and achievements

needs and group goals. It has been determined that in many English-speaking countries, **individualism** is central to the culture — that is, a concern for personal needs, interests, goals, and achievements. In other countries, particularly those in Eastern Europe and Asia, central to the culture is **collectivism** — a concern for group needs, interests, goals, and achievements. These cultural differences help set the stage for ease in collective or group goal setting and group goal achievement. The group, rather than the person, is the primary functional unit. As the motor behavior professional considers these two cultural approaches when dealing with groups, it is important to determine how individuals view themselves based upon culture as well.

GROUP COHESION AND GROUP PERFORMANCE

Team cohesion
the relative strength of a group to remain focused and together in its attempt to achieve group goals

Group performance in sport has been studied in great detail through team cohesion. **Team cohesion** refers to the relative strength of a group to remain focused and together in their attempt to achieve group goals. Several factors affect group cohesion in sport (Carron, 1982):

- Environmental factors
- Personal factors

- Team factors
- Leadership factors

Environmental factors involve those that are supplemental or tangential to the group. Scholarships, contracts, eligibility rules, codes of behavior, age, sex, or sexual orientation can all be considered environmental factors that influence group cohesion.

Personal factors can include an individual's motives for belonging to the group as well as an individual's orientation to task cohesion and social cohesion (Williams & Hacker,

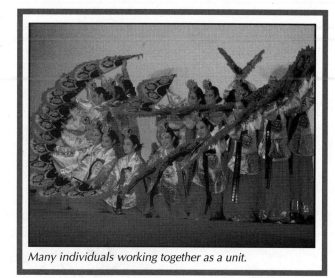

Many individuals working together as a unit.

1982). If an individual is attracted to attempting and completing group tasks, the group's task cohesion will be enhanced. If an individual is attracted to belonging to the group, social cohesion will be enhanced.

Team factors include those that make team sports just that: working together as a group, willingness to assist in group success, contributing to the development of team norms, and being interdependent.

Leadership factors focus upon styles of leadership that are exhibited through behaviors. Relationships are then established within the group based on leadership style.

One of the ways in which group cohesion and group performance can be measured involves sociometry. **Sociometry** is the measurement of how group members feel about something or why they performed a particular behavior. A **sociogram** is a method of diagramming the relationships among members of a group. Figure 12.1 represents a sociogram of a twelve-person team. Those persons who are most often chosen as most liked by others could be placed in the center of the diagram; the least often selected could be placed on the periphery. Further identification could be provided to categorize those who are *stars* (#7 in Figure 12.1) or highly popular; *pairs* (#2 and #3 in Figure 12.1), two who have reciprocal bonds, and *chains* (#9, 10, 11) as subgroups or cliques. The number of times an individual is chosen (choice status), the number of times an individual is rejected (rejection status), the relative number of mutual pairs in a

Sociometry
the science studying how group members feel about something or why they behave as they do

Sociogram
a graphic figure depicting the relationship and status between members of a group

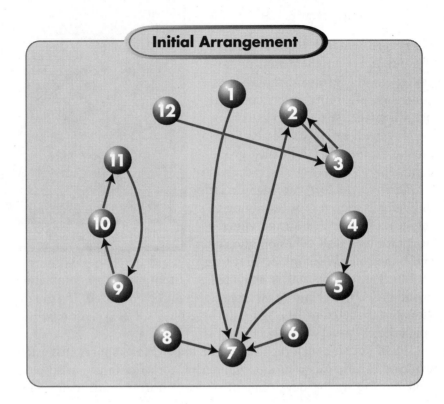

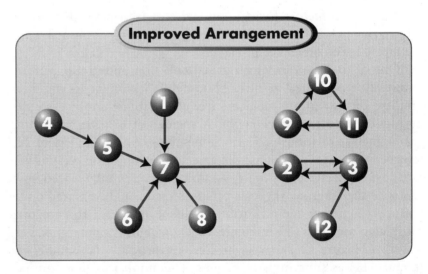

*Sample
sociogram*

group (cohesion status), and the relative number of isolates (group integration status) can all be determined through the use of a sociogram (Moreno, 1960). This can be particularly helpful when the motor behavior professional is trying to create groupings for optimal learning environments. The following learning lab is an example of a questionnaire that can be devised to reflect group member relationships.

Several investigations (Fiedler, 1954; Myers, 1962; Lenk, 1969) tried to determine the effect of team cohesion on group performance. Generally, it was found that the more successful the team, the less important it was for members to like one another. On more successful teams, the best teammate seemed to be one who was less emotionally involved with others on the team; on less successful teams, the best teammate seemed to be one who was more emotionally involved with others on the team. Additionally, competition brought an unexpected dimension to the fold: those groups that experienced any type of competition developed better interpersonal relations than those that did not experience competition, regardless of how successful the team was. It was also determined (McGrath, 1962; Landers & Leuschen, 1974) that teams that focused on developing strong interpersonal relations did not improve in motor skill performance. It could be said, then, that the effect of performance on cohesion is stronger than the effect of cohesion on performance.

Other investigations, however, have found the opposite. Teams with high levels of cohesion performed better than those with low levels of team cohesion (Klein & Christensen, 1969; Bird, 1977; Martens & Peterson, 1971). This conclusion was based upon collective efficacy (how well teammates expected the group to perform) and upon the group's perception of member closeness within the group.

Group cohesion and its relationship to performance might also be sport-specific (Steiner, 1972). When the requirements of the sport demand coordination and cooperation between team members, team cohesion positively affects team success. For example, in basketball, volleyball, team handball, or ice/field hockey, team members are *interactive* (meaningful interaction is required of team members to produce team success) and interdependent for team success. When the sport requires little or no interdependence, team cohesion may have a strong relationship to team success. Archery, gymnastics, biathlon, pistol shooting, tae kwan do, or bowling provide opportunities for **coaction** — individuals perform together but independently of other team members. It would seem logical, then,

Coaction
little interaction of team members required to produce team success

LEARNING LAB

This is a questionnaire that has been devised to facilitate the use of sociometry and to assist in revealing relationships within groups. Complete this learning lab by collecting data and analyze the results by developing a sociogram.

Questionnaire

Directions: Please remain anonymous by not signing this questionnaire. The information you provide will be kept confidential. Complete the blanks with the names of members on your team who fit the question. Provide first and second choices to each. Use only the names of others on your team, not your own. You may use the same team members' names as many times as you like, but only once per question.

1. On our road trips, which team members would you room with if you had a choice?
   _____ and _____

2. On our team, which team members are the most fun to be around?
   _____ and _____

3. On our team, which team members are the best students in the classroom?
   _____ and _____

4. On our team, which team members do not apply themselves in practice?
   _____ and _____

5. On our team, which team members apply themselves the most in practice?
   _____ and _____

6. On our team, which team members know the most about strategy and game plays?
   _____ and _____

7. On our team, which team members do you have the most confidence in when situations get tough?
   _____ and _____

8. On our team, which team members do you like the least?
   _____ and _____

9. On our team, which team members would run a practice if the coach did not show up?
   _____ and _____

10. On our team, which team members would you look to for guidance if the team was disoriented during play?
   _____ and _____

that those team sports that have both coactive and interactive demands (like cricket, baseball/softball, doubles tennis, doubles badminton) may have a component of team cohesion, but the extent to which cohesion plays a role has yet to be fully understood (Hanrahan & Gallois, 1993). Additional investigations must be conducted to test the viability of this concept.

STRATEGIES FOR BUILDING TEAM COHESION

The motor behavior professional can play an important role in building team cohesion. Members of the team and support staff can also facilitate team cohesion. Several guidelines have been developed to assist in the process (Anshel, 1990; Carron, 1982; Weinberg & Gould, 1995).

One of the most important components in building team cohesion is that of efficient and effective communication (the sharing of meanings). The motor behavior professional must work on communicating clearly what is required to be a member of the team, to contribute to the team, and to be supportive of the team. Team members need to feel comfortable with their roles on the team. Motor behavior professionals must work to ensure that those whose roles are substitutes feel valued in the total team experience and total team success.

The distinctiveness of the team and its parts is important to team cohesion. For example, the defensive line in American football could be referred to as "The Wall," giving it a distinctiveness that builds solidarity within a portion of the team.

Team goals that produce challenges and that are attainable with solid effort have an impact on the development of team cohesion. The development of a slogan like "What have you done today to prepare for the 2000 Olympic Games in Sydney?" can promote a team identity in combination with a team goal that is challenging and attainable.

Team meetings can be held for purposes of communication, reshaping goals, and conflict resolution. The goals for each meeting might include the production of strategies and a willingness to commit to actions that will resolve conflicts.

Each person in the group must feel special. Knowing birthdays, anniversaries, siblings' names, and where people have lived can provide details from which to build caring, concern, and compassion that can support behaviors that indicate an interest in the individual as a person, not only as a member of a team.

Team members can also facilitate team success through team cohesion. They can contribute to creating a shared goal or mission that everyone agrees to and is committed to accomplishing. By their behaviors, they can help to build a climate of trust and openness where individuals feel comfortable to learn and grow. There must be a freedom to express ideas, where no idea is considered a bad one. Diversity must be a valued asset, whereby the greater good of the team is benefitted by divergent thinking when solving challenges.

Because many motor skills are performed in a group environment, understanding the nature of groups, how individuals relate to groups, and how groups influence motor behavior leads to a better understanding of the impact social perspective has on motor behavior, from learning to performance. The contributions of social interactions to motor behavior are still in the process of being fully understood.

KEY POINTS

- Human movement relates not only to the individual, but also to the interaction and interdependence of individuals as they move through multidimensional time and space.

- A group is not just a collection of individuals. One of its distinctive markers is the characteristic of interdependence.

- Other characteristics of a group can include interaction, structure, size, goals, unity, and temporal change.

- There are four stages in the process of team development: forming, storming, norming, and performing.

- Actual productivity = potential productivity − losses through faulty group process

- The Ringelmann effect involves the notion that when people perform motor skills in a group, individual performance is decreased.

- Social loafing refers to an individual's decrease in performance, which may be attributed to that person's allocation of effort strategy or minimizing strategy.

- Once individuals become members of groups, their perceptions of personal responsibility may decrease (diffusion of responsibility).

- Attributions are the explanations people create for the causes of behaviors and events.

- Significant others play important roles in influencing achievement motivation and achievement attributions.

- The phenomenon of social facilitation affects motor performance.

- Goal setting is another means of achieving group success.

- Team cohesion refers to the relative strength of a group to remain focused and together in their attempt to achieve group goals.

- Numerous strategies have been devised to build team cohesion. They include efficient and effective communication, distinctiveness, team goals that are challenging and attainable, team meetings, and feeling special as a result of being in the group.

DISCUSSION QUESTIONS

1. What is social facilitation theory? How can this theory be applied in the practice environment?

2. Using the example of the village as a model, devise a group of fifty members on a coed track and field team. Describe ways to build team cohesion.

3. Using Steiner's model for determining group performance, provide an example of the actual productivity of a ten-person bowling team.

4. Determine at least two more internal and external factors relating to sport attribution theory. State your rationale for their selection.

5. Three basic questions were listed involving goal setting. List them and then use them to develop three specific goals for a practice session in a favorite activity.

ADDITIONAL READINGS

Brawley, L. R., Carron, A. V., & Widmeyer, W. N. (1987). Assessing the cohesion of teams: Validity of the Group Environment Questionnaire. *Journal of Sport Psychology, 9,* 275–294.

Reis, H. T., & Jelsma, B. (1978). A social psychology of sex differences in sport. In W. F. Straub (Ed.), *Sport psychology: An analysis of athlete behavior* (pp. 276–286). Ithaca, NY: Mouvement.

Zander, A. (1975). Motivation and performance of sports groups. In D. M. Landers (Ed.), *Psychology of sport and motor behavior II* (pp. 25–29). University Park: Pennsylvania State University Press.

REFERENCES

Albrecht, T. L., & Adelman, M. B. (1984). Social support and life stress: New directions for communication research. *Human Communication Research, 1,* 3–22.

Allport, F. H. (1920). The influence of the group upon association and thought. *Journal of Experimental Psychology, 3,* 159–182.

Anshel, M. (1990). *Sport psychology: From theory to practice.* Scottsdale, AZ: Gorsuch Scarisbrick.

Biddle, S. J. H., & Hill, A. B. (1988). Causal attributions and emotional reactions to outcome in a sporting contest. *Personality and Individual Differences, 9,* 213–223.

Bird, A. M. (1977). Development of a model for predicting team performance. *Research Quarterly, 48,* 24–32.

Bird, A. M., Foster, C. D., & Maruyama, G. (1980). Convergent and incremental effects of cohesion on attributions for self and team. *Journal of Sport Psychology, 2,* 181–194.

Bond, C. F., & Titus, L. J. (1983). Social facilitation: A meta-analysis of 241 studies. *Psychological Bulletin, 94,* 264–292.

Brickner, M. A., Harkins, S. G., & Ostrom, T. M. (1986). Effects of personal involvement: Thought-provoking implications for social loafing. *Journal of Personality and Social Psychology, 51,* 763–770.

Bukowski, W. M., & Moore, D. (1980). Winners' and losers' attributions for success and failure in a series of athletic events. *Journal of Sport Psychology, 2,* 195–210.

Carron, A. V. (1982). Cohesiveness in sport groups. Interpretations and considerations. *Journal of Sport Psychology, 4,* 123–138.

Deaux, K. (1984). From individual differences to social categories: Analysis of a decade's research on gender. *American Psychologist, 39,* 105–116.

Duda, J. L. (1986). Perceptions of sport success and failure among white, black, and Hispanic adolescents. In J. Watkins, T. Reilly, & L. Burwitz (Eds.), *Sport science* (pp. 214–222). London: E. & F. N. Spon.

Fiedler, F. E. (1954). Assumed similarity measures as predictors of team effectiveness. *Journal of Abnormal and Social Psychology, 49,* 381–388.

Hanrahan, S., & Gallois, C. (1993). In R. N. Singer, M. Murphey, & L. K. Tennant (Eds.), *Handbook of research on sport psychology* (pp. 623–646). New York: Macmillan.

Harkins, S. G., Latane, B., & Williams, K. D. (1980). Social loafing: Allocational effort or taking it easy? *Journal of Experimental Social Psychology, 16,* 457–465.

Horn, T. S. (1985). Coaches' feedback and changes in children's perceptions of their physical competence. *Journal of Educational Psychology, 77,* 174–186.

Huddleston, S., Doody, S. G., & Ruder, M. K. (1985). The effect of prior knowledge of the social loafing phenomenon on performance in a group. *International Journal of Sport Psychology, 16,* 176–182.

Ingham, A. G., Levinger, G., Graves, J., & Peckham, V. (1974). The Ringelmann effect: Studies of group size and group performance. *Journal of Experimental Social Psychology, 10,* 371–384.

Jackson, J. M., & Williams, K. D. (1990). *A review and theoretical analysis of social loafing.* Belmont, CA: Brooks & Cole.

Johnson, L., & Biddle, S. J. H. (1988). Persistence after failure: An exploratory look at "learned helplessness" in motor performance. *British Journal of Physical Education Research Supplement, 5,* 7–10.

Kerr, N. L. (1983). Motivation losses in small groups: A social dilemma analysis. *Journal of Personality and Social Psychology, 45,* 819–828.

Kerr, N. L., & Bruun, S. E. (1981). Ringelmann revisited: Alternative explanations for the social loafing effect. *Personality and Social Psychology Bulletin, 7,* 224–231.

Klein, M., & Christensen, G. (1969). Group composition, group structure, and group effectiveness of basketball teams. In J. W. Loy & G. S. Kenyon (Eds.), *Sport, culture, and society* (pp. 397–408). New York: Macmillan.

Kluka, D. (1991). Volleyball P.R.ide — Pass it on! *Coaching Volleyball Journal, 8*(5), 17–18.

Kluka, D. (1996). The Olympic spirit: Reflection, perspectives, and possibilities. *ICHPERSD Journal, 23*(2), 8–10.

Landers, D. M., & Leuschen, G. (1974). Team performance outcome and the cohesiveness of competitive coacting groups. *International Review of Sport Sociology, 9,* 57–71.

Latane, B., & Darley, J. M. (1970). *The unresponsive bystander: Why doesn't he help?* New York: Appleton-Century-Crofts.

Latane, B., Williams, K. D., & Harkins, S. G. (1979). Many hands make light the work: The causes and consequences of social loafing. *Journal of Personality and Social Psychology, 37,* 823–832.

Lenk, H. (1969). Top performance despite internal conflict: An antithesis to a functionalistic proposition. In J. W. Loy & G. S. Kenyon (Eds.), *Sport, culture and society* (pp. 393–397). New York: Macmillan.

Lewin, K. (1948). *Resolving social conflicts: Selected papers on group dynamics.* New York: Harper.

Mackie, D. M., & Goethals, G. R. (1987). Individual and group goals. *Review of Personality and Social Psychology, 8,* 144–166.

Martens, R. A., & Peterson, J. A. (1971). Group cohesiveness as a determinant of success and member satisfaction in team performance. *International Review of Sport Sociology, 6,* 49–61.

McGrath, J. E. (1962). The influence of positive interpersonal relations on adjustment and effectiveness in rifle teams. *Journal of Abnormal and Social Psychology, 65,* 365–375.

Mento, A. J., Steel, R. P., & Karren, R. J. (1987). A meta-analytic study of the effects of goal setting on task performance: 1966–1984. *Organizational Behavior and Human Decision Processes, 39,* 52–83.

Moreno, J. L. (Ed.). (1960). *The sociometry reader.* Glencoe, NY: Free Press.

Myers, A. E. (1962). Team competition, success, and adjustment of group members. *Journal of Abnormal and Social Psychology, 65,* 325–332.

Read, P. P. (1974). *Alive.* New York: Avon.

Roberts, G. C. (1993). Motivation in sport and exercise: Conceptual constraints and convergence. In G. C. Roberts (Ed.), *Motivation in sport and exercise.* Champaign, IL: Human Kinetics.

Rudisill, M. E. (1988). Sex differences in various cognitive and behavioural parameters in a competitive setting. *International Journal of Sport Psychology, 19,* 296–310.

Simmel, G. (1902). The number of members as determining the sociological form of the group. *American Journal of Sociology, 8,* 1–46, 158–196.

Steiner, I. D. (1972). *Group process and productivity.* New York: Academic Press.

Travis, L. E. (1925). The effect of a small audience upon eye-hand coordination. *Journal of Abnormal and Social Psychology, 20,* 142–146.

Triplett, N. (1898). The dynamogenic factors in pacemaking and competition. *American Journal of Psychology, 9,* 507–533.

Tuckman, B. W. (1965). Developmental sequence in small groups. *Psychological Bulletin, 63,* 384–399.

Weinberg, R., & Gould, D. (1995). *Foundations of sport and exercise psychology.* Champaign, IL: Human Kinetics Publishers.

Weiner, B. (1979). A theory of motivation for some classroom experiences. *Journal of Educational Psychology, 71,* 3–25.

Weiss, M. R., McAuley, E., Ebbeck, V., & Wiese, D. M. (1990). Self-esteem and causal attributions for children's physical and social competence in sport. *Journal of Sport and Exercise Psychology, 12,* 21–36.

Wheeler, L., Reis, H. T., & Bond, M. H. (1985). Collectivism-individualism in everyday social life: The middle kingdom and the melting pot. *Journal of Personality and Social Psychology, 57,* 79–86.

Whitehead, J. (1986). A cross-national comparison of attributions underlying achievement orientations in adolescent sport. In J. Watkins, T. Reilly, & L. Burwitz (Eds.), *Sport science* (pp. 297–302). London: E. & F. N. Spon.

Williams, J. M., & Hacker, C. M. (1982). Causal relationships among cohesion, satisfaction, and performance in women's intercollegiate field hockey teams. *Journal of Sport Psychology, 4,* 324–337.

Wood, W. (1985). A meta-analysis review of sex differences in group performance. *Psychological Bulletin, 102,* 53–71.

Zander, A. (1982). *Making groups effective.* San Francisco, CA: Jossey-Bass.

Zajonc, R. B. (1965). Social facilitation. *Science, 149,* 269–274.

Performance Perspectives

The 1996 Olympic Games held in Atlanta produced record-breaking performances in a variety of sports. Accounts of superlative performances were documented throughout the Games. The road to the Olympic Games for many individuals reflected fascinating perspectives on performance. One such individual was Michele Smith, Olympic Gold Medalist and pitcher for the USA Softball Team, with a batting average of .325 and Olympic record of 2–0.

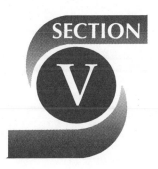

As a youngster, Smith began to excel in basketball, softball, and field hockey. She participated in all three in high school, and made All-State Softball and All-Conference basketball and field hockey. After a near-fatal automobile accident in 1986 at age 15, Smith underwent intensive rehabilitation on her pitching arm and came back stronger than ever. While on a full softball scholarship at Oklahoma State University, she led the nation in home runs, had an 82-20 record as a pitcher, made All-Big Eight Conference Tournament, All-Academic Big Eight, President's Honor Roll, was the Broderick Award Runner-Up, and was selected the State of Oklahoma College Athlete of the Year by USA Today. She earned the Canada Cup Most Valuable Player and Most Valuable Pitcher Awards, USA Softball's Bertha Tickey Award, was selected as the United States Olympic Committee Softball Sportsperson of the Year, and was a member of gold medal teams at the Intercontinental Cup, Softball World Championships, and Pan American Games.

What are some of the factors that may have contributed to Smith's performance success? How were many of these performances measured to reflect performance excellence?

275

Scientific Measurement and Motor Behavior

CHAPTER 13

- Performance curves to determine learning
- Basic procedures of data collection and statistical analysis in motor behavior investigations
- Various assessment categories that have been used in motor behavior investigations

The acquisition of motor skills implies that humans establish behavioral repertoires that can be observed. It is important to understand how motor behavior is assessed through performance measurements, the meaning of some of those measurements, and the types of instruments that have been used to research observable motor behavior.

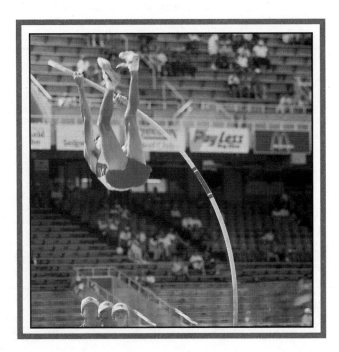

MOTOR BEHAVIOR
AND PERFORMANCE MEASUREMENTS

Motor skill acquisition has traditionally been documented by measurements of performance. These measurements, when systematically recorded, give field-based professionals indicators of changes in behavior. These "snapshots" of performances over time can be referred to as **performance curves**. Motor behavior researchers have traditionally used performance curves when documenting the effect of various instructional strategies on the learning of motor skills (Bryan & Harter, 1897; Godwin & Schmidt, 1971; Franks & Wilberg, 1982). Smith's batting average over several seasons exemplifies performance snapshots that could easily be used to create a performance curve. Because learning, as earlier defined, cannot be directly viewed, performance measures show behavior changes through practice over time. With a performance curve, the results generally indicate improvement over time as well as consistency of improvement. If volleyball serving success is determined by the number of serves completed over the net and in the court out of five pretrial, the percentage of successful serves should increase over time. Consistency should also be noted. Figure 13.1 reflects this type of performance curve. In graphing this type of curve, performance used to assess the skill is placed on the vertical axis (y axis),

Performance curves
"snapshots" of performances over time displayed in a graph format

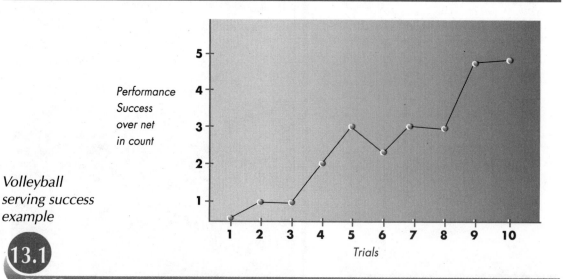

Volleyball serving success example

13.1
FIGURE

while the time or trials over which the performance occurred is placed on the horizontal (x axis). The intersection of the x and y axes is always marked 0,0 (zero, zero), and time is always represented in equal units, increasing from zero. Additionally, each trial is linked to each performance by the intersection of the two points on the graph. Generally, the intersection is marked by a dot that is then connected to other dots by a line. The resulting line is what is referred to as the actual performance curve.

CHANGES IN PERFORMANCE AS A RESULT OF PRACTICE

Objective: To observe changes in practice of a motor skill through repeated trials.

Equipment and Preparation: Three tennis balls; stop watch; data sheet; microcomputer graph application program or graph paper; partner; cleared area, 10' by 10'

Experience: Using three tennis balls to juggle, hold two tennis balls in one hand (Balls 1 and 3) and one in the other (Ball 2). Toss number 1 into the air. Just prior to catching 1, toss 2 into the air. Then toss 3 up into the air just before catching 2. Continue this pattern so that one of the balls is in the air continuously while one ball is being grasped in each hand.

With a partner, practice the process of juggling for two minutes (timed by the partner). At the end of two minutes of practice, the partner says "go" to begin each juggling trial. While juggling, the partner records the number of successful times a ball is caught. (A ball is caught when the person grasps the ball in one hand.) At the end of two minutes, the partner says "stop." The number successfully completed is recorded. The partner now begins the same procedure. Each partner completes five trials of two minutes. After both partners are finished and before leaving class, secure the results from five other members of the class.

Assignment: Find the overall mean for all of your trials. Find the overall mean for each of the other peoples' trials. Find the overall group mean for all trials. Find the group mean for each trial. Using a line graph computer applications program, enter the data into a separate file. Once the data have been entered, each person's overall mean, the overall group mean for all trials, and the group mean for each trial can be plotted.

Discuss what you found as a result of the overall means for the group, each person's overall mean, and the group mean for each trial. What do these performances mean relative to the learning of a motor skill? What effect, if any, did practice have? What effect, if any, did rest have?

THE MEANING OF PERFORMANCE CURVES

Linear curve
a graphical, proportional measure of performance over time

Positively accelerated curve
graphic depiction showing little improvement initially and performance improvement during later trials

Negatively accelerated curve
an indication of rapid improvement in early trials and stabilized performance soon thereafter

S-shaped curve
a combination of linear, positively accelerated, and negatively accelerated curves

To repeat, a performance curve usually shows improvement in performance scores over time. There are four basic types of performance curves commonly observed in typical motor behavior research. These are illustrated in Figure 13.2. Each is displayed as an equal amount of increase in performance for each time interval. A **linear curve** represents performance increases over time that are proportionate. As the number of trials increases, performance increases proportionately. In a **positively accelerating curve**, little improvement is recorded over the initial trials, and performance improves during later trials; that is, the rate of learning increases over time. A **negatively accelerating curve** indicates that rapid improvement is made in the early trials, and performance stabilizes soon thereafter; that is, the rate of learning decreases over time. An **S-shaped curve** (ogive curve) is a combination of positively accelerating and negatively accelerating curves. In some cases, improved performance would really be indicated by a reduction in time or in error; therefore, the direction of the slope is down rather than up. For example, when recording performances of 200 m freestyle in swimming,

Performance curves

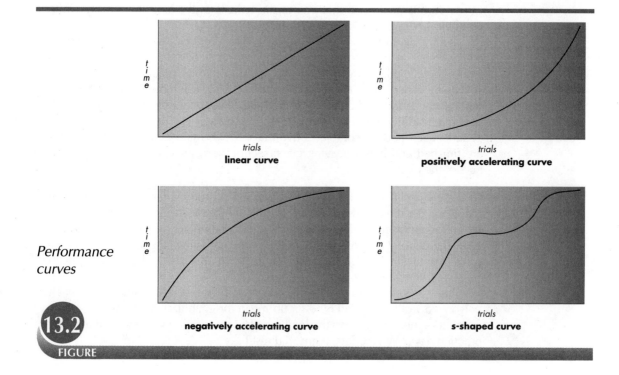

13.2
FIGURE

performance times should decrease with subsequent trials. Similarly, the recording of typing errors should exhibit a decrease in errors.

Schmidt (1991), Newell (1991), and Shea, Shebilske, and Worchel (1993) have criticized the use of performance curves as a measure of learning. Difficulties have arisen when performance scores have been used to determine learning, because performance curves have generally been developed in a short period of time (e.g., minutes, hours, or days) and/or through repeated and blocked trials (e.g., sixty trials with the same goal). Learning is equivalent to retention or transfer, so this must be tested for if learning is to be measured. Blocked trials have been represented as a single average, thereby losing fluctuations exhibited during the learning process.

Additionally, performance curves established for groups have sacrificed individual differences, taking individual scores that were higher on some trials and averaging them with individual scores that were lower, thereby making the average of scores provide a picture that could be misleading to the professional interpreting the performance curve to infer learning. A method of analysis used by the motor behavior professional to assess motor performance involves the use of statistics.

LAB EXERCISE

TYPES OF INSTRUMENTATION

Objective: To devise instruments that can be used to assess one of the following conditions, assess individuals, determine and descriptively interpret the results:

(a) coincidence anticipation time

(b) reaction time

(c) perception

(d) selective attention

(e) feedback

(f) transfer

Equipment and Preparation: Using equipment that is found at Walmart, K-Mart, or similar stores, construct an instrument that can be used to assess one of the above motor behaviors.

Assignment: Using this instrument, assess two groups of people, 10 in each group. Using descriptive statistics, describe the results of each group. Devise a performance curve based upon each group's results and compare the curves. Interpret the results.

BASIC STATISTICS: THEIR USE IN MOTOR BEHAVIOR PERFORMANCE ASSESSMENT

While performance curves provide visual images of data, the data are more easily understood when they are organized and summarized. Collecting and recording data are valuable as well. Instrumentation used in data collection and recording will be discussed later in the chapter. An understanding of a few basic statistical terms and procedures will be helpful to interpreting the results.

Untreated individual scores that are collected are referred to as **raw data**. Raw data are used to calculate measures that describe elements more effectively (**descriptive statistics**) or use samples of a population to test presumptions, or hypotheses (**inferential statistics**).

One technique used to describe a set of data is **central tendency**. Central tendency simply means the determination of a number that is a cluster point for the data examined. Two measures of central tendency commonly used in motor behavior descriptive statistics are mean and median.

The **mean**, or the arithmetic average, is calculated by adding all of the scores and dividing by the total number of scores (M = Mean; Σ = Sum of; X = raw score; N = total number of scores). The mean is affected by every score's size.

$$\text{Mean } (M) = \frac{\text{Sum of the raw scores } (\Sigma X)}{\text{total number of scores } (N)} \text{ or } M = \frac{\Sigma X}{N}$$

Sometimes it is helpful to determine the median rather than the mean. The median can be determined when there seem to be a few scores that are substantially different. The **median** is the middle of the scores or the fiftieth percentile and is affected by the position of scores to one another. To calculate the median, all raw scores must be ranked in order (e.g., smallest to largest, where time is the score). The score that is in the exact middle is the median score. When the total number of scores is even, the two middle scores are averaged to determine the median score.

To determine whether to use the mean or median score, the following example may prove helpful. If an individual's scores on a test involving length of lateness in anticipation time were 0.002, 0.003, 0.003, 0.004, 0.008, 0.009, 0.010, 0.010, 0.011, 0.012, 0.012, 0.013, 0.013, 0.015, 0.020, the mean score would be 0.009. The median score would be 0.010. If the first and last scores were changed

Raw data
scores collected on subjects in a research investigation

Descriptive statistics
mathematical means for detailing information from a group

Inferential statistics
mathematical means for sampling a population to test hypotheses

Central tendency
the determination of a number that is a cluster point for the data examined

Mean
the arithmetic average

Median
the middle of a set of scores or the 50th percentile; affected by position of scores to one another

to 0.001 and 0.050, respectively, the median would still remain at 0.010, but the mean would change to 0.012. The mean, in the second case, shows more appropriately the central tendency of scores.

While central tendency refers to the common tendencies of scores, the **standard deviation** refers to how scores differ from one another, or their **variability**. In the case of standard deviation, the mean serves as a "standard" by which all other scores are measured. The difference between each score and the mean is the deviation from the mean. In general, the smaller the standard deviation, the more homogeneous (similar) the sample is. The larger the standard deviation, the more heterogeneous (dissimilar) the sample is.

To calculate the standard deviation (sd), place the scores in a column (x); add the scores in the column (Σx); divide Σx by the total number of scores (n) to get the mean; determine how much each score deviates from the mean (column d); square the column d; calculate the sum of d^2 (Σd^2); place answers in the formula; calculate the formula.

> **Standard deviation**
> a statistical depiction of how scores differ from one another
>
> **Variability**
> how scores differ from one another

$$sd = \frac{\Sigma d^2}{n - 1}$$

A **normal distribution** of scores is illustrated in Figure 13.3. It represents a symmetrical distribution, where the mean, median, and mode (most common score) are the same. Typically, about two-thirds (68 percent) of all scores fall within one standard deviation of the mean. Only about one-sixth of the scores (13 percent) are more than one standard deviation below or above the mean. Only 3 percent are two standard deviations above or below the mean. For example, dart throwing accuracy was measured on a group of thirty individuals, ten trials each. Distance from the center of the bull's-eye was recorded. Using Figure 13.3 as a model, if the mean for the group was 15 mm and the standard deviation was 5 mm, an individual having a score of 18 mm and another having a score of 13 mm would both have average scores (within 68 percent).

> **Normal distribution**
> symmetrical distribution of scores, in which the mean, median, and mode are the same

Another useful statistic is the **range**. It is calculated by subtracting the lowest score from the highest one. It is a coarse, but simple, way to determine how different the scores are within groups. The larger the range, the more heterogeneous the group.

> **Range**
> a numerical representation of the spectrum of scores

When comparing performance measurements between groups of individuals, samples of populations are used to estimate the overall population. Inferential statistics can be used to help determine

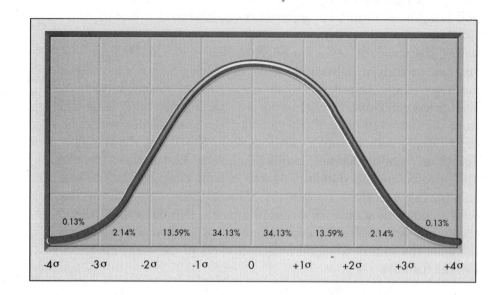

A normal distribution of scores

0.13%   2.14%   13.59%   34.13%   34.13%   13.59%   2.14%   0.13%

-4σ   -3σ   -2σ   -1σ   0   +1σ   +2σ   +3σ   +4σ

13.3
FIGURE

Correlation
a statistic used to determine the relationship between variables

Coefficient of correlation
a numerical value ranging from +1 to −1, used to indicate a relationship

differences (i.e., no statistical significance) and similarities (i.e., relationships) between groups.

One of the statistical procedures most commonly used to determine if there is a relationship between variables is the **correlation**. Simply, it is used to determine the strength of their interrelatedness. The **coefficient of correlation**, a numerical value ranging from +1 to −1, is used to indicate the relationship (Figure 13.4). If the coefficient is +1.00, there is a linear relationship, meaning that as one variable increases, the other increases in direct proportion. When a 0.00 coefficient exists, there is no relationship between the two variables. When the coefficient is −1.00, there is a direct linear relationship whereby when one variable increases, the other variable decreases in direct proportion. The closer the coefficient is to ± 1.00 (e.g., ± .75), the more closely the variables are related. For example, if the coefficient is between 0 and 0.20, a weak relationship exists; between 0.21 and 0.40, a low relationship; between 0.41 and 0.60, a moderate relationship; between 0.61 and 0.80, a high relationship; and between 0.81 and 1.00, a very high relationship.

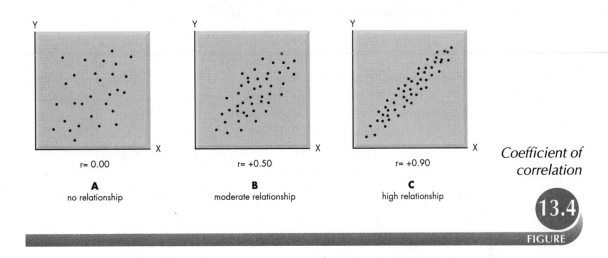

Coefficient of correlation

13.4
FIGURE

It is also possible to determine if differences, rather than relationships, exist between groups. Two statistical procedures commonly used in motor behavior investigations are t-tests and analyses of variance. The **t-test** is generally used to determine if two means are significantly different from one another. A t-test is a ratio of the difference between means and sample size variability. It helps us to determine if the difference between two groups is large enough not to have occurred by chance. It is most appropriate when only one variable is of interest. For example, an investigator might wish to determine if there was a significant difference between two groups when one group was presented with knowledge of results when learning a task, while the other group was not. In this case, the presence or absence of knowledge of results could account for the difference in scores between groups.

The ratio that is attained from the differences between the two group means and standard deviations is referred to as a **critical ratio**. This numerical value, when compared to values found in statistical tables (tabled values), displays the **level of significance** (e.g., .05 or .01) that five times out of one hundred or one time out of one hundred the results discovered would occur by chance. The **level of confidence,** on the other hand, represents the number of times the results would occur (e.g., .95 or .99). In general, if the calculated-t value is less than or equal to the tabled-t value, the groups are significantly different.

T-test
a statistical procedure to determine if two means are significantly different from one another

Critical ratio
the ratio attained from the differences between the two group means and standard deviations

Level of significance
the level at which the number of times the results will occur by chance can be predicted

Level of confidence
the level at which the number of times the results will occur can be predicted with some accuracy

UNDERSTANDING OTHER PERFORMANCE MEASUREMENTS

Retention tests
tools used to determine how much has been retained as a result of block-type information presented

Absolute retention scores
scores indicating that which has been retained

Relative retention scores
scores that indicate how much information was retained or lost as a result of comparing the difference between the score attained in the skill acquisition portion on the last trial and what was attained on the first trial of a retention test

Savings scores
scores that reflect the rate at which a given level of performance of a skill returns when the skill has not been practiced for some of time

Transfer tests
measurement of the skills learned in one situation in a different practice setting

The measurement of retention of motor skills is another way to determine the level of learning. **Retention** testing is used often by field-based professionals to determine how much has been retained from block-type presentations (such as a unit in swimming, modern dance, or low-impact aerobics). Retention testing also provides the field-based professional with information about instructional strategies used. This measurement approach fits well in assessing motor learning. Motor learning, a multifaceted set of internal processes through which there is a relatively permanent change in human performance through practice, by definition involves a change in behavior that is more or less permanent. Sometimes a pretest is given at the beginning of the unit, with the same test used as a posttest to determine performance increases. A third administration of the test should be given at some designated time after the skills are no longer practiced to determine if motor skills were retained. The scores earned from the third test are called **absolute retention scores** (Christina & Shea, 1988), because they indicate that which has been retained. In addition to the calculation of absolute retention scores, relative retention scores and savings scores have recently emerged as other measures suitable for analyzing retention (Christina & Shea, 1993). **Relative retention scores** indicate how much information was retained or lost as a result of comparing the difference between the score attained in the skill acquisition portion on the last trial and what was attained on the first trial of the retention test. **Savings scores** also reflect the rate at which a particular level of performance of a skill returns when the skill has not been practiced for a period of time. It is calculated by adding the number of trials it takes to reach the level of skilled performance achieved at the end of the acquisition portion.

Another way to measure learning involves testing for transfer. For many field-based motor behavior professionals, not only is retention an issue of importance, but skills being transferred to other settings is also important. The skills individuals have practiced in one situation should be transferable to different situations. **Transfer testing** occurs when the skills performed in one situation are assessed in another practice setting. For example, a series of skills tests have been devised to assess the overhead volleyball pass, the serve, the forearm pass, and the spike. To test for transfer, the same skills could be performed and assessed under gamelike conditions.

The notion of transfer was discussed in Section I. Two basic types of transfer tests exist in the motor learning literature: intratask transfer and intertask transfer. An *intratask transfer test* compares the performance of a specific motor skill in one environment under a specific set of conditions to the performance of the same skill under a different performance condition. For example, a female gymnast has performed giant swings successfully on high bar; she must then transfer them to the high bar on unevens. The *intertask transfer test*, conversely, assesses two different motor skills that may have some common elements. After learning a smash in badminton, the individual must perform a spike in volleyball. Both are quite dissimilar in technique. The individual must try to use cognitive strategies to transfer basic concepts from one skill to the other in two different environments.

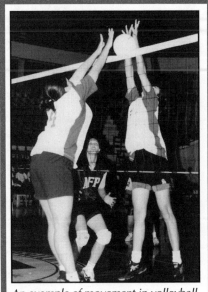

An example of movement in volleyball.

Memory recall tests add to the mixture of assessments used to determine performance. Also known as pattern recognition tests, these assessments identify short-term perceptual strategies and characteristics of individuals. For example, these tests are typically used to identify the perceptual strategies used by skilled and unskilled persons. Chunking, the process of grouping meaningful information into manageable bits, can be inferred based upon the notion that those who chunk better can remember better. Researchers (Chase and Simon, 1973) found that skilled chess players were able to recall the positions of chess pieces within gamelike situations significantly better than less skilled players. There was no difference, however, between skilled and unskilled players when chess pieces were randomly placed on the board. This result implies that skilled chess players used chunking strategies that were recalled within the context of the chess game. Using a more physically dynamic environment to assess the same concept, researchers developed slides of specific and random basketball (Allard, Graham,

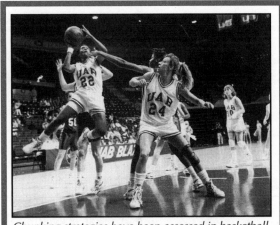

Chunking strategies have been assessed in basketball.

& Paarsalu, 1980), field hockey (Starkes & Deakin, 1984), and volleyball (Abernethy, Burgess-Limerick, & Parks, 1994) offensive and defensive situations and showed them to collegiate and recreational players. Similar results were found: when the collegiate players viewed specific plays, they recalled those plays significantly better than the recreational players; when both groups were shown random formations, no significant difference was noted.

This type of testing is not without challenges. Questions have been raised periodically about the nature of using static tests when dynamic information is sought (Abernethy, Burgess-Limerick, & Parks, 1994). Static photos, impressions, are limited in providing information, as they provide isolated frames of the environmental picture; that which can provide meaningful information to the performer (movement dynamics) is absent. A second issue raised is somewhat like the question of what came first, the chicken or the egg — do experienced athletes already possess better perceptual strategies or does experience contribute to enhancing those perceptual strategies? A third portion of the debate includes the issue of the extent to which enhanced perceptual abilities contribute to superior motor behavior. Enhanced perceptual abilities may be the result of contextual experience rather than a contributing factor.

KEY POINTS

- Motor skills have traditionally been observed by measuring performance.
- "Snapshots" of performances over time can be compiled into performance curves.
- There are four basic types of performance curves: linear, positively accelerated, negatively accelerated, and S-shaped.
- Descriptive and inferential statistics are categories of statistics used to assist in the interpretation of scores.
- The mean, median, and standard deviation are used to describe data.
- A normal distribution represents a symmetrical distribution of scores, where the mean, median, and mode are the same.
- A t-test is commonly used to determine if two means are significantly different from one another.

- Retention testing is used to determine how much has been retained as a result of block-type information presentation.

- Transfer testing is used when the skills performed in one situation are used in another setting.

- Memory recall tests are typically used to determine perceptual strategies used by skilled and unskilled individuals.

DISCUSSION QUESTIONS

1. Discuss the value of performance curves in the learning process.

2. What do the following curve categories mean to the field-based motor behavior professional: linear curve, positively accelerated curve, negatively accelerated curve, S-shaped curve?

3. Describe the differences between inferential and descriptive statistics. Explain the differences between mean, median, mode, and standard deviation.

4. What do the following performance measures assess: retention testing, transfer testing, pattern recognition testing? Why are they important in motor behavior assessment?

ADDITIONAL READINGS

Christina, R. W. (1992). The 1991 C. H. McCloy Research Lecture: Unraveling the mystery of the response complexity effect in skilled movements. *Research Quarterly for Exercise and Sport, 63*(3), 218–230.

Shea, C. H., Shebilske, W. L., & Worchel, S. (1993). *Motor learning and control.* Englewood Cliffs, NJ: Prentice-Hall.

REFERENCES

Abernethy, B., Burgess-Limerick, R., & Parks, S. (1994). Contrasting approaches to the study of motor expertise. *Quest, 46,* 186–198.

Allard, F., Graham, S., & Paarsalu, M. E. (1980). Perception in sport: Basketball. *Journal of Sport Psychology, 2,* 14–21.

Bryan, W. L., & Harter, N. (1897). Studies in the physiology and psychology of the telegraphic language. *Psychological Review, 4,* 27–53.

Chase, W. G., & Simon, H. A. (1973). Perception in chess. *Cognitive Psychology, 4,* 55–81.

Christina, R. W., & Shea, J. B. (1988). The limitations of generalization based on restricted information. *Research Quarterly for Exercise and Sport, 64,* 2, 217–222.

Christina, R. W., & Shea, J. B. (1993). More on assessing the retention of motor learning based on restricted information. *Research Quarterly for Exercise and Sport,* 64(2), 217–222.

Franks, I. M., & Wilberg, R. B. (1982). The generation of movement patterns during the acquisition of a pursuit tracking task. *Human Movement Science, 1,* 251–272.

Godwin, M. A., and Schmidt, R. A. (1971). Muscular fatigue and discrete motor learning. *Research Quarterly, 42,* 374–383.

Newell, K. M. (1991). Motor skill acquisition. *Annual Review of Psychology, 42,* 235–244.

Schmidt, R. (1991). *Motor learning and performance: From principles to practice.* Champaign, IL: Human Kinetics.

Shea, C. H., Shebilske, W. L., & Worchel, S. (1993). *Motor learning and control.* Englewood Cliffs, NJ: Prentice-Hall.

Starkes, J., & Deakin, J. M. 1984). Perception in sport: A cognitive approach to skilled performance. In W. F. Straub and J. M. Williams (Eds.), *Cognitive Sport Psychology* (pp. 115–228). Lansing, NY: Sport Science Associates.

Types of Psychological and Physiological Instrumentation

*N*ow that you have an understanding of performance curves, retention tests, and transfer tests, we proceed to the numerous methods and types of instrumentation that have been used to systematically record performance and infer motor learning. Early investigations were generally conducted with little or no instrumentation, perhaps more qualitative than quantitative in design. Early

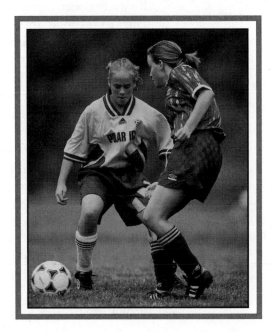

methods of measurement were used to determine outcomes; the research designs focused on the use of experimental variables that could be manipulated. More recent investigations using dynamic systems theory have focused on how the responses were achieved, rather than solely on outcome.

Psychological and physiological measurements and combinations of both have been used. Psychological methods used to assess behavior have involved reaction time and errors in performance.

One of the most popular measurements of human movement is the quantifiable length of time it takes an individual to begin a movement. **Reaction time** is the time from the onset of a stimulus to the initiation of a movement. It does not include the movement, only the time it takes to begin the movement once the stimulus has been displayed. Typically, when reaction time is measured, three events transpire: warning signal, stimulus signal, and beginning of response. The warning and stimulus signals are generally under the control of the investigator, while the initiation of a response is the responsibility of the performer.

The warning signal, if used by the investigator, allows the performer to get ready for the appearance of the stimulus signal. The warning signal may be varied or randomized. This period of time is referred to as the foreperiod. A randomized foreperiod means that the amount of time that the warning signal is displayed varies randomly between trials. The stimulus signal lets the performer know when to respond and is generally in the form of a sensory alert of a light, a sound, or a shock. The actual response can be in the form of almost anything that is action. For example, the individual might press a button with the thumb or finger, or move an arm, leg, or the entire body from one point to another.

Reaction time measurements have been the focus of numerous investigations (Henry & Rogers, 1960; Kelso, 1977; Christina & Rose, 1985), particularly in the 1960s and 1970s. Reaction time (RT) represents the time between the unanticipated presentation of a stimulus and the initiation of movement. Responses to a starter's gun in a sprint is a field example of reaction time. This type of RT is known as **simple reaction time** (SRT), because there is only one possible reaction to only one possible stimulus. RT is also embedded in other activities, such as baseball or softball batting. It has already been determined by the coach and the hitter that when certain conditions exist certain responses will be conducted. If a fastball is thrown, the hitter will hit away; if an inside curve is thrown, the

Reaction time
the interval between the unanticipated presentation of a stimulus and the initiation of movement

Simple reaction time
the time that it takes to react to one possible stimulus

hitter will let it go; if a changeup is thrown, the hitter will bunt. This type of RT is referred to as **choice reaction time** (CRT), because the hitter has more than one signal to which must a response must be made, and each signal has a specific response. The third type of RT is known as **discrimination reaction time** (DRT). In this case, there are a number of possible stimuli but the performer has only one response. The individual will suppress the response unless the correct stimulus occurs. These types of reaction time measurements were used to determine the time required to process information.

Choice reaction time
the interval between the presentation of a stimulus that competes with other stimuli so that the individual must choose and the initiation of movement

Discrimination reaction time
the interval between the presentation of a stimulus that is paired with a response and the initiation of movement

Hick's law (Hick, 1952) emerged from detailed investigations involving choice reaction time. This law states that as the number of stimulus-response choices increases, reaction time will increase, logarithmically. Specifically, the following equation summarizes the law: $RT = K \log2 (N + 1)$. (RT = reaction time; K = a constant, usually simple reaction time; N = the number of choices). There is, then, a linear relationship between the number of choices and the amount of time it takes an individual to select and respond. More specifically, the increase in reaction time and the increase in information possibilities to be transmitted are results of the log2 function. Log2 is used to provide information in the form of a bit (having a yes/no answer choice). There are two choices in a one-bit scenario, four choices in a two-bit, and eight choices in a three-bit. The number of bits delimits the least number of choices available to the individual.

Hick's Law
as the number of stimulus-response choices increases, reaction time will increase logarithmically.

Hick's law is important to sport and physical activity, particularly when individuals are provided with options in open environments. When players in ice hockey perform a faceoff, they are presented with several options: to hit the puck to a teammate, to an opponent, or to allow the opponent involved in the faceoff to hit the puck. The more choices available to the player, the longer the reaction time. From a practical standpoint, to decrease reaction time, the choices must be limited.

Another part of the response time equation includes **movement time**. Response time is the total of reaction time and movement time. Movement time (MT) is measured from the initiation of the overt movement to the end of the movement itself. It can be symbolically stated as: $ResT = RT + MT$, where $ResT$ = Response Time; RT = Reaction Time; and MT = Movement Time. Response time should not be considered the same as reaction time, but rather the time it takes to complete both RT and MT.

Movement time
the interval from the initiation of the movement to the end of the movement itself

Speed/accuracy tradeoff
as distance of targets increases, movement time increases; as target size decreases, movement time increases

Fitts Law
there is a tradeoff between speed and accuracy: when speed is emphasized, accuracy is reduced; when accuracy is emphasized, speed is reduced

Fractionated reaction time
reaction time that has several component parts

Premotor time
the interval from stimulus presentation to the first recorded change of electrical activity in the primary agonist muscle involved in the movement

Motor time
the interval from when the first recorded change of electrical activity in the primary agonist muscle occurs and is completed when the movement begins

Movement time measurement has been frequently used in the assessment of speed and accuracy. It appears to be governed by a concept known as the **speed/accuracy tradeoff**, which works according to **Fitts' law,** based on the work of Paul Fitts (1954). Essentially, when speed is emphasized, accuracy is reduced. When accuracy is emphasized, speed is reduced. The speed/accuracy tradeoff will occur when both movement distance and target size can vary. Movement time is equal to the log2 of twice the movement distance divided by the target width: $MT = a + b \log2 (2D/W)$. MT = movement time; a and b = constants; D = movement distance; W = target size. As a law, there is little or no discussion as to the viability of this tradeoff. The question remains as to how the motor control system operates in movement environments requiring the tradeoff.

In many sport situations, it is necessary to move quickly and accurately to be successful. When performing a compound attack in foil, the fencer must orchestrate accurate manipulative movements of the foil hand (fingers, hand, arm) with large movements of the lower body (hips, upper and lower legs, feet) in combination with speed in order to successfully beat an opponent's parry or defensive movement. The assessment of MT would provide helpful information to determine the effectiveness of power/biomechanical concepts being employed. The question as to whether the fencer plans the entire attack sequence in advance or plans part of it and builds upon it as play develops was difficult to answer based upon MT assessments alone.

During the 1980s (Anson, 1982; Christina, Fischman, Vercruyssen, & Anson, 1982), reaction time was measured more completely through the use of **fractionated reaction time** (FRT). FRT involves an even more precise method of measuring cognitive processes: using surface electromyography (EMG) to divide time into **premotor time** (PreMot) and **motor time** (MoT). Premotor time, directly observable, assesses the time from stimulus presentation to the first recorded change of electrical activity in the primary agonist muscle involved in movement. For example, in performing a bicep curl, the biceps brachii is considered the primary agonist during the flexion phase of the movement, while the triceps brachii would be considered the primary agonist during the extension phase. Premotor time represents the time necessary for a stimulus to be received and interpreted to initiate a voluntary contraction of the corresponding musculature for appropriate movement. Motor time, not directly observable, is initiated when the first recorded change of electrical activity in the primary agonist muscle occurs and is completed when the movement begins. MoT can be determined by subtracting Pre-Mot from ResT. It can be represented as:

$$ResT - PreMot = MoT$$

By measuring FRT, researchers (Christina, 1992; Christina & Rose, 1985) have been able to discern differences between movements themselves and that which contributes to the actual movements. This type of research has also provided distinct thoughts on delays in movement initiation as they relate to cognitive processing complexities or biomechanical and physiological factors.

Response time performance errors have traditionally been a source of information for individuals interested in various perspectives of performance accuracy. This performance accuracy has been divided into two parts: **spatial accuracy** and **temporal accuracy**. Spatial accuracy refers to how closely an individual's movement is to a specific target. Temporal accuracy refers to how accurately an individual moves in a specific amount of time. The biathlon event involves both spatial and temporal accuracy. It is helpful to know whether the biathlete has overshot or undershot the target; it is also helpful to know how quickly the biathlete traversed the course between segments of shooting and how quickly and accurately the athlete was able to shoot while lying in a prone position. By knowing this information, one can make adjustments in response accuracy by altering spatial and temporal components.

Through the use of **chronometry** (measuring time accurately), the amount of error made when attempting to achieve temporal accuracy can be measured. The types of scores that are generally used to assess performance errors include absolute error (AE), constant error (CE), and variable error (VE), absolute constant error (|CE|), and total error (E). These scores provide interesting information from slightly different perspectives. **Absolute error** (AE) simply means the amount of algebraic error in a performance, regardless of sign (e.g., $+1$ or -1 $= 1$). It provides general information about performance as it relates to the goal or target. **Constant error** (CE) delineates directionality as well as amount of error, thereby providing response bias. It is calculated as the average of algebraic errors. **Variable error** (VE) provides yet another piece of information. This indicates the consistency of performance, or conversely the variability in a performance. VE is the standard deviation of algebraic error. The higher the standard deviation, the more variability in performance; the lower

Spatial accuracy
how closely an individual's movement is to a specific target

Temporal accuracy
how quickly an individual moves in a specific amount of time

Chronometry
methods of measuring time accurately

Absolute error
the amount of algebraic error in a performance, regardless of sign

Constant error
delineates directionality as well as amount of error, thereby providing response bias

Variable error
indicates the consistency of performance, or the variability in a performance

Absolute constant error
the absolute value of the constant error

Total error
exposes variability and response bias equally

the standard deviation, the more consistent the performance. **Absolute constant error** (|CE|) is the absolute value of the constant error. This represents response bias without directionality. It has been offered as an alternative performance error score to counterbalance response bias in groups, thereby being a more valid measure of performance error (Henry, 1974; Schutz and Roy, 1973). Simply consider the number of +'s and −'s for CE scores for each individual in the group. **Total error** (E) exposes variability and response bias equally. It provides a more complete picture of the total variability of performance error than any other measure.

In the air pistol event (.177 caliber pistols from 10 m), for example, one shot is fired per target. The course of fire is 60 shots in 1 minute and 45 seconds for men and 40 shots in 1 minute and 15 seconds for women. Where the shot is placed on each target is important. A perfect score is 600 for men and 400 for women. Absolute error scores would provide the coach and athlete with a general impression of shots that missed the targets' centers. Constant error scores would provide meaningful information if shots were clustering or randomly distributed off-target. Variable error scores would provide an understanding of performance consistency, if the athlete was making the same performance errors. Absolute constant error scores would be a viable measure when comparing the air pistol team's scores, to counterbalance response bias in the group. Total error scores would provide information about where shots on the targets were recorded and how consistent performances were. From this information, specific strategies could be constructed by the coach and the biathlete to enhance future performance.

PHYSIOLOGICAL MEASURES

Physiological measurements detect the body's responses to performance demands. For example, the results of pupillary measurement during competition infer the level of anxiety of the individual. Changes in heart rate, increases in lactate levels, or the lowering of skin temperature all indicate changes associated with motor behavior acquisition. These types of physiological measurements are known as physiological correlates. Although these correlates can be linked to motor behavior acquisition, they should not be considered primary methods for measurement. In the 1920s, the **electroencephalogram** (EEG) was developed to record graphically the waves of electrical activity during activities. By means of surface electrodes,

Electroencephalogram (EEG)
a representation of brain wave activity

brain waves were monitored to detect normal and abnormal brain activity. Other technology began to emerge as viable for the measurement of the brain in the 1970s. **Computerized axial tomography** (CAT) scanners are present in many hospitals in the United States. As an X ray scans the brain, a computer generates pictures of the brain and its structures. This technique can provide a representation of brain structures without surgery or pain. By the 1980s, PET (**positron emission tomography**) scans had been developed to determine the most active areas of the brain during various activities. Radioactive sugar, injected into the individual, was traced in the brain to find patterns of absorption. To date, the most promising type of measurement for motor behavior investigations is the MRI (**magnetic resonance imagery**) technique. The MRI provides color-coded information by sensing heat that is generated throughout the brain while the individual is actually moving specific body parts. The apparatus allows scientists to record brain activity as it occurs. The position, intensity, and duration of brain activity can be discovered in real time. This could be particularly meaningful in answering questions about retention and retrieval or motor program initiation. Because of the cost of this equipment, few motor behavior researchers have conducted investigations using the device, which presently provides the most detailed information available about brain activity during performance.

As is evident in this and the previous chapters, scientific measurements in motor behavior are becoming more exact. Advances in technology within the last two decades have provided opportunities for investigations that are more quantitatively based. Scientists want to measure that which is meaningful. Acceptance by the scientific community of case studies, small numbers of subjects, and applied field research data collection has substantially assisted those professionals conducting meaningful research in the area of motor behavior. As technology and research designs become more sophisticated and discriminating, increasingly meaningful data will become available to support or refute previously held theories and models.

Computerized axial tomography (CAT)
a computer-generated pictorial representation of the brain and its structures

Positron emission tomography (PET)
a scan of the brain to find patterns of absorption of radioactive sugar which is injected into the individual

Magnetic resonance imaging (MRI)
color-coded information by sensing heat that is generated throughout the brain while the individual is actually moving specific body parts

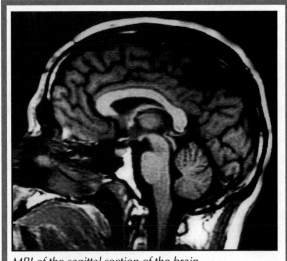
MRI of the sagittal section of the brain.

KEY POINTS

- Reaction time measurements have been the focus of numerous investigations.

- Simple reaction time, choice reaction time, and discrimination reaction time have been used to determine the time required to process information under different circumstances.

- Movement time, which is a part of response time, has been used in the study of speed and accuracy.

- Fractionated reaction time is divided into premotor time and motor time.

- Temporal accuracy refers to response time performance errors.

- Absolute, constant, variable, absolute constant, and total error refer to chronometric measures of the amount of error made when attempting to achieve spatial or temporal accuracy.

- The electroencephalogram, computerized axial tomography, positron emission tomography, and magnetic resonance imaging techniques have been used to gain information about physiological processes that relate to motor behavior.

DISCUSSION QUESTIONS

1. Why are there differences in the measurement devices used for psychological and physiological measurements of motor behavior?

2. Describe the differences between simple reaction time, choice reaction time, and discrimination reaction time as they relate to the assessment of reaction time.

3. Why is the speed/accuracy tradeoff of interest to motor behavior professionals?

4. Through the use of chronometry, what information is provided about spatial and temporal accuracy?

ADDITIONAL READINGS

Kluka, D., & Love, P. (1990). The study of eye movements related to sport: A review of the literature. *Sportsvision, 6*(1), 23–29.

Snyder, C. W., Jr., & Abernethy, B. (1998). *Understanding human action through experimentation.* Champaign, IL: Human Kinetics.

REFERENCES

Anson, J. G. (1982). Memory drum theory: Alternative tests and explanations for the complexity effects on simple reaction time. *Journal of Motor Behavior, 14,* 228–246.

Christina, R. W. (1992). The 1991 C.H. McCloy Research Lecture: Unraveling the mystery of the response complexity effect in skilled movements. *Research Quarterly for Exercise and Sport, 63,* 3, 218–230.

Christina, R. W., Fischman, M. G., Vercruyssen, J. J. P., & Anson, J. G. (1982). Simple reaction time as a function of response complexity: Memory drum theory revisited. *Journal of Motor Behavior, 14,* 301–321.

Christina, R. W., & Rose, D. J. (1985). Premotor and motor reaction time as a function of response complexity. *Research Quarterly for Exercise and Sport, 56,* 306–315.

Fitts, P. M. (1954). The information capacity of the human motor system in controlling the amplitude of movement. *Journal of Experimental Psychology, 47,* 381–391.

Henry, F. M. (1974). Variable and constant performance errors with a group of individuals. *Journal of Motor Behavior, 6,* 149–154.

Henry, F. M., & Rogers, D. E. (1960). Increased response latency for complicated movements and a "memory drum" theory of neuromotor reaction. *Research Quarterly, 31,* 448–458.

Hick, W. E. (1952). On the rate of gain of information. *Quarterly Journal of Experimental Psychology, 5,* 11–26.

Kelso, J. A. S. (1977). Motor control mechanisms underlying human movement production. *Journal of Experimental Psychology: Human Perception and Performance, 3,* 529–543.

Schutz, R. W., & Roy, E. A. (1973). Absolute error: The devil in disguise. *Journal of Motor Behavior, 5,* 141–153.

Appendix
Answers to Lab Exercises

CHAPTER 7 — Somatosensory Receptors — Monosynaptic Stretch

Answer: The time interval between the tap of the tendon and the initiation of the kick has been assessed as approximately 50 ms (Bennett, 1977). It would take considerably longer (at least another 150 ms) for sensory information to travel to the brain and then for motor neurons to relay the information back to the muscles involved. The motor impulse, "reflected" back to the muscle, is referred to as a "reflex."

CHAPTER 7 — Audition/Vestibular Apparatus

Answer: The glass will, at first, remain stationary. The glass moves with respect to the water it contains. Eventually, the water will begin rotating with the container. When the turntable is turned off, the water will continue to rotate.

CHAPTER 8 — Visual/Perceptual Skills — Fusion and Peripheral Vision

Answer: The finger will appear to be hotdog-shaped, with a fingernail on each end. It will seem to float in the air.

By focusing on the poster at a distance, the visual/perceptual skill of fusion is unable to be utilized efficiently. The left eye's image of the left finger and the right eye's image of the right finger overlap so that the hotdog appearance is perceived. Because the peripheral system detects motion, movement will become even more blurred. During the performance of a motor skill, movement may occur within three feet of the performer. Because the visual/perceptual skill of fusion requires extremely quick eye movements to adjust, the performer may miss information when focusing at a distance. For example, a baseball batter, playing in a summer league, focuses on the release point of the pitch. Simultaneously, a small wasp flies within 18 inches of his nose. As the pitch approaches, he is stung in the back of the neck by the wasp. He later stated that he never saw the wasp.

CHAPTER 8 — Eye Movements and Perceptual Processing

Answer: The individual who does not notice that there are two "THE" words tends to view patterns of things as wholes, rather than viewing things individually. Individuals who view patterns may need to work on isolating parts of movement in order to identify movement inefficiency.

CHAPTER 8 — Occlusion of Vision and Apparent Motion Experience

Answer: The fan appears to be either relatively stationary, or slowly moving in the direction of its spin, or moving opposite to the direction of its spin. These results happen because the fan is seen only at regularly spaced moments. Through the visual occlusion of the plate, the fan is not seen in between. This concept is similar to the use of stroboscopes (strobe lights) or movies/videos, where a series of images are chained evenly together to produce apparent motion when shown on a film projector or VHS machine.

CHAPTER 8 — Eye (Sighting) Dominance Experience

Answer: The eye that "sees" the square is the one that is the dominant eye. If the dominant eye is different at distance than near, what may be the reason for the difference?

CHAPTER 8 — Vestibular/Ocular Sensory System Experience

Answer: It should be easier to keep the scene appearing steady the faster the jumps.

CHAPTER 8 — Pathway of the Visual Fields Experience

Answer: The pupil of the eye not receiving the light will constrict. When the light is removed, both pupils will dilate back to their original appearance.

Glossary

A

Ability an aptitude or trait that is a component of skilled performance

Absolute constant error true value of the constant error

Absolute error the amount of algebraic error in a performance, regardless of sign

Absolute retention scores scores indicating that which has been retained

Accessory optic nuclei nuclei located in the brainstem that coordinate eye movements that compensate for head movements

Accommodation adjustment of the eye's lens to obtain clarity of an object, controlled by ciliary muscle contraction

Achievement motivation an individual's efforts to behave competently, taking pride and displaying excellence in that competence, and overcoming adversity to do so

Action potential the point of instantaneous firing of neurons

Acuity dominance describes the eye that is more accurate on measures of static visual acuity

Adaptation sensory receptors changing to meet the needs of the stimulus

Adequate (sufficient) stimulation specific thresholds of specific sensory receptors for conductance of electrical energy

Advanced stage of learning the level of freedom at which joints and body segments are most coordinated

Afferent neurons that carry sensory information to the brain and spinal cord

Alertness the state of mental preparation at which an individual can activate and sustain discrete performance

Allocational strategy a technique whereby individuals make a total effort when working alone and mask individual performance when working in a group

Alpha motor neuron a nerve cell that innervates skeletal muscle

Ambient vision peripheral vision used in localizing objects, which is not central

Amblyopia farsightedness

Anticipation coordination of a motor response to coincide with an external event

Anterograde amnesia inability to remember events that transpire after an injury to the brain

Apparent motion an illusion that perceives motion as the result of viewing appropriately timed sequences of stationary stimuli

Applied research an experiment to determine an answer to a specific question for the field-based professional

Aqueous humor a nutrient chamber at the front of the eyeball

Arousal a state of internal excitement or alertness

Associative attentional strategy focusing on items that associate with a motor behavior, such as heart and breathing rates as well as muscular tension, while running a marathon

Associative stage of learning the level at which learners understand how parts of the movement relate to one another and develop the ability to identify inappropriate performances and preliminarily provide solutions in subsequent trials of the skill in dynamic environments

Attention processing information by focusing on relevant stimuli; alertness; selectivity

Attentional cueing a strategy that provides opportunities for practicing an entire skill while concentrating on only one or two parts of it

Attentional focus a state of focus in which irrelevant stimuli are removed and relevant ones are enhanced

Attribution theory what individuals attribute their successes or failures to

Auditory/vestibular system receptors of the body, involving the ears and their mechanisms, that facilitate hearing and balance

Augmented feedback feedback that is provided externally to the individual

Automatic processing a method of information that requires little attention and is fast, parallel, and involuntary

Autonomous stage of learning the level at which a learner's movements appear automatic, stable, and somewhat effortless

Axon transmitting pole of a neuron

B

Basal ganglia an area of the brain, located near the center of the forebrain, that facilitates movement involving power, speed, direction, and amplitude in preparation of movement

Basic research an experiment to determine additional information to contribute to a theory

Bilateral transfer a concept that holds that performing a motor skill using one side of the body will also increase performance when using the other side of the body to perform the same movement

Binocular vision the eyes receiving information from slightly different angles, producing two distinct images

Biofeedback the immediate display of an individual's biological signals through specialized electronic equipment

Biofeedback training programs that have been designed to alter or maintain biosignals

Blocked practice training in which individuals practice many repetitions of the same skill before going on to another skill

C

Central nervous system the brain and spinal cord of the human body, composed of two types of cells — neurons and neuroglia

Central tendency the determination of a number that is a cluster point for the data examined

Cerebral cortex a portion of the brain that contains two cerebral hemispheres and accounts for nearly 80 percent of the weight of the brain

Choice reaction time the interval between presentation of a stimulus that competes with other stimuli, form which the individual must choose and initiation of movement

Choking when motor performance repeatedly deteriorates in crucial situations, characteristics of which include increased heart rate, sweating, breathing rate, and muscular tension; inappropriate situational flexibility, narrow focus, internal focus; disruption of coordinated movement, increased muscle tension and fatigue, timing detriment, and relevant cues unattended to

Chromatic vision sight in which the cones provide the highest acuity and color vision

Chronometry method of measuring time accurately

Chunking grouping meaningful information into manageable bits

Ciliary muscles muscles that change the shape of the lens to focus light onto the retina

Classical conditioning shaping the relationship between stimulus and response, how a stimulus or a response is associated with another stimulus, and the conditions under which stimulus and response are independently assessed

Closed loop theory a paradigm that compares feedback against a reference to explain human movement

Closed skills skills characterized by a stable environment, little change in environmental conditions, and the individual control of the spatial environment

Coaction little interaction of team members required to produce team success

Coding categorizing sensory transmission into the central nervous system, which can be designated through intensity or frequency

Coding frequency the firing rate of each type of photoreceptor for sensory transmission into the central nervous system

Coding intensity the number of each type of photoreceptor for sensory transmission into the central nervous system

Coefficient of correlation a numerical value ranging from +1 to +11, used to indicate a relationship

Cognitive memory memory responsible for storaging neural images that link individual memory experiences

Cognitive stage of learning level at which learners initially attempt to form the overall concept of a specific motor skill by gaining information through the senses in the form of sensory feedback by observing, getting verbal feedback from others, or through muscle spindles that detail each movement internally

Cognitive theories paradigms that explain that an additional step is present before information can be made meaningful to guide movement

Cohesiveness close linking of group members

Collectivism concern for group needs, interests, goals, and achievements

Color deficiency a condition in which sensitivity of cones is not sufficient to stimulate color discrimination; generally, an inability to perceive correctly one or more of the primary colors

Color perception the ability to identify a spectrum of colors, thereby using chromatic vision

Competitiveness achievement motivation in the context of motor behavior with social evaluation

Computerized axial tomography (CAT) a computer-generated pictorial representation of the brain and its structures

Concentration focusing attention on relevant environmental cues and maintaining that focus

Cones color receptors in the eye that provide chronomatic vision and facilitate the highest acuity

Consistency of movement close similarity over a series of performances

Constant error delineates directionality as well as amount of error, thereby providing response bias

Contextual interference the use of different contexts through practice

Continuous skill a series of movements that are repetitive or linked with other parts of skills to achieve a goal

Contrast sensitivity function the ability to process or filter spatial and temporal information about objects and their backgrounds under varying lighting conditions

Control arriving at total body movement based upon the degrees of freedom for each segment

Control group a group designated in a research design that is given no treatment

Controlled processing a method of information gathering marked by serial processing, which is slow, is under voluntary control, and requires attention

Coordination effectively and efficiently patterning body movements by constraining the available degrees of freedom to achieve the goal of the skill

Cornea a fluid-filled nutrient chamber at the front of the eyeball

Correlation a statistic used to determine the relationship between variables

Critical ratio the ratio attained from the differences between the two group means and standard deviations

Cue utilization theory a paradigm in which the breadth of stimuli to which an individual can attend is narrowed when arousal is high and ability to determine relevance of the stimuli is lower

Cutaneous receptors somatosensory mechanisms categorized in three areas: thermoreceptors, mechanoreceptors, and pain receptors

D

Declarative knowledge an understanding of factual information and what to do with it

Degrees of freedom (of movement) the options or possibilities available within the human body to perform a movement

Dendrite a receiving pole of a neuron

Dependent variable the variable that is measured in an experimental investigation (in contrast to the independent variable, which is not)

Descriptive statistics mathematical means for detailing information from a group

Diffuse attention a wider span of the attentional field with less vivid details

Diffusion of responsibility decreased perceptions of personal responsibility once individuals become members of groups

Disassociative attentional strategy focusing on items separate from motor behavior, such as denying physiological feedback from the body to cope with fatigue, abdominal cramping, or "hitting the wall" when running a marathon

Discrete skill a skill in which the movement has a specific beginning and a specific ending

Discrimination reaction time the interval between presentation of a paired stimulus and initiation of movement

Distractor an irrelevant cue or a cue that takes attentional focus away from object of interest

Distributed practice practice that contains rest components between attempts so the practice of specific skills has no noticeable breaks

Dorsal column route one of two routes over which electrical impulses travel to the brain

Dual-systems theory a paradigm that explains the two systems responsible for learning and memory: cognitive memory and habit memory

Duration how long something occurs

Dynamic stereopsis gauging the distance of objects in relative motion

Dynamic systems theory a paradigm that describes the control of coordinated movement and its dynamic relationship between the environment and the individual

Dynamic visual acuity clarity of eyesight when there is relative motion

E

Ecological theory a paradigm explaining human movement, in which the individual interacts with the environment and interaction that is based upon the individual's perception

Effector level one of two levels in an open-loop system that organizes the muscles and joints to produce the preplanned movement

Electroencephalography (EEG) electronic recording of brain wave activity

End bulbs of Krause body units that restrict blood circulation

Engram a memory trace

Episodic memory system a system of storing an individual's events with time relevance

Equipotentiality principle the concept that certain tasks related to a sensory system are stored in a sensory region of the brain rather than at a specific location; hence, the region has an equal potential for storing memory

Excitation-contraction coupling the conversion of electrical to chemical energy, followed by an action potential that sets up the opportunity for proteins to interact and create muscular force

Executive level one of two levels in an open-loop system, which determines the movement to make, which muscles to contract, when they contract, and in what order they contract

Experimental group the component of a research design that is given a treatment to determine the effects of that treatment

Expert-novice paradigm a model by which researchers assess characteristics of elite athletes and their novice counterparts

Expert stage of learning the level at which the movement produces efficiency as well as effectiveness through reorganization and addition of degrees of freedom

Exproprioception the visual system providing information about body position in the environment, using the dimensions of time, force, and flow to influence movement

Externally paced activities activities that are influenced by another person (partner/opponent), or an object

Exteroception information that is derived from outside the body

Extinction the process of phasing out a behavior; the length of time between presentation of the original stimulus to evoke a response and the new stimulus to evoke the same response

Eye dominance (sighting dominance; sensory dominance; acuity dominance)—the preferred eye; the eye that holds monocular images the longest; the eye that is more accurate on measures of static visual acuity

Eyes sensory receptors sensitive to light waves of varying length and frequency

F

Feedback sensory information obtained about movement

Feedforward the process of launching signals prior to movement that gives meaning to information as a result of movement

Fitts Law a principle involving the tradeoff between speed and accuracy: When speed is emphasized, accuracy is reduced; when accuracy is emphasized, speed is reduced

Fixation/diversification stage of learning the level at which the movement is consistent within the presented environments (fixation) and adapting (diversification) the movement enough to perform successfully in the environment

Fixed rate reinforcement a type of schedule of reinforcement that is given after predesignated trials

Flexibility of movement the ability to accomplish a task using a variety of musculoskeletal resources

Focal attention attending to a small field with vivid details

Focal vision conscious and central eyesight used in identifying objects

Forebrain the part of the brain composed of cerebral hemisphere, basal ganglia, hypothalamus, and thalamus

Forming the first stage in team development, in which individuals must make decisions as to whether they want to belong to a group

Fovea the center of clearest visual acuity in the eye

Fractionated reaction time reaction time that has several component parts

Fractionation dismantling the coordination of a skill into several parts

Free nerve endings the most widespread somatosensory receptors in the skin and throughout the body that can detect light touch and pressure

Free-rider effect the concept that some individuals in a group work only as hard as they perceive that others in the group work

G

Gamma motor neuron highly specialized neuron, located in contractile fibers of skeletal muscles, that carries messages to muscle spindles

General space in Laban Notation terms, space that is outside the personal reach of the body

Generalized motor program a program that produces novel and flexible movement in various dimensions

Generator potential neurons receptor cells which raise or lower the probability that a sensory neuron axon will fire

"Getting the idea" stage of learning the phase at which the learner understands how the movement must be organized to accomplish the goal of the skill

Glare recovery the time required to redefine an object after bright light has bleached out the rods and cones of the eyes

Goal setting translating vision into achievable action

Golgi tendon organs stretch receptors located in the junction between skeletal muscles and their tendons

Group dynamics the influential processes within groups

H

Habit memory memory that facilitates skilled behaviors that appear automatic

Hick's Law as the number of stimulus-response choices increases, reaction time will increase logarithmically

Hierarchy theory a concept of motor control based on a hierarchy that begins with the brain and its neocortex and operates in a hierarchical fashion to orchestrate lower areas of the central nervous system in performance

Hindbrain the part of the brain consisting of pons, cerebellum, and medulla

Hyperopia increasing difficulty of the lens of the eye to focus on near objects as a result of diminishing flexibility as the individual ages

Hypothesis an "educated guess" designed to be logically developed to predict the change in outcome

I

Identical elements theory a concept holding that learning is quite specific based upon components of the learning that were exact

Illusion a visual cue involving spatial and temporal decision making that is uncertain and subject to misinterpretation

Impulsive learning style a way of learning that reflects reactivity rather than proactivity to the environment (externally paced activities)

Independent variable the variable in a research design that is manipulated or changed (in contrast to the dependent variable)

Individualism concern for personal needs, interests, goals, and achievements

Inferential statistics mathematical means for sampling a population to test hypotheses

Innervation the stimulation of a muscle by nerves

Intensity the depth to which something occurs

Interaction the ways in which group members influence each others' behaviors

Interdependence mutual influence of two or more individuals in a relationship

Interference theory a paradigm supporting the notion that people forget because other memories preclude or interfere with memory

Interneurons neurons that synapse with alpha motor neurons and help to create opportunities for excitation or inhibition throughout the spinal cord

Intertrial rest interval the duration of rest between attempts

Inverted-U hypothesis a paradigm that attempts to explain the relationship between arousal levels and performance

Iris the colored ring of the eye

J

Joint receptors the parts of joint capsules and ligaments that provide information about movement and limb position

K

Kinesphere in Laban Notation, space within personal reach of the body

Kinesthesis movement sensation; the conscious appreciation and identification of movement and position of limbs

Knowledge base memory long-term memory

L

Laban Notation a classification system of movement according to the type of exertion or effort and the type of spatial adaptation or shape used

Labeling providing a short, meaningful image to a movement through verbalization

Lateral geniculate nucleus portion of the brain where the optic nerves enter and become the optic tracts

Lens a portion of the eye that allows light to enter and is refracted and focused onto the retina

Level of confidence the level at which the number of times the results will occur can be predicted with some accuracy

Level of significance the level at which the number of times the results will occur by chance can be predicted

Levels of processing theory a paradigm explaining that the individual, through attentional control, determines the depth of processing by determining its significance and linking it to previously remembered information

Linear curve a graphical, proportional measure of performance over time

Long-term memory the type of memory that stores information rather permanently

M

Macula the portion of the eye located near the center of the retina where vision is clearest

Magnetic resonance imaging (MRI) a method of gaining color-coded information by sensing heat generated throughout the brain while the individual is moving various body parts

Magno system a classification system identified by its peripheral, depth perception, movement identification, low luminance, high contrast sensitivity, rapid response, and low spatial frequency

Massed practice practice that involves little or no rest between attempts and functions rather continuously

Mean the arithmetic average

Mechanoreceptors skin receptors that involve pressure-mechanical deformation of the skin

Median the middle of a set of scores or the 50th percentile; affected by position of scores to one another

Meissmer's corpuscles cells in the fingertips, the lips, and other areas where distinguishing subtle differences in touch is important

Memory (sensory; short-term; working) a component of information processing that stores information for retrieval

Memory trace the memory mechanism that selects and initiates a movement

Merkel's disks the structural parts found near Meissner's corpuscles to transmit long-lasting signals that permit tolerance of constant contact with the skin

Midbrain the part of the brain consisting of the superior colliculi and inferior colliculi

Minimizing strategy a technique whereby individuals within the group save energy because they believe their lack of effort will go undetected

Mnemonics memory strategies

Mode the most common score in the data set

Modifiability of movement the explanation for a person's ability to alter a movement during its performance

Monochromatic vision eyesight that is unable to detect color, just blacks, whites, and shades of gray

Motivation the effort applied to direct and energize behavior

Motor behavior all human movements and postures; also, the processes that lead to relatively permanent changes in performance

Motor control human performance and postures and the internal processes that command them

Motor learning a multifaceted set of internal processes that effect relatively permanent change in human performance through practice, provided the change cannot be attributed to a human's maturation, temporary state, or instinct

Motor neuron pool a set of motor units that is recruited for use in a voluntary movement

Motor program a plan or program determined in advance, stored in the brain, and run through the rest of the body system

Motor skill performance with a goal, accomplished by voluntary body movement

Motor stage of learning autonomous stage in the Fitts and Posner model of 1967

Motor time the interval between the first recorded change of electrical activity in the primary agonist muscle and the time the movement begins

Motor unit consists of one motor neuron, its axon branches, and all of the muscle fibers it innervates

Movement time the interval between initiation of the movement and the end of the movement

Multistore model a paradigm of memory structure using a computer hardware and software analogy as under an individual's control, facilitating the flow of information stored and retrieved

Muscle spindles body structures responsible for providing detailed information and having the ability to ascertain subtle and gross changes in muscle length; they stretch when the muscle lengthens and shortens when the muscle relaxes

Myelination a protective sheath of myelin that insulates each axon from other neural paths

Myopia nearsightedness

N

Need achievement theory an interactive paradigm in which personal and situational characteristics serve to predict behavior

Negative reinforcement rewards that that the recipient perceives as unpleasant

Negative transfer interference by a skill with the learning of another skill

Negatively accelerated curve an indication of rapid improvement in early trials and stabilized performance soon thereafter

Neuromuscular junction a motor end plate

Neuron an elongated cell designed to transmit excitation by receiving and conducting impulses

Neutral transfer learning in which one learned skill has no influence upon the learning of another skill

Normal distribution symmetrical distribution of scores, in which the mean, median, and mode are the same

Norming the third stage in team development, when group members begin to get a sense of ease so they can perform at a given level and work together

Novice stage of learning the phase at which individuals try to simplify the degrees-of-freedom issue by increasingly reducing them

Nuclear bag one of two types of muscle spindles, having a 5:2 ratio with nuclear chains

Nuclear chain one of two types of muscle spindles

O

Observation viewing a movement another person performs before initiating that movement

Open skills skills in which the relationship between the environment and the individual or object changes; the individual must determine the spatial and temporal demands and match them with the environment

Optic array ambient light reflected from objects, presenting a unique texture to the brain at each point of observation

Optic disk the area in the eye where no receptors are located

Optic radiations a portion of the brain where axons stemming from the optic nerves run through to the primary visual cortex in the brain's occipital lobes

Optical tau a mathematical formula that details the time an object travels to contact a given point in space

Optic tracts optic nerves after entering the brain and extending to the lateral geniculate nucleus of the thalamus

Organic sensitivity receptivity to stimuli surrounding internal organs

Orders of neurons the first, second, and third orders of neurons in the dorsal column and spinothalmic route that facilitate input from receptors to the brain

Outcome orientation the perspective that determines the worth of one's performance by comparing it to the performance of others

Overlearning (overpractice) practice time spent above the amount of time needed to attain a level of performance based upon preestablished criteria

P

Pacinian corpuscles cells that provide sensitivity to deep pressure sensations

Pain receptors receptors that determine intensity sufficient to cause tissue damage

Part task practice motor skills presented and practiced in parts

Parvo system a model characterized by central, texture, shape, color-sensitive, high luminance, low-contrast sensitivity, high spatial frequency, and sustained response

Perceived confidence perception of ability determined through orientations which mean success

Perception the application and interpretation of sensory-stored information

Perceptual anticipation the point at which the individual is able to see the approaching object of interest consistently

Perceptual trace the mechanism used to compare the movement being performed with its internal memory reference

Performance an act at a moment in time

Performance curves "snapshots" of performances over time displayed in a graph format

Performing the last stage in the process of team development when focus and actions envelop the notion of team success and team members function well in roles

Peripheral vision eyesight outside approximately 3° of the visual spectrum

Phasic motor units motor units of large fiber size that produce large action potentials with high conduction velocities

Photopigments chemicals of opsin and retinal used in the initial transduction of light in the eye

Positive reinforcement rewards that the recipient perceives as pleasurable

Positive self-talk silent speaking to oneself that assists in focusing thoughts on the present through motivational or instructional elements

Positive transfer learning a new skill facilitated by performing a previous skill

Positively accelerated curve graphic depiction showing little improvement initially and performance improvement during later trials

Positron emission tomography (PET) a scan of the brain to find patterns of absorption of radioactive sugar injected into the individual

Practice environment the surroundings and conditions used for rehearsal of motor behavior performances

Practice variability changes in the practice environment to provide variety

Premotor time the interval between stimulus presentation and the first recorded change of electrical activity in the primary agonist muscle involved in the movement

Pretectum pathway portion of the brain near the superior colliculus that assists in controlling size of pupils of the eye

Primary neurons rapid-firing neurons also known as Group Ia

Primary visual cortex main area of visual perception, located in occipital lobe of brain

Proactive inhibition interference of new learning by old memories

Procedural knowledge an understanding of how to do something

Procedural memory system information storage about motor skills that pertains to how to do something

Proprioception internal sensory information providing messages about movement and limb position

Proprioceptors sensory receptors that provide information about the status of the body

Pupil the dark center of the eye that regulates the amount of light entering the retina

Pupillary size diameter of the pupil of the eye determined by sphincter and dilator muscles of the iris, dependent upon the individual's arousal level and the amount of light falling on the retina

Pursuit rotor an instrument designed to assess learning and performance using a record player type of turntable that revolves clockwise or counterclockwise

R

Range a numerical representation of the spectrum of scores

Raw data scores collected on subjects in a research investigation

Reaction time the interval between the unanticipated presentation of a stimulus and the initiation of movement

Recall schema a set of rules that selects parameter values for specific movement and initiates the goal-directed performance

Receptor anticipation expectation based on when the individual is unable to constantly see the approaching object of interest, based on pieces of information and past experiences

Receptor potentials a type of receptor, having no axon, transmitted to other neurons having axons that are capable of producing action potentials

Receptors specialized nerve cells in each sensory system that respond to certain changes in the individual or in its environment and transmit these responses to the nervous system

Reflective learning style the propensity to react to the environment proactively rather than reactively (self-paced activities)

Reflex theories paradigms that explain behavior as the use of stereotyped, involuntary, and rapid responses to stimuli

Reflexes responses that are mediated at the spinal cord level and require no conscious effort

Rehearsal active performance of a movement

Relative retention scores scores that indicate how much information was retained or lost as a result of comparing the difference between the score attained in the skill acquisition portion on the last trial and what was attained on the first trial of a retention test

Relevant cues pieces of information that are meaningful to the individual

Response recognition schema a set of rules used to assess and compare the outcome with parameters selected, using sensory information to store future corrections

Retention tests tools used to determine how much has been retained as a result of block-type information presented

Retina a thin membrane of receptor cells located on the back of the eyeball

Retroactive inhibition new learning interference with already established memories

Retrograde amnesia inability to remember events that transpired prior to brain injury

Ringelmann effect member's performance in each group decreases as group size increases; the basis for the term "social loafing"

Rods long, slender cells located primarily in peripheral areas of the eye that are unable to detect color

Ruffini endings body cells that produces sweat to cool the body

S

Savings scores scores that reflect the rate at which a given level of performance of a skill returns when the skill has not been practiced for some of time

Schedule of reinforcement a program to selectively reinforce through positive and negative rewards

Schema a set of rules that guide decision making relative to the goal

Schema theory a paradigm that explains the rules governing movement

Sclera white, opaque, outer covering of the eye

Scotopic vision night vision

Secondary neurons slow-firing neurons that connect only to nuclear chain fibers; also known as Group II neurons

Segmentation dividing skills into parts based upon temporal and spatial characteristics and levels of performance; then combining each of the parts with other parts, leading to performance of the entire skill

Self-organization the interaction or coordination of smaller systems within dynamic systems theory

Self-paced activities activities in which individuals can participate at their own rate that involves a relatively stable environment, predictable situations, and little need for rapid changes

Self-talk silent monologue that enables a person to shape emotional responses that factor into multidimensional learning through motor behavior

Semantic memory system storage of information about the general environment that has developed over time

Sensory dominance refers to the eye that holds monocular images longer

Sensory memory brief holding of sensory information just before it is processed into short-term memory

Sensory transduction electrical charges that change firing patterns in axons that lead into the central nervous system

Short-term memory a passive rehearsal buffer for information

Sighting dominance the eye that is preferred through behavior

Simple reaction time the time required to react to one possible stimulus

Simplification modifying movements to the simplest basics of the skill within a particular environment

Size principle the concept holding that the size of the motor unit innervating the muscle group will determine its length of activation; the larger the motor unit, the shorter is its firing duration

Skill a goal-oriented action; a qualitatively assessed performance

Skilled motor behavior a performance wherein environmental parameters have been selected and degrees of freedom condensed to produce an appropriate action

Social facilitation competition with someone else rather than with time to improve performance

Social inhibition an audience's producing a level of arousal in the individual that detracts from performance

Social loafing performance of each group member decreases as the number of individuals within the group increases

Sociogram a graphic figure depicting the relationship and status between members of a group

Sociometry the science studying how group members feel about something or why they behave as they do

Soma a cell body of a neuron

Spatial accuracy an individual's closeness of movement to a specific target

Spatial summation a stimulus that causes the initial number of proprioceptors to fire

Speed/accuracy tradeoff An increase in movement time as distance of targets increases and a decrease in movement time as target size decreases

Spinothalamic route one of two paths over which electrical impulses travel to the brain

Sports vision an interdisciplinary area of sport science, initiated by optometrists, ophthalmologists, and sport science researchers who were interested in the relationship of vision to sport performance from perspective of vision correction, vision enhancement, and ocular injury perspectives

S-shaped curve a combination of linear, positively accelerated, and negatively accelerated curves

Standard deviation a statistical depiction of how scores differ from one another

Static visual acuity clarity of features distinguished by the eyes under high-contrast conditions

Stereopsis the ability to see objects in depth

Storming the second, "testing-of-power" stage in the process of team development involving discussions about decisions, conflicts, and disharmony as roles, responsibilities, and status are established within the group

Strabismus a condition in which one eye is turned in or out, preventing binocular vision

Strategic knowledge an understanding of the general principles that facilitate what to do and how to do it

Stretch reflex a short-loop reflex, involving a single synapse that adjusts the position of the skeleton continuously by contracting, through muscle spindles

Stroop phenomenon the tendency for objects to be depicted in opposites, which produces longer reaction times, thereby displaying parallel processing

Sufficient (adequate) stimulation the specific thresholds of specific sensory receptors necessary to conduct electrical energy

Synapse the junction between two neurons involved in transmitting of action potentials

T

Task orientation the use of prior personal performances as the yardstick by which success is measured

Team cohesion the relative strength of a group to remain focused and together in its attempt to achieve group goals

Temporal accuracy how quickly an individual moves in a specific amount of time

Temporal summation a stimulus that causes more frequent firing of proprioceptors

Thalamus portion of the brain involved with visual perception

Theory/Theoretical model a succinct way of explaining a concept

Thermoreceptors receptors that involve temperature

Tonic motor units motor units that have smaller fiber size, slower conduction velocity, and a high threshold to electrical stimuli

Total error statistical concept that exposes variability and response bias equally

Trace decay theory the notion that a person can forget when the neural connections involved in memory are not strong enough and "decaying" of the connection occurs over time

Transfer the influence of one skill on the learning of another

Transfer tests measurement of the skills learned one situation in a different practice setting

Trichromatic spectrum the range of primary, secondary, and tertiary colors

Trigger words key terms that centralize attention

T-test a statistical procedure to determine if two means are significantly different from one another

U

Uniqueness of movement The relative movement occurs, even more variables are added, thereby making movements identical impossible

V

Variability how scores differ from one another

Variable that portion in an experimental investigation which needs to be controlled to determine the effect of the experiment

Variable error indicates the consistency of performance, or the variability in a performance

Variable rate reinforcement a schedule of reinforcement after an average of trials, thereby making the rate varying

Verbal/motor stage of learning the cognitive and associative stages were combined from the Fitts and Posner model, while devulging an association between the cognitive and motor aspects in the initial stage of learning

Vergence (convergence; divergence) the ability of the eyes to follow an object moving toward or away from the body

Vertigo severe disorientation combined with nausea

Video overlay technique which produces live video images shown on a screen with various measurements specific to a sport

Visual acuity (static; dynamic) the ability to visually discern detail of objects

Vitreous humor After leaving the lens, light travels through the main chamber of the eye which contains pressurized fluid that maintains the shape of the eyeball

W

Withdrawal reflex a long-loop reflex which is a result of body parts being quickly withdrawn as a result of intensely painful stimuli

Whole task practice motor skills presented and practiced as an entire unit

Working memory the active part of long-term memory which can temporarily hold small bits or chunks of information

Author Index

Subject Index